Divine Doctors and Dreadful Distempers

Clio Medica: Perspectives in Medical Humanities

91

Divine Doctors and Dreadful Distempers

How Practicing Medicine Became a Respectable Profession

Christi Sumich

Amsterdam - New York, NY 2013

Cover illustration: The Water Doctor, 1685. Courtesy of the Wellcome Library, London.

The paper on which this book is printed meets the requirements of "ISO 9706:1994, Information and documentation - Paper for
documents - Requirements for permanence".

ISBN: 978-90-420-3688-8
E-Book ISBN: 978-94-012-0947-2
© Editions Rodopi B.V., Amsterdam – New York, NY 2013
Printed in The Netherlands

Always laugh when you can. It is cheap medicine.
– Lord Byron

This book is dedicated to my family, whose laughter has proven the best medicine for whatever ails me.

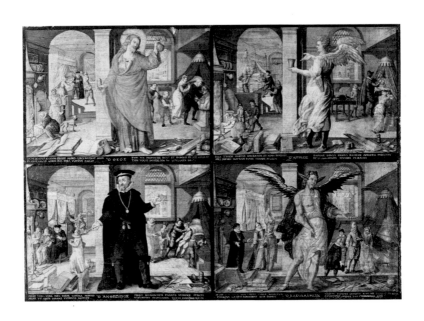

Figure 2: The physician as god, angel, man and devil
Courtesy of Wellcome Library, London

Table of Contents

Acknowledgements

I write this as Hurricane Isaac passes over the city of New Orleans, and I am reminded of all the obstacles that have stood in the way of this book's completion. It began as my dissertation and was rudely interrupted by both Hurricane Katrina and the lightning strike that devastated our home. My documents and notes have survived wind, water, and fire, and so it seems appropriate that I conclude the writing phase amidst one last challenge. Any reasonably sane person might interpret the slew of natural disasters that have accompanied this project as a sign from the universe, but I'm stubborn. Instead, I'll thank all those who have helped this book see the light of day. I am grateful to my dissertation advisor, Dr. Linda Pollock, and my committee members for assisting me in the early days of the project. The archival collections of the British Library, the Huntington, and the Wellcome Library were all immensely helpful to my research. The Wellcome also generously allowed me to use images from their collection for this book. My colleagues at Loyola have been incredibly helpful, especially Dr. Sara Butler, who graciously read a draft and offered comments, and Dr. Melanie McKay, who is supportive of all my professional endeavors.

On a personal note, I would like to thank my parents and my in-laws for the countless hours of babysitting, without which I would not have been able to work efficiently. My children, Jason, Hayley, and Kaitlin, have been more than patient. They have accepted the appendage that has been my laptop for the past several years, and they have pretended to find subjects like plague interesting for my sake. No child should have to discuss buboes at the dinner table, but I am thankful that they humored me. Most of all I would like to thank my husband, Leni Sumich II, for supporting me, and for always believing that I could accomplish any goal, no matter what the daily consequences would mean for him. There is no way I would have completed this book without his unfaltering support. All of the above-mentioned individuals deserve my appreciation, and I will be forever grateful for their contributions.

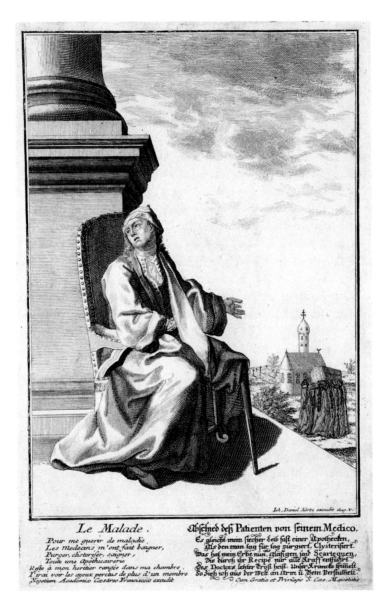

Le Malade.

Pour me guerir de maladie,
Les Medecins m'ont fait baigner,
Purger, clisterisier, saigner,
Toute une apothicairerie
Reste à mon heritier rangée dans ma chambre.
J'irai voir les ayeux perçus de plus d'un membre
Negotium Academiæ Cæsareo Franciscea excudit

Abschied deß Patienten von seinem Medico.

Es gleicht mein siecher Leib fast einer Apothecken,
Als den man tag für tag purgiert, Clysterisiert.
Was hat mein Erbe nur, glaß gen und Scartequen,
Die durch ihr Recipe nur alle Kraff entfuhrt.
Des Doctors letzter Trost heist: Unser Krancke stirbt,
So zieh ich aus der Welt, in strm ü. Pein versumelt.
Cum Gratia et Privilegio S. Cæs. Majestatis.

Figure 3: A sick man lamenting the uselessness of his physicians
Courtesy of Wellcome Library, London

Introduction

'Physick keeps her very bare'[1]:
Why Would Anyone See a Doctor in the
Seventeenth Century?

Disease and illness were an inevitable part of life in early modern England, a necessary component of the human condition. Hamlet described disease as 'the thousand natural shocks that flesh is heir to.'[2] It was man's legacy after the fall from grace to endure sickness and suffering, ideally with pious resignation. It is easy for us to forget just how fundamental the threat of ill health was to the consciousness of early modern individuals. John Donne's frustration over the chaos and havoc disease could wreak is indicative of contemporary fears of ill health:

> We study *Health*, and we deliberate upon our *meats*, and *drink*, and *Ayre*, and *exercises*, and we hew, and wee polish every stone, that goes to that building; and so our *Health* is a long & a regular work; but in a minute a Cannon batters all, overthrows all, demolishes all; a *Sickness* unprevented for all our diligences, unsuspected for all our curiositie; nay undeserved, if we consider only *disorder*, summons us, seizes us, possesses us, destroyes us in an instant.[3]

Donne's tone of defeatism stems from a sense of futility in a world where disease seemed always lurking in the shadows.

Yet there is a second emotion present: indignation that the sickness was undeserved in light of the sufferer's defense against ill health. Trying to stave off illness was an activity early modern people took seriously. Healthcare was not a last resort—a quick fix to quell disease. Most people afforded good health its due diligence. They were not resigned to the fatalistic notion that disease would find them, no matter what. They took ownership of their health and invested time and money to maintain it. They monitored their health and made changes accordingly. Preventative measures for sound health were not dissimilar to those espoused by most modern healthcare professionals. Indeed, as foreign as the early modern conceptual framework of disease seems to us today, some of the basic tenets of good health (fresh air, ample rest, and avoidance of extremes in diet and physical activity) are quite familiar to us. Similarly, physicians complained then, as some do now, that patients were too inclined to self-diagnose and inform their physicians of what measures needed to be taken to provide a cure for their ailment. Patients' primary resources were medical manuals written for the lay public rather than the internet, but the result could prove equally frustrating for physicians.

The key difference, of course, is the incidence of disease in the early modern era. It is not hyperbole to suggest that death and disease were omnipresent. Approximately eighty-five per cent of the population was faced with chronic ill health as well as frequent acute illness.[4] Along with horrifying outbreaks of plague, a myriad of assorted deadly epidemics, contagious diseases, and fevers threatened people's health. In addition, the aches and pains of everyday life, childbearing, and aging led seventeenth-century men, women, and children to encounter illness on a regular basis. Most people did not expect to feel good most of the time: diarists often recorded days when their health was good, implying that good health was more an aberration than the norm.[5]

Monitoring one's health, therefore, was imperative. This included paying close attention to the six nonnaturals: air, diet, exercise, evacuations, sleep, and mental and emotional stimulation. If any of these changed too rapidly, if they became corrupted, or if the patient got too little or too much of something, the four humours (black bile, yellow bile, phlegm, and blood) would be out of balance, and illness could ensue. There was no single regimen to ensure that nonnaturals would be properly regulated or the humours balanced, as each person possessed a unique humoral makeup. As a result, the quest to achieve and preserve health was an ongoing activity, requiring diligence from the patient and a carefully constructed course of therapy devised by a learned physician.

This was the ideal; however, studies focusing on the patient's perspective of illness remind us that most people did not consult a physician when they became ill, and they certainly did not do so when they were healthy. Most people treated themselves when sick, or they received treatment from family members, neighbors, or friends, any of whom could draw from the vast amount of lay medical knowledge that was widely available.[6] Furthermore, it was not physicians who bore the brunt of caring for illness in early modern England, especially outside the Royal College of Physician's seven-mile radius of jurisdiction.[7] Barber-surgeons, apothecaries, and myriad empirical and lay healers took on this responsibility.[8] Historians have concluded that there were many similarities in the methods of treatment and remedies prescribed for patients by most healers, whether they were learned physicians or popular healers. Doreen Nagy has described seventeenth-century medicine as an 'untidy mixture of folklore, superstition, Galenic theory, herbal tradition, astrology and, eventually, chemical medicine,' and it was into this concoction that both licensed and unlicensed practitioners indiscriminately dipped.[9] Although physicians put forth great effort in convincing the public that their knowledge and remedies were superior to other available alternatives, they generally were not, nor were they always distinct from what other healers were offering, as physicians borrowed treatments from folk medicines. The great variety of lay and empiric healers resulted in a disparity in skill level, though no doubt some were at least as effective as physicians were, possibly more so, and nearly all charged less. The public respected lay healers. They were deemed a reasonable option for health care, as evidenced by the accounts of some people who had the access and means to pay physicians but who chose lay or popular healers instead.

There were, in fact, numerous reasons to account for the decision to eschew a physician in favor of an empiric or lay healer. Physicians did not save lives more consistently than other healers did, although this expectation was not nearly so entrenched then as it is now. University-educated physicians were scarce, particularly outside of London, and those granted a license to practice medicine by the Royal College of Physicians were even more so. Perhaps the most compelling reason to forgo the assistance of physicians lay in their hefty fees, which meant they were not an option for the majority of patients.[10] Even those who could afford the fees complained about them, and others struggled to pay for the medication required for the course of treatment.[11]

The heavy costs associated with engaging a physician led to an unsavory reputation of physicians as greedy, a reputation furthered by the actions of the Royal College of Physicians. While the College has at times been presented by historians in a favorable light, more recent historiography has reconsidered the actions and motivations of this group.[12] Particularly damning was the tendency of previous historians to forward 'Whiggish' interpretations of the Royal College of Physicians as a group trying to carve out a niche for scientific professionals amidst a superstitious public who would have preferred

3

purchasing amulets and cure-all powders from itinerant healers, rather than listen to their sage advice, garnered from years of study.[13] Some historians have called such interpretations into question. They have instead presented the Royal College of Physicians as a rather paranoid group of elite intellectuals who jealously guarded their privileges, bestowed upon them by the crown, and who sought to control the current state and future of medicine, quite possibly to the detriment of the country as a whole. The result has been some rather negative portrayals of the inchoate profession of medicine. For example, Harold Cook has delineated the diminishing regulatory power of the College and the decline of traditional Galenic medicine in general by the close of the seventeenth century, citing various social, political, and economic changes influencing the medical marketplace. His assessment of physicians and their professional identity is decidedly negative, causing one to wonder how such a miserable little group of complainers ever survived the seventeenth century.[14] Margaret Pelling and Joseph Birken have both demonstrated that physicians as a group were plagued with issues of low social status, a fact that explained their aggressive attitude when faced with competition.[15]

These and other reassessments of seventeenth-century medicine represent the physician as having little to offer. This is said to explain his antagonistic stance towards all other competitors, who are often depicted as providing comparative remedies at a lower cost, with less unwarranted erudite advice to boot.[16] In fact, Margaret Pelling has argued that the College defined itself by prosecuting those whom it considered to be irregular practitioners, to the extent that it was 'parasitic for its own identity in the confrontations with irregulars.'[17] The work of Pelling and other historians constitutes an important reassessment of overly complimentary portrayals of physicians wherein the rise of their professional status seemed inevitable. Such work has also been helpful in redefining the medical scene and who was involved in healing, as well as demonstrating that the success of physicians was anything but a forgone conclusion in the seventeenth century.

These studies suggest that university-trained physicians did not possess practical advantages over lay or empirical healers. Why, then, would people engage the services of a physician in the seventeenth century? The question is a deceptively simple one, and its answer lies in contemporary ideas about illness and patient expectations of medicine and healing. Simply put, those who employed physicians did so because they believed physicians offered them the best chance of a favorable outcome in dealing with their health concerns. Those concerns could range from providing a cure for a disease

4

to maintenance of good health. There have been excellent studies on lay conceptions of medicine and healing options, while others have shed light on the complex and diverse medical marketplace of seventeenth-century England.[18] This book builds upon all of these, while also considering studies related to Calvinism's influence on healing, the manner in which knowledge about diseases was constructed, and the importance of rhetoric in the healing process, in order to argue that physicians were able to present a convincing enough portrayal of themselves as respectable and their services as valuable in a century when there was precious little more than perception to recommend them. They were able to differentiate themselves from their competition as a result of specific actions: a self-fashioning of their profession that stood in contrast to the traditional criticism of physicians as greedy atheists, a presentation of their offerings as unique and essential, and a view of the public health and their vital role in it.

All of the above actions were informed by lay perceptions of illness that greatly influenced the way physicians offered their services. People increasingly wrote about sickness and their reactions to being ill during the seventeenth century, greatly simplifying the historian's task of discerning what contemporaries thought about illness. There are first-hand accounts from sufferers as well as expressions of suffering in drama and poetry. Illnesses of all kinds were being catalogued, pondered, and discussed in unprecedented numbers over the course of the seventeenth century. The combination of these voices has led historians to conclude that early modern patient expectations of medical intervention are far different then today. For example, people did not necessarily expect physicians to cure them any more than they expected medicine to make them feel better.[19] Such notions were not nearly so entrenched then as they are now. The definition of a successful consultation with a physician is not uniform but is culturally determined, just as the way in which individuals experience illness and pain is culturally determined.[20]

In the seventeenth century, not all suffering was equal. There was, in a sense, a hierarchy of illness and pain in early modern English culture. Gout was an affliction reserved primarily for the wealthy and could therefore connote affluence, while syphilis was largely ignominious. Some suffering, like the aches associated with old age, was thought to be inevitable. At the end of a life, dying the good death, in which a person bore pain nobly, could solidify his or her reputation and was considered a sign of great piety and personal strength. The various facets that defined individual sufferers affected the way

5

they were treated and were dependent upon a host of factors, ranging from their socioeconomic status to their level of piety, as sickness was often considered to be sent directly from God as a punishment, test, or for some other divinely ordained purpose.

The manner in which the pain and discomfort associated with illness was interpreted was heavily dependent upon religious beliefs. Work on Calvinism has demonstrated that the increasing focus on individual, everyday suffering stemmed from perceptions of a religious dimension to illness. The godly greatly valued inward experience, and they were encouraged to record all afflictions and deliverance from illness as testaments of God's mercy and justice.[21]

Religion also affected ideas about collective health. Illness for the lay population typically was not seen as a random accident striking from the outside, but as a deeply significant life event, integral to the sufferer's whole being—spiritual, moral, and physical. The belief that God punished sin, both on an individual and a collective basis, was omnipresent in both secular and religious writing of the time and became particularly acute during periods of epidemic disease such as plague outbreaks. Health was a shared concept, not just in terms of individual notions about what led to disease, but also because miasmas of a sinful population could affect and quite literally *infect* the health of the entire nation. The nation's health depended upon the morality and spiritual fitness of its people; conversely, those individuals' wellbeing was comprised of physical as well as spiritual health.

The inroads made by learned medicine were largely dependent upon physicians' conception of health as a combination of physical and spiritual factors: specifically, the association of the university-trained physician with moral authority, as well as his association with the divine (as God's ordained healer). These provided the grounds upon which physicians felt they had a claim to public trust, as the most logical choice for caring for the entire patient, whose body housed the soul. Physicians' success, therefore, was dependent upon collectively held ideas about body/soul duality and the interconnection of medicine and religion in a society that interpreted all phenomena in terms of moral agency.

It might seem counter-intuitive that physicians differentiated themselves from less educated healers by basing their ideas about health and medicine on Divine Providence and retribution, yet by doing so, they were reflecting lay beliefs about disease and healing. The claim that physicians were in step with common cultural and spiritual beliefs constitutes a reassessment of physicians as a backward group clinging stubbornly to Galenic medicine and resistant to changes in the medical marketplace that altered the way medicine was offered.[22] Physicians' contributions brought even a new disease like the pox, and an epidemic like bubonic plague, into Galenic theory. They furthermore proved capable of adjusting to and capitalizing upon changes in the medical marketplace, such as the dissemination of medical knowledge to the public through the printing press and providing confidentiality for venereal patients.

Physicians used their university education and training to present themselves as knowledgeable about diseases and remedies and to occupy the role of moral guardian over the health not only of individual patients, but also of the nation as a whole. Their role meshed seamlessly with a lay culture of illness characterized by Roy and Dorothy Porter as one in which 'mind, mentality, morals, and medicine were mutually defining.'[23] Medicine as practiced by physicians fit this description as well. In fact, core ideas about the interconnection of morality and medicine were fairly consistent whether they appeared in a sermon, a medical treatise, or a diary. Lay beliefs regarding illness do not change greatly over the course of the century, nor do they vary widely according to the patient's religious beliefs. As Raymond Anslement has concluded, the majority of people in the seventeenth century readily assented to the traditional belief that sickness was the visitation of God, and none disputed the corollary that health was His blessing.[24] Physicians espoused these beliefs as well. Among other reasons, it was financially prudent for them to do so. David Harley has argued that presenting medical ideas in an open market required them to connect with the core beliefs of a substantial group of potential patients.[25] It was also essential that they convince potential patients that their services were preferable because they included moral authority that was so closely associated with a university education. Moral authority was valuable because it conveyed a sense of trustworthiness to the patient. As chapters three and four will demonstrate, trustworthiness, along with physicians' construction of knowledge about disease and treatment, were both essential components in delineating a successful outcome of medical intervention in the seventeenth century. The definition of a successful outcome varied according to the patient and the complaint. It did not necessarily mean that a patient was cured in our modern sense of the word. For example, it could indicate a treatment that elicited a satisfactorily evident response from the body rather than the absence of any symptoms.

Roger French has argued that many medieval and early modern physicians were successful from a contemporary viewpoint, in that they were able to meet society's expectations. They achieved this, at least in part, by helping to *create* those expectations.[26] David Harley has argued that in the realm of patient expectations, mental processes are not separate from bodily functions, but that trust and expectation have physiological effects that are required for successful healing. Harley defines healing as a 'social construction that requires a plausible practitioner who can deploy a credible system in a successful negotiation that brings order to the patient's experience.'[27] The manner in which physicians represented their offerings was crucial to their ability to differentiate themselves from their competition. Physicians' rhetoric was an important element in their self-representation to each other and their patients, a fact more readily recognized by practitioners in the past than by historians of medicine.

For seventeenth-century physicians, rhetoric included the struggle for plausibility that links medical theories, education, and licensing. Much of the evidence presented in this book is physicians' rhetoric. How they conceptualized their profession is an essential component to understanding how they were able to attract patients.[28] Roger French has described the culmination of their collective efforts as The Good Story. This was their means of persuading patients, pupils, and those in power that physicians were effective practitioners. It encompassed notions about the efficacy of their medicines as well as their right to practice medicine.[29]

What physicians were really offering was perception: the perception that they possessed the knowledge, judgment, and moral probity to be entrusted with a person's health. Many seventeenth-century physicians perceived of themselves as godly physicians, within whose practice medicine and religion did not simply coexist, but complemented one another. It was these perceptions that differentiated the university-educated physician from all other healers. Specifically, physicians capitalized on the parallel between personal and spiritual health as well as between individual and public health in order to distinguish their profession from all other healers, as one that was of prime importance to the physical and spiritual health of the nation. Their efforts helped frame them as both medical and moral authorities, a duality that greatly improved their chances of gaining in status. They used their esoteric knowledge to their advantage by developing medical theories that supported public efforts as diverse as moral reform campaigns aimed at curbing the spread of venereal disease to controlling the sinful behavior of the masses during times of plague.

Public perception was key to the medical profession, yet there were numerous examples in popular culture of physicians exhibiting dubious practices and motivations. Physicians were eager to rehabilitate their image by stressing their piety. Chapter one will therefore define the image of the pious physician that members of the profession constructed, partly in response to criticisms that they were avaricious and atheistic. This self-fashioning was a reaction to negative portrayals in popular culture. It was ultimately beneficial to the profession in that it forced them to articulate their offering and to argue that the contemporary belief in the antagonism of medicine and theology was misinformed: piety and healing came together in the godly physician and offered the best chance of success for their patients. Chapter two explores how in defining their image, physicians received help from religious sermons that employed metaphors to compare Christ with a physician. The sermons integrated the tenets of Christianity with the principles of the practice of medicine. Ideas about the connection between religion and medicine were echoed in the writings of the lay population and were promulgated by physicians, providing them with a way to differentiate their services from those offered by their competition.

This idea of competition is taken up in chapter three, with physicians' attempts both to professionalize and to distinguish themselves from alternative practitioners by offering services that they considered both unique and marketable. They touted their university education and attempted to close ranks against those who practiced medicine without an education or on a part-time basis. Part of their efforts to distinguish themselves depended upon convincing the public of the superior efficacy of orthodox versus unorthodox medical care. This chapter also explores issues of status that were acute to the medical profession in the early seventeenth century due to women practicing midwifery and the tradition of elite women providing medical services for the poor. Chapter four continues the consideration of how competition from unlicensed and part-time practitioners effected the medical profession by focusing on the potential crisis of the dissemination of medical knowledge through the printing press. The new media threatened to devalue university-educated physicians by making advice on medical matters readily available to an increasingly literate public. Physicians eventually responded by using the printing press to their advantage by marketing their self-fashioned image through their own publications. They also used the printing press to convince the public of the connections between learning and morality that lay behind their claims to professional authority while simultaneously deriding their competition.

Chapters five and six focus on one specific disease: syphilis, or the pox, in order to illustrate the manner in which physicians exploited the connection between medicine and morality to champion themselves as superior healers. In chapter five, the effects of the pox on the growth of the medical profession are analyzed. Contemporaries considered the pox a new disease, and therefore physicians had to construct knowledge about it and attempt to fit it into the Galenic model. Their remedies were not substantially different from empiric remedies, but physicians argued that their learned counsel and sage advice yielded the safest course for a dangerous treatment. Chapter six delves into the repercussions of physicians' choosing to associate the disease and its mode of transmission with illicit sexual behavior, specifically prostitution. Stressing the sexual component of the disease led physicians to moralize in their medical writings and navigate a fine line wherein they blamed women for spreading the disease while simultaneously treating infected men with sympathy. The chapter also highlights the difference in the way gender and socioeconomic factors were influential in determining how a sufferer was treated.

The final chapter focuses on plague outbreaks throughout the seventeenth century to continue the examination of the unique offering of physicians: their moral as well as physical healing advice in times of epidemic disease outbreaks. It was through physicians' attempts to control and cure bubonic plague that a new concept of the public health of the nation emerged. Physicians offered comprehensive advice for controlling the behavior of those thought most likely to spread disease: the urban poor. They recommended that the vices of the poor be curbed for the purpose of protecting the public health of the majority. This advice meshed with commonly held beliefs that both disease and vice were harbored in the crowded and unsanitary suburbs of London and other urban centers throughout England. Their suggestions for controlling public behavior in times of epidemic outbreaks and beyond bolstered their position as authority figures and helped them professionalize. The physician's expanded role in regulating public behavior, particularly for those disenfranchised members of the public most often associated with disease of both the physical and spiritual kind, figures prominently in physicians' conceptualization of public health.

The idea that the poorer sort were responsible for spreading disease and therefore must be compelled to remain clean in both a physical and moral sense was influential in determining some physicians' recommendations about what measures should be taken to improve the public health for everyone.

Physicians made notable inroads in the seventeenth century in convincing the public that they could be trusted with the health of the body and the soul. In early modern England, bodily health and the health of one's soul were inexorably entwined. It was therefore imperative that physicians present themselves as capable of caring for both in order to be trusted with the whole health of the individual. Their ability to embrace the nexus of physical and spiritual health is what began to set the learned physician apart from all other types of healers over the course of the seventeenth century. They were able to combine the legacy of their university training with an emerging sense that their skills were divinely ordained to cure disease, particularly disease considered punishment for sin, in order to present themselves as protectors of a bodily health that was dependent on both physical and spiritual wellness.

In a society in which disease was largely interpreted in terms of moral agency, and the physical and spiritual world were so intimately connected, the responsibility of caring for the entire patient, both body and soul, was a matter of public trust. To assume such trust required the highest degree of moral authority, a trait that physicians argued was connected to being learned. Their ability to convince the public of their moral authority is what ultimately proved to be their most powerful weapon against lay and popular healers at a time when there were so many other feasible options for healthcare.

Notes

1   F.P. Verney and M.M. Verney (eds), *The Verney Memoirs. 2 Vols.* (London: Longmans, Green and Company, 1925), 1660. Cited in A. MacFarlane (ed.) *Diary of Ralph Josselin 1616-1683* (London: Oxford University Press, New Series, 1976), 643.

2   W. Shakespeare, 'Hamlet,' in A. Harbage (ed.), *The Complete Pelican Shakespeare* (New York: Viking Penguin, 1969), 3.1.

3   J. Donne, *Devotions Upon Emergent Occasions* (1623), 33.

4   D. Nagy, *Popular Medicine in Seventeenth-Century England* (Bowling Green: Bowling Green State University Popular Press, 1988), 20.

5   L. Beier, 'In Sickness and in Health: A Seventeenth Century Family's Experience,' in R.Porter (ed.), *Patients and Practitioners: Lay Perceptions of Medicine in Pre-Industrial Society* (Cambridge: Cambridge University Press, 1985), 5. Studies of the diary entries of Samuel Pepys and Ralph Josselin support this contention. See R. Latham and W. Matthews (eds), *The*

Diary of Samuel Pepys, 11 vols. (London: Bell & Hyman, 1970-83) and in particular Roy Porter's comments on Pepys in R. Porter, 'The Patient in England, C. 1660-C. 1800,' in A.Wear (ed.), *Medicine in Society* (New York: Cambridge University Press, 1992), 98-99. For commentary on Ralph Josselin's views see L. Beier, 'In Sickness and in Health: A Seventeenth Century Family's Experience' and A. MacFarlane (ed.), *Diary of Ralph Josselin 1616-1683* (London: Oxford University Press, New Series, 1976).

6   See for example L. Beier, *Sufferers and Healers: The Experience of Illness in Seventeenth-Century England* (New York: Routledge, 1987); A. Wear, 'Interfaces: Perceptions of Health and Illness in Early Modern England,' in R. Porter and A. Wear (eds), *Problems and Methods in the History of Medicine* (London: Groom Helm, 1987); and R. Porter, 'The Patient's View: Doing Medical History from Below,' *Theory and Society* 14, no. 2 (1985).

7   The Royal College of Physicians was a tiny group, so I prefer to delineate as physicians those who received a university education, as they comprised a much larger group of practitioners who viewed themselves as a distinct, professional group. Therefore, when I refer to a 'physician' I am indicating an individual who received a university education in medicine, but not necessarily a license from the College of Physicians. For more on this see H. Cook, 'Good Advice and Little Medicine: The Professional Authority of Early Modern English Physicians,' *The Journal of British Studies* 33, no. 1 (January 1994); D. Nagy, *Popular Medicine in Seventeenth-Century England* (Bowling Green: Bowling Green State University Popular Press, 1988); M. Pelling, 'Irregular Practitioners: A Wilderness of Mirrors,' in M. Pelling (ed.), *Medical Conflicts in Early Modern London: Patronage, Physicians, and Irregular Practitioners, 1550-1640* (Oxford: Clarendon Press, 2003); R. Porter, *Disease, Medicine, and Society in England, 1550-1860* (Basingstoke: Macmillan, 1987); and R. Porter and D. Porter, *In Sickness and in Health: The British Experience 1650-1850* (London: Fourth Estate, 1988).

8   The tripartite system of medicine in early modern England placed the physician at the top, followed by the barber-surgeon (and later just the surgeon), then the apothecary. There were many quarrels among these groups, as has been well documented by historians. This book, however, focuses on physicians' struggles to distinguish themselves from part-time healers, empirics, and women healers. In chapter three

12

I will argue that it was a lack of regulation of these practitioners that concerned physicians.

9   D. Nagy, *Popular Medicine in Seventeenth-Century England*, 2 and M. Pelling, *The Common Lot: Sickness, Medical Occupations and the Urban Poor in Early Modern England* (New York: Longman, 1998), 244.

10 Peter Lewis Allen notes that in seventeenth-century England, a single appearance by a physician might cost twenty times the daily income of a poor family. P. L. Allen, *The Wages of Sin: Sex and Disease, Past and Present* (Chicago: University of Chicago Press, 2000), 56. D. Nagy estimates the cost of a London physician in the first half of the seventeenth century to range from 6s 8d to 10s. D. Nagy, *Popular Medicine in Seventeenth-Century England*, 21. For contemporary comment on physicians' fees, see C.D., *Some Reasons, of the Present Decay of the Practise of Physick in Learned and Approved Doctors* (1675) and E. Chamberlayne, *Angliae Notitia, or the Present State of England* (1682).

11 Sir Ralph Verney's sister, Betty Verney, fell heavily into debt, due in part to medical expenses following an illness, causing Sir Ralph Verney to comment, 'Physick keeps her very bare.' F. P. Verney and M.M. Verney (eds), *The Verney Memoirs. 2 Vols.* (London: Longmans, Green and Company, 1925), 1660. Cited in A. MacFarlane (ed.), *Diary of Ralph Josselin 1616-1683* (London: Oxford University Press, New Series, 1976), 643.

12 N. Moore, *The History of the Study of Medicine in the British Isles* (Oxford: Clarendon Press, 1908). The seminal work is Sir G. Clark, *History of the Royal College of Physicians of London* (Oxford: Clarendon Press, 1964). For commentary on and a reassessment of Clark's work, see R.S. Roberts, 'The Royal College of Physicians of London in the Sixteenth and Seventeenth Centuries,' *History of Science* 5 (1966), 87-100.

13 H. Cook, 'Policing the Health of London: The College of Physicians and the Early Stuart Monarchy,' *Social History of Medicine* 2 (1989); C. Webster, 'The College of Physicians: "Solomon's House" In Commonwealth England,' *Bulletin of the History of Medicine* 51, no. 5 (2003); F. Dawbarn, 'Patronage and Power: The College of Physicians and the Jacobean Court,' *BJHS* 31 (1998); and W.J. Birkin, 'The Royal College of Physicians of London and Its Support of the Parliamentary Cause in the English Civil War,' *The Journal of British Studies* 23, no. 1 (1983). These historians have contended that past work on the history of medicine focused too narrowly on the activities of the Royal College

of Physicians, a minuscule group when compared to all other healers.

14   H. Cook, *The Decline of the Old Medical Regime in Stuart London* (Ithaca: Cornell University Press, 1986).

15   M. Pelling, 'Compromised by Gender: The Role of the Male Medical Practitioner in Early Modern England,' in H. Marland and M. Pelling (eds), *The Task of Healing: Medicine, Religion and Gender in England and the Netherlands 1450-1800* (Rotterdam: Erasmus Publishing, 1996), 102 and W. Birken, 'The Social Problem of the English Physician in the Early Seventeenth Century,' *Medical History* 31 (April 1987), 62. See also J. Axtell, 'Education and Status in Stuart England: The London Physicians,' *History of Education Quarterly* 10, no. 2 (Summer 1970).

16   For some examples see H. Cook, *The Decline of the Old Medical Regime in Stuart London* (Ithaca: Cornell University Press, 1986); R. Porter, *Health for Sale: Quackery in England 1660-1850* (Manchester: Manchester University Press, 1989); and D. Nagy, *Popular Medicine in Seventeenth-Century England*.

17   M. Pelling, *Medical Conflicts in Early Modern London: Patronage, Physicians, and Irregular Practitioners, 1550-1640*, 332-3.

18   For example, on the culture of illness from patients' perspectives, see R. Porter, 'The Patient's View: Doing Medical History from Below'; R. Porter, *Health for Sale: Quackery in England 1660-1850*; R. Porter, 'The Patient in England, C. 1660-C.1800,' in A. Wear (ed.), *Medicine in Society* (New York: Cambridge University Press, 1992); L. Beier, *Sufferers and Healers: The Experience of Illness in Seventeenth-Century England*; M. Pelling, 'Irregular Practitioners: A Wilderness of Mirrors'; and M. Pelling, *Medical Conflicts in Early Modern London: Patronage, Physicians, and Irregular Practitioners, 1550-1640*.

19   M. Pelling, *The Common Lot: Sickness, Medical Occupations and the Urban Poor in Early Modern England* (New York: Longman, 1998), 5.

20   R. Anselment, *The Realms of Apollo: Literature and Healing in Seventeenth-Century England* (Newark: University of Delaware Press, 1995), 17, 11.

21   R. Anselment, *The Realms of Apollo: Literature and Healing in Seventeenth-Century England*, 16.

22   See for example H. Cook, *The Decline of the Old Medical Regime in Stuart London*; F. Dawbarn, 'Patronage and Power: The College of Physicians and the Jacobean Court,' *BJHS* 31 (1998); and C. Hill, 'The Medical Profession and Its Radical Critics,' in C. Hill (ed.), *Change and Continuity in Seventeenth-Century England* (London: 1774).

23 R. Porter and D. Porter, *In Sickness and in Health: The British Experience 1650-1850*, 72. The Porters give credit for these ideas to D. King-Hele, *Doctor of Revolution: The Life and Genius of Erasmus Darwin* (London: Faber, 1977), 255.

24 R. Anselment, *The Realms of Apollo: Literature and Healing in Seventeenth-Century England*, 30.

25 D. Harley, 'Rhetoric and the Social Construction of Sickness and Healing,' *The Society for the Social History of Medicine* (1999), 414.

26 R. French, *Medicine Before Science: The Rational and Learned doctor from the Middle Ages to the Enlightenment* (New York: Cambridge University Press, 2003), 1.

27 D. Harley, 'Rhetoric and the Social Construction of Sickness and Healing,' 434.

28 D. Harley, 'Rhetoric and the Social Construction of Sickness and Healing,' 434.

29 R. French, *Medicine Before Science: The Rational and Learned doctor from the Middle Ages to the Enlightenment*, 2.

PART I

THE DOCTORS

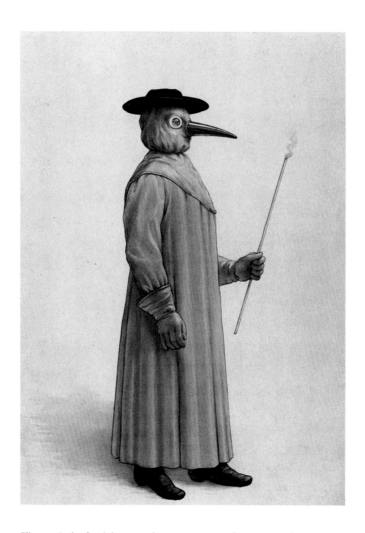

Figure 4: A physician wearing a seventeenth-century plague
preventive costume
Courtesy of Wellcome Library, London

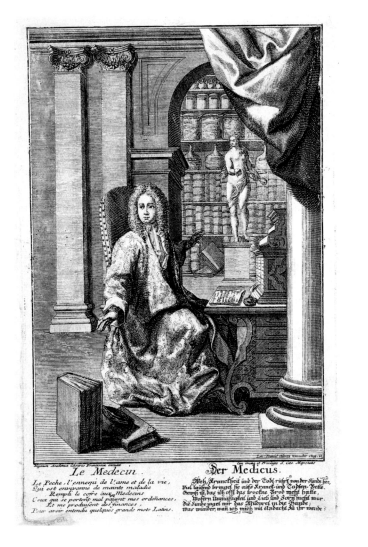

Figure 5: A physician in his study, turning to the viewer to exploit illness arising from sin
Courtesy of Wellcome Library, London

1

'God heals, and the Doctor takes the fee'[1]:
Combatting the Negative Reputation

People fall into the Doctor's hand, and so consequently into the Lord's…Ten Tyburns cannot turn men over the perch so fast as one of these brewers of purgations…an Art to make poor souls kick up their heels. Insomuch that even their sick grunting patients stand in more danger of M. Doctor and his drugs than of all the Cannon shots which the desperate disease itself can discharge against them.[2]

Thomas Dekker, *The Gull's Hornbook* 1609

A Good Physitian comes to thee in the shape of an Angell, and therefore let him boldly take thee by the hand, for he has been in Gods garden, gathering herbes: and soveraine rootes to cure thee.[3]

Thomas Dekker, *The Plague Pamphlets* 1603

These two powerful statements about physicians were written during the same decade by the same author, yet they present the image of the physician in contradictory ways. How can we account for these divergent strains? Which one should be used as evidence of the manner in which seventeenth-century society regarded the physician? The profession of medicine was not viewed uniformly throughout society, at the beginning of the century, or at any other time. Attitudes toward physicians can be unearthed through an array of source material, but perhaps one of the most useful is popular drama, as it is a media that reflected values and commonplace beliefs of society at large. The representation of physicians on the stage was overwhelmingly negative, as well as prolific, in the first half of the century. This representation stands in stark contrast to physicians' writing about the profession of medicine. Their incarnations of the ideal physician are remarkably homogenous in their assertion that he possessed the moral authority central to engendering trust in his patients. This proved a hard sell for physicians, as they were attempting to buck two firmly entrenched beliefs consistently alluded to on stage: that the profession was intrinsically immoral, perhaps even atheistic, and equally damning, that physicians' services were wholly irrelevant to the lives and healthcare needs of the vast majority of the population.

Recent studies of the history of medicine, often from the patient's perspective, have yielded valuable insight into the ways in which patients viewed their health and the options available to them when they became ill. These historians agree that the majority of healing was done by family members, empirics, or gentlewomen. They have concluded that the university-educated physician was largely superfluous to the popular culture of healing in seventeenth-century England.[4]

This culture of illness is typically described as one in which licensed physicians were few, employing them could be cost-prohibitive, and a hierarchy of resort was normal procedure for dealing with illness. The hierarchy of resort is a concept developed by anthropologists and utilized by historians to describe how a suffering individual sought help. The individual's first response to signs of illness was to reflect on previous personal experience and then to compare notes among family and friends. As concern escalated or the condition proved stubborn, one recourse after another was tried, eventually leading to consultation with a practitioner. Generally, the practitioner was a last resort, and sometimes he was not consulted at all. This hierarchy was at least in part geographical, since licensed physicians could be difficult to find in more remote areas.[5]

The implication of such arguments is that the lay community did not see the value in consulting physicians for most of their ailments. However, not employing a physician did not necessarily correlate with a lack of respect for the profession or a lack of trust in the efficacy of their healing. Instead, the reasons why many people did not employ physicians when they became ill tended to be practical rather than principled. Neither Samuel Pepys nor Ralph Josselin regularly consulted physicians, yet in both cases the motivation was not ideological. Samuel Pepys felt he could handle most of his ailments on his own although he counted physicians among his friends and acquaintances. Ralph Josselin could not afford to employ a physician for much of the timespan covered in his diary writing, so he and his wife treated their family's illnesses, even the most serious cases.[6] In fact, when it became financially feasible for the Josselins to hire a physician, they began doing so, going so far as to consult one even when they were healthy. Josselin even recorded his criticism of a woman whom he believed could afford the help of a physician but elected instead to pay a poor woman two shillings to ask a doctor for advice rather than have him consult with her directly.[7] Failure to consult physicians, therefore, does not imply the public's lack of respect or skepticism about their expertise.

Yet negative stereotypes of the physician abounded in popular culture. They were anything but new during the early modern period. The trope of the atheistic and greedy physician was deployed as early as the Middle Ages, and depictions in seventeenth-century drama and literature generally impugned physicians on similar grounds.[8] They were often derided for their propensity to use indiscernible Latin terms in order to cloak a suspicious lack of knowledge about the conditions they charged so much to cure. In John Earle's *Microcosmographie* the physician's learning is limited to his 'reckoning up the hard names of diseases, and the superscriptions of Gallypots in his Apothecaries Shoppe, which are rank't in his shelves and the Doctors memory.' He 'speaks Greeke many times when he knows not.'[9] In Thomas Middleton's *A Fair Quarrel*, the medical man is continually asked to speak in plainer terms until he is forced to admit that he does not understand the patient's disorder:

> Marry, in plainer terms I do not know what to say to him; the wound, I can assure you, inclines to paralism, and I find his body cacochymic…
> I nourish him altogether with viands refrigerative, and give for potion the juice of savicola dissolved with water cerefolium; I could do no more, lady, if his best ginglymus were disseuered.[10]

Although the physician may be eager to impress his patient, his enthusiasm is reserved only for the wealthy, as evidenced by the following sardonic comment in Ben Jonson's *The Poetaster*: 'You make no more haste now, than …a physician to a patient that has no money.'[11]

These greedy pseudo-intellectuals are portrayed as causing more harm than good. Thomas Dekker's *Fortunatus* includes the following wry observation: 'Hunger is an excellent physician, for he dares kill anybody.' In the same play, a character declares: 'I am a true doctor indeed, that tie up my living in the knots of winding sheets.'[12] In Ben Jonson's *Volpone,* doctors are accused of being 'the greatest danger / And worse disease to escape.'[13] Shakespeare's *Timon of Athens*, meanwhile, contains the following admonition: 'Trust not

21

the physician / His antidotes are poison, and he slays / More than you rob.'[14]

It is not surprising, then, that the characters who become ill in these works are leery of submitting to the care (and fees) of the physician. Massinger asserts that the physician's skill is 'to make sound men sick, and sick men kill,'[15] while the lead character in *Perkin Warbeck* exclaims that he would rather be executed than 'Be massacred alive / By some physician, for a month or two.'[16] Worse still, there is some insinuation that at times the physician, out of avarice, might hasten a patient's death. Ben Jonson's *Volpone* and *The Silent Woman*, as well as in Lyle's *Campaspe*, allude to such fears.[17] All suggest how unwise it is to make one's physician one's heir. The most complete and utter impugning of the character of the physician, however, appears in John Ford's *The Lover's Melancholy*:

> Thou art in thy religion an Atheist, in thy condition a cur, in thy diet an epicure, in thy lust a goat, in thy sleep a hog; thou takest upon thee the habit of a grave physician, but thou art indeed an imposturous empiric. Physicians are the cobblers, rather the botchers, of men's bodies; as the one patches our tattered clothes, so the other solders our diseased flesh.[18]

It is not just the technical skill and the erudite learning of the physician that this diatribe calls into question but his character as well.

Such descriptions would seem to imply that the physician was held in contempt in early Stuart society, but why? There was a widespread feeling that the profession was untrustworthy, arising from specific instances of high profile physicians acting in a morally suspect manner. An example was Dr. Roderigo Lopez, Elizabeth I's physician, who was executed for an alleged conspiracy to poison the queen. The scandal was still remembered by Stuart society. Physicians like George Bate, Peter Chamberlen, and William Stanes, all of whom suggested that they had speeded Oliver Cromwell's death, perpetuated this image of untrustworthiness, particularly the association of the physician with poisons.[19] They were mirrored by characters administering poisons on the stage, such as the physician Eudemis in Jonson's *Sejanus*, Dr. Julio in Webster's *The White Devil*, and Doctor Lecure in Beaumont and Fletcher's *The Tragedy of Thierry and Theodoret*.[20] Webster's *Duchess of Malfi* questions the efficacy of the physician's medicine: 'She'll use some prepared antidote of her own, Lest the physicians should re-poison her.'[21] Whether intentional or through gross incompetence, the result would be the same:

grievous harm at the hands of a physician.

There was also a lack of morality, or 'odour of impiety,' that surrounded the profession. This stemmed from the popular belief that physicians were naturally atheists. The medieval tag *ubi tres medici, duo athei*—where there are three physicians there are two atheists—provides telling evidence of long-standing popular attitudes.[22] In the seventeenth century, suspicions continued to dog the profession, as the following passage in the Reverend John Ward's diary illustrates: 'One told the bishop of Glocester not long since, that hee imagined that physitians, of all other men, were the most competent judges of all others in affairs of religion; and his reason was, because they are wholly unconcerned in the matter.'[23] This supposed impiety had its roots in traditional medicine's theoretical foundations resting on the teachings of Hippocrates and Galen. While the theories of these Pagan healers might be sound, they were an uncomfortable fit in a Christian world that deemed sickness to be sent by God. All too often the physician was seen ignoring such religious considerations and treating sickness in an entirely naturalistic way.[24]

Not surprisingly, physicians vehemently disagreed with this assessment of their role. Physicians argued that they were not treating sickness as a purely natural phenomenon and that there existed no inherent conflict between the practice of medicine and religion. Physicians did not feel constrained by religious teaching, nor did they believe that their actions were in conflict with religious doctrine.[25] In fact, medical practitioners were as frightened of atheism as anyone else in seventeenth-century society was, and they were equally concerned with matters of religion and religious orthodoxy both in their personal lives and in their practice of medicine.[26]

Physicians had not been hesitant in the past to take up their pens in defense of physic. There existed in the seventeenth century a long tradition of writing medical rhetoric. There were orations, dedicatory letters, elegies, and complimentary poems, all in praise of medicine and physicians. The writers could call upon a compilation of commonplaces about medicine's origins, nobility, and usefulness. Indeed, many of them were conveniently collected in various encyclopedic compendiums from which they could draw inspiration.[27]

When physicians addressed the issue of medicine and religion in their writing, they acknowledged the negative stereotypes in society but defended their profession against them. The physician Edmund Gayton acknowledged that "tis true, that Sir Jeffry Chaucer had but an ill opinion of my Faculty, when he saith of a Doctor of Physick, "His meat was good and digestible,

/ But not a word he had o' th' Bible."' Such images of physicians compelled him to pen his meditations 'To wipe off that stain and aspersion…to shew the World, that it is possible for a Physician of the Lower Form to be Theologue,' and he pointed out that Saint Luke was a 'Physician, an Apostle and Evangelist.'[28] Although Gayton would have liked to convince the world of the piety of physicians, it is unlikely that many people outside of the medical community read his meditations. Far more were exposed to popular drama, yet in their writing physicians were clarifying, at least for themselves, an ideal of the godly physician and how he should practice medicine.

In his *Anatomy of Melancholy*, Robert Burton argued that the model practice united medicine and religion: 'We must use prayer and physicke both together; and so no doubt but our prayers will be available, and our physicke take effect.'[29] The physician Thomas Browne ruminated on the relationship between physicians and religion in his *Religio Medici*, and he concluded that the profession as a whole was working against medicine's 'odour of impiety,' which some considered to be the 'general scandal of [the medical] profession,' although Browne insisted that religion and medicine were complementary.[30] Browne even claimed that the study of medicine should lead physicians away from atheism by allowing them to study and gain respect for God's creation. He asserted that God entrusted the physician with the care of 'the masterpieces of the Creator.' A healer's awesome responsibility placed him in a unique position to appreciate the divinity in nature and man's singular role in the chain of being. A member of the College of Physicians, Browne had participated in dissections, a controversial practice in terms of Christian morality. Yet Browne argued that anatomizing a human body had allowed him to 'contemplate God's wonder in miniature.' By studying the microcosm, he was able to gain perspective on his own mortality within God's grand plan, an endeavor that led him even closer to God.[31] Physicians such as Browne stressed the compatibility of devout Christian faith with scientific investigation, making it clear that one could and should be a pious Christian as well as a physician. In doing so, these writers helped form the ideal of the godly physician, within whose practice medicine and religion did not simply coexist but complemented one another.

This perceived interconnection of medicine and religion was part of a greater discussion stretching beyond England. Continental physicians, both Catholic and Protestant, presented models of how religious faith should affect the morals and personal character of the practitioner. The Catholic physician Caspar Bartholin encouraged anyone who was a student of the art of physic to be a moral, honest Christian who 'every single morning, after prayers [should] read one or two chapters from Holy Scripture, not superficially but carefully and reflectively; and in such a way that each and every year he runs through the whole Bible and completes it.' His view of the intrinsic nature of religion in the practice of medicine was summed up in the following advice aimed at those considering entering the profession: 'First and foremost, therefore, I commend to you piety, an unblemished life, daily prayers, love of the Word of God and heed for it: If God is not present and pours strength into herbs, what use, I ask, ...is panacea?'[32] This type of godly physician was determined to be the ideal practitioner by seventeenth-century European physicians.[33] The Catholic physician Girolamo Bardi asserted that such medical practitioners 'carry with them a panacea not so much to counter diseases as to eradicate sins by the roots.' Bardi stressed that since God created medicine, ideal physicians should be 'learned men, who practice sacred medicine with holiness and devoutness.'[34]

Both Catholic and Protestant physicians agreed that because religion played an integral role in the practice of medicine for the pious physician, Jewish physicians were problematic, in some cases suggesting that they endangered their patients' souls.[35] The seventeenth-century physician Scipion Mercurio wrote against Jewish physicians for this reason. He remarked that some people (he mentions specifically heathens and Jews) undertook the study of medicine without piety but would have difficulty succeeding in the profession because it was one 'fraught with difficulty and anxiety,' in which only God can help.[36] The Hamburg physician Jacob Martini claimed that a physician was concerned not only with what related to health, but with what related to the conscience as well. He concluded that a Jewish physician was not capable of being trusted with these.[37] The Jewish physician Benedict a Castro responded to such claims:

> Physicians do not concern themselves with conscience, with the health of the soul, but the health of the body and the remedy and cure of diseases, and thus he [the writer] should have found fault with Jewish physicians not for their Jewishness (for that is a question of religion), but for some supposed lack of learning and an ineptitude for the art of medicine.[38]

25

Castro's remarks attempted to refute common thinking: that medicine was entwined with Christianity, just as the body was entwined with the soul. Jewish physicians practicing in Christian countries, therefore, faced an uphill battle in arguing that there was no intrinsic connection between medicine and Christianity. Castro acknowledged the connection just as he argued against it: 'If I should ask you why you practice the art of medicine, you would say without doubt, because as a doctor, you are a Christian. But this assertion is stupid and of no moment.'[39] The frustrated tone of Castro's defense illuminates the entrenched assumption among Christian physicians of the connection between their practice of medicine and their practice of religion.

For the godly physician, there was no friction between religion and the practice of medicine. It was an inherent part of how the profession defined not only their personal character but also their professional history. Religious doctrine, in particular Calvinisim, gave its moral approval to godly practitioners and proved a boon to the image of the godly physician. By rejecting the miraculous efficacy of sacraments and relics, Calvinists saw God as operating almost exclusively through secondary causes. As chapter three will demonstrate, this view was favorable to the advancement of medical knowledge and the medical professions. It encouraged regular practitioners to take pride in their profession as a calling, and it gave them the moral imperative in challenging their competitors, who, unlike physicians, were seeking only a monetary reward. Calvinism's effect on the practice of medicine outlived its tenure. Even when Providentialism significantly eroded after 1660, many of the moral attitudes associated with it survived among non-conformists and pious Anglicans.[40]

Such was the arsenal of the pious physician, and while the majority of English physicians were not penning meditations on religion, they were incorporating these values into their medical writings. The overwhelming majority of physicians' treatises written in the seventeenth century included ready references to the healing power of God, biblical quotations, prayers, and notations that they were publishing for the needy, even sometimes indicating that their works were to be distributed free of charge to the poorer sort. In light of the aforementioned lampooning of physicians, these inclusions may be more than mere lip service. The image of the godly physician helped combat the mockery of atheistic, greedy physicians in drama. Focusing on their connection with religion helped dispel what physicians considered to be the myth of their 'odour of impiety.' It is this image that would come to define the medical profession's unique offering of a healer capable of caring for the whole individual, body and soul. It was an image whose influence proved exceedingly helpful to the moral authority of the seventeenth-century physician.

Physicians' writing throughout the century stressed the Providential nature of disease, the centrality of the physician in God's plan for healing, and the connection between body and soul in the health of the individual. Medical treatises acknowledged that bodily sickness was sometimes God's mode of instruction. Robert Burton concluded that 'Sickness may be for the good of their souls; 'tis parcel of their destiny; the flesh rebels against the spirit; that which hurts the one must help the other. Sickness is the mother of modesty, and putteth us in mind of our mortality.'[41] Scipion Mercurio, a physician writing in Padua in the early seventeenth century, asserted that all diseases were 'ordained by divine providence,' for a variety of reasons. Disease could be God's punishment on His enemies or the consequence of sin. Its purpose often was to lead sinners to repentance, so that 'removing the cause of the punishment...might also remove the punishment itself.'[42] Such reasoning made the duty of the physician all the more important, as he must consider not only what disease ailed a patient, but also why God chose to send it to that patient at that particular time.

Nicholas Culpeper referred to health as 'the greatest of all Earthly Blessings.'[43] His assertion is indicative of the message that many physicians espoused in their writing: disease was sent from God, health was His blessing and medicine His gift to mankind. Seventeenth-century physicians were consistent in stressing their association with the divine. Medical tracts often began with biblical passages that emphasized the role of God in the art of physic. The tracts often included prayers and an acknowledgment that all remedies worked only through the grace of God.[44] Even if such inclusions were merely customary, they were nevertheless indicative of a culture of healing, extending throughout the century, and espoused by physicians, which assured that God was intrinsically involved.[45]

Additional evidence that physicians found an ideological place for God in their healing throughout the century exists in the numerous and at times lengthy discussions about the association of sin and disease in otherwise secular medical treatises. In 1617 the physician William Vaughan discussed the issue at length and finally remarked, 'For who can count all the diseases which the Justice of *God* hath heaped upon man for sinne?'[46] A physician in 1700 stressed that members of his profession should never forget where their healing power originated: 'The right Phisician is indeed made of God

27

for the health of Mankind.'[47] Physicians therefore stressed the proper usage of their talents, urging others of their profession to 'Use our Labors with Diligence, Care, Ingenuity, Compassion towards the sick, and in the fear of God. Attribute the Success and Honor of all thy Endeavors to him.'[48] Doreen Nagy has argued that late in the century authors of medical tracts 'co-opted the Divine to establish their legitimacy in the treatment of illness.'[49] Evidence of this lies in late seventeenth-century medical treatises, which stressed the need to receive God's blessing as part of a plan for preventative medicine: 'Above all things, devoutly invoke God for his benediction without which neither Paul, nor Apollo, Galenist nor Chymist, Food nor Physick can do anything.'[50] God was the ultimate source of all healing, as physicians were quick to acknowledge.

As Robert Burton stated in *The Anatomy of Melancholy*: 'For all the physick we can use, art, excellent industry, is to no purpose without calling upon God…we must use prayer and physick both together: and so no doubt but our prayers will be available, and our physick take effect.'[51] It was both logical and pragmatic for physicians to cling to the association between medicine and religion for as long as possible because it offered them a cultural sanction that complemented their expertise. While God ordained sickness and health, He also endowed the physician with the ability to affect well-being.

Many medical writers also found it prudent to remind the public of the biblical references to the physician, which may account for the quoting of biblical passages on so many front-pages of physicians' medical writing. In 1622, Richard Banister quoted Ecclesiastes 38:4 on his title page: 'God hath created medicines of the earth, and he that is wise, will not condemn them.'[52] Some physicians quoted the passage in its entirety to justify employing a physician when illness occurred, such as Alexander Read whose title page read: 'Honour the Physician with that honour that is due unto him because of Necessity: for the Lord hath created him. For of the most High cometh healing…The Lord hath created medicines, etc.'[53] Thomas Brugis reproduced the same passage and concluded that the physician, whom he described as 'God's Hand,' was only marginally less important than God himself in the treatment of illness.[54] This biblical quotation appeared again on Peter Leven's title page, coupled with the admonition 'Give unto the Physician, that unto him belongeth.'[55]

An anonymous seventeenth-century commonplace book of medical quotations and anatomical notes declared 'The short life of our Saviour… was, as it were, as spiritual caring, and healing of the Soul, and afterwards of the Body also; such physitians afterwards were his apostles.'[56] These quotations and statements alluded to the natural connection between God and the physician and the latter's necessity in healing with the blessing of the former.

Physicians considered themselves the heirs of God's healing power, and as such, they could never be interested exclusively in physical healing but must consider the health of the soul as well. As the physician Girolamo Bardi avowed, ideal physicians 'carry with them a panacea not so much to counter diseases as to eradicate sins by the roots, prepared both for the office of priests and physicians.'[57] Seventeenth-century physicians stressed the necessity of maintaining the health of body and soul alike. The physician William Parke offered his medical treatise as a 'panacaea of both soul and body.'[58] Edmund Gayton modeled proper health maintenance for his patients: he had not neglected his body or his soul, as such 'ought to be the care of every man, much more of a Christian.'[59] Their connection with God lay in a healing power that was ordained by Him and was therefore appropriate for healing the whole patient, both body and soul. However, physicians were careful to disentangle their intended services from those of the minister: they were meant to care for the body first and foremost, and the healthy soul was a by-product:

> 'Tis certain, according to practice, our Art doth not so much intend the amendment of the soul as of the body… But to say precisely and peremptorily, that the Physician hath nothing to do in respect of the soul is more than can be justified: for the physic of the body is but a preparative for the bettering of the soul, which is highly eased and fitted for Divine contemplation, by emptying a Plethorick cask.[60]

Nevertheless, as these tracts demonstrated, it was not only sermon writers who explored the importance of both body and soul to the overall health of the individual. In fact, the linking of body and soul would prove a crucial argument in physicians' efforts to present themselves as caretakers of the health of the entire individual.

Physicians even considered the function of the soul in anatomical terms, as evidenced by the following dissection tract, wherein the author discussed the anatomical significance of the size of man's liver in relation to its spiritual purpose:

29

It is bigger in man than any other living creature, if you consider the proportion of his body; for it was fit so to bee, [so that] man was to have greatest store of bloud, lest spirits should faile in performing the functions of the soule, wherewith man is most copiously furnished.[61]

Medical writers scientifically delineated the link between body and soul in order to assert the association between God and the physician. Another physician wrote of the centrality of the soul to the body: 'For, this I see, that the soule quickeneth these mortall bodies, and giveth life to them, so long as it remaineth therein.' This system was ordained by God, 'who maintaine and keepe this orderly course of the whole world.'[62]

Yet just as the soul could imbue the body with life, so could the soul, if diseased, debilitate the body. The French physician Jacques Ferrand listed the most common and troubling diseases that afflicted the soul as 'Forgetfulnesse of God, Torment of Conscience, and Despair of Mercy.'[63] Although the diseases Ferrand described were spiritual, just as they were in sermons, physicians argued they had a physical, debilitating effect on the body. Physicians' publications emphasized that an unclean soul could lead to a distracted mind, which could have serious repercussions for one's health: 'for the Body being diseased adds grief to the mind, the mind being distracted encreaseth the Disease, so both being oppressed…till at length you must die.'[64] William Cole elaborated on how all elements were entwined:

For as when the body is diseased, the spirit is presently sad, or hindred from its action: so when the spirit is ill disposed, the minde cannot performe its functions dextrously: as we may see in drunken, melancholie, mad-men, *&c*. Hence it is, that the gifts of the minde follow the temperature of the body.[65]

It was through the health of both that a man 'shall become excellent in all conditions…and lead his life with health of body and mind.'[66] William Cole discussed the importance of maintaining the soul as part of overall bodily health. He described the soul as the 'Seate of a distemper' that could infect the rest of the body.[67] If the soul were in poor health, the body would suffer illness as well.

In essence, seventeenth-century physicians elaborated on a long-standing concept of total-body health that encompassed body and soul, and in doing so, their writing melded neatly with religious sermons that were explaining health in precisely the same terms. The medical explanation was in fact so similar to those espoused in sermons that the divine Thomas Adams actually used medical theory in his sermon *Diseases of the soule a discourse diuine, morall, and physicall*. When he described the '*Sickenesses* in mens *Soules*' that 'are bred like diseases in naturall, or corruptions in ciuill bodies' he 'borrow[ed] so much Timber out of *Galens* wood, as shall serue me for a scaffold to build vp my Morall discourse.'[68] Conversely, the Catholic physician Scipion Mercurio used medical theory to prove that the sacrament of reconciliation could aid a patient's physical recovery. The day after confession, the patient would experience improvement in his or her pulse, urine, sputum, and excrements. If the patient confessed early in the course of illness, he or she could lessen the severity of illness. Although confession was not an option in Protestant England, Catholic as well as Protestant physicians seemed to have agreed upon the idea that a guilty conscience could negatively affect the body. Richard Palmer has noted that this explanation actually stemmed from the Galenic tradition of medicine, which held that lessening psychological stress (which confession did for many patients) led to improvement in the patient's symptoms.[69]

According to medical men, nothing increased psychological stress more than a guilty conscience. In his section on distressed consciences, David Irish reasoned that if the guilt 'proceed from a consideration of things done that are really sinful in themselves, such Trouble has its *[reign]* from *Conscience*,' and accordingly, negative health consequences would ensue, as no man was so 'Mean, Illiterate, or Rude' as to be immune to the 'ill effects of a *Guilty Soul*.' There was help for those suffering from a guilty conscience, in the form not only of the minister, but also of the Godly physician. Irish reassured those who were sick that they 'ought not to dispair, nor distrust God's ability, with means used to restore you to Health and Peace of Conscience' because 'we see by the goodness of God, with the discreet applications of knowing and honest Phisicians, many reap great benefit, being by them wonderfully restor'd to their former health and strength.'[70]

Irish's tract was typical of medical treatises because he attempted so much more than merely dispensing medical advice. He expounded on the expertise of the physician, assumed his authority derived from God, combined the body and soul in his concept of health, and offered both medical and moral advice. He managed to advertise these varied interests in his title, which is worth quoting in its entirety:

> *Levamen infirmi: or, cordial counsel to the sick and diseased Containing I. Advice concerning physick, and what a physician ought to be; with an account of the author's remedies, and how to take them. II. Concerning melancholy, frensie, and madness; in which, amongst other things, is shew'd, how far they differ from a conscience opprest with the sense of sin, and likewise how they differ among themselves. III. A miscellany of pious discourses, concerning the attributes of God; with ejaculations and prayers, according to scripture rule. Likewise an account of many things which have happen'd since the creation. To which are added several predictions of what may happen to the end of the world. The whole being enrich'd with physical, pious, moral & historical observations, delightful to read, & necessary to know.*

Irish's writing is indicative of physicians' attempts to infuse their tracts with morality in addition to medicine. The fact that the publication date of this tract is 1700 is also significant in that it serves as a reminder not to place too much emphasis on the scientific revolution or the even more nebulous 'secularization of medicine' as factors that successfully separated religion from medicine in the seventeenth century.[71] Although medicine certainly was changing in the seventeenth century, even at the close of the century, despite inroads of Newtonian science, both sermon and medical writers did not ignore an overarching divine wisdom.[72] Physicians were reflecting common lay beliefs in their writing about the intersection of the divine and medicine. As Nancy Sirasi has suggested, in spite of specialized learning and the professional self-consciousness of university-educated physicians, a significant portion of early modern medicine involved knowledge and attitudes shared with and highly dependent upon broader society.[73] University-educated physicians did not consider themselves at odds with the major cultural or religious beliefs of society at large. While their education might set them apart intellectually, they were eager for the public to consider them mainstream in their religious beliefs.

It was necessary to emphasize that religion and healing could peacefully coexist in physicians' practices because their professional authority depended upon this assumption. As Harold Cook has demonstrated, physicians early in the century linked their professional authority to two key concepts, judgment and advice. These concepts were attributes of character at least as much as knowledge. It would not suffice to possess knowledge by itself. Good judgment and advice must be tempered with inner discipline and deep consideration. This was, in part, what a university education yielded to physicians, and it is what separated them from all other medical practitioners. Their formal education aimed to transform students of medicine into physicians of good character, deserving of the public's trust and capable of exercising good judgment and advice.[74] Patients who employed physicians wanted them to make predictions about the course and outcome of an illness. The prognosis was valued in a system where diagnosis tended to be sketchy and medical practitioners' curative skills were lacking.[75] Predicting the course an illness might take and advising the patient on a carefully considered health and diet regimen depended upon the sound judgment of the physician.

In addition to prognosis, the physician's task, as he understood it, was to offer wise council about health. The early modern physician was a lifestyle advisor more so than a slayer of disease. He tailored his advice to each patient. Doing so necessitated judgment of the unique qualities of each person. Consequently, physicians gave counsel, restoring health to their patients and persuading them to change their habits, rather than simply administering medicines to them. This persuasion included stressing the connection between health and virtue, making it even more essential that the physician possess excellent character as well as knowledge.[76]

Historians of medicine have searched in vain for a code of early modern medical ethics. As Harold Cook has pointed out, they have found only medical etiquette, but etiquette *was* a form of professional ethics as understood in the period.[77] For physicians their outward appearance, their dignified and grave demeanor, their erudite advice, and their moral character functioned as their code of ethics. This is why physicians of the period were so interested in delineating the characteristics of a good physician and why excellent character was an unwavering element in their compendium of desired qualities. The moral authority that they claimed was an inherent part of their profession and was as important as their long robes and caps in identifying them as physicians. Their dress instantly signified them as physicians on the Elizabethan stage, with or without their iconic urine flask.[78] This was, of course, part of why they made such an attractive target for on-stage parodying. The formal dress, the elaborate jargon, and the serious demeanor of physicians all lent themselves to caricature.

These readily identifiable features of the physician also worked to his advantage in the early seventeenth century. They disentangled the learned physician from his competitors, a concept discussed in chapter three. It could also be argued that these external trapping of erudite language and distinctive garb could aid efficacy in patient care. Trust in the ability of the healer was key to a successful encounter, and the identifiable features of the physician helped to engender such a trust. As David Harley has demonstrated, the process of establishing trust with the patient turned upon the physician having a good reputation, behaving in a way that the patient considered appropriate, and giving an account of the disease that either impressed or made sense to the patient. The presence of a trusted and authoritative healer was essential because patients brought their attitudes and beliefs with them to the healing process, as they continue to do in the present, and this could affect the outcome. The practitioner's persona was inseparable from successful healing, just as a white coat and stethoscope today symbolize access to science and hidden knowledge.[79] The specific trappings or qualities that create confidence in the patient are culturally constructed and changeable. The self-fashioned image of the early modern learned medical professional hinged on a moral authority intended to encourage trust in his patients of his judgment and ability, and thereby offer them the best chance for a satisfactory medical encounter.

'Send them [physicians] packing…beat not your brains to understand their parcel-Greek, parcel-Latin gibberish.'[80] The purposely-convoluted terminology that signified the erudite learning of the medical profession was often mocked, but physicians envisioned their university education as an intrinsic element necessary in the performance of their subscribed duties of wise judgment and good counsel, both of which formed the core of their moral authority. While it is easy to default to citing pithy jabs at physicians in plays and rhymes in order to claim that the seventeenth-century physician was much maligned, there are more voices to be heard, among them the physicians' themselves. The atheistic physician was a stock character, and as such should be handled cautiously. Most people probably did not take literally the suggestion that physicians were atheists, but the hyperbole of the atheistic physician suggested a much more plausible truism: that the study of science in general, and medicine in particular, was not compatible with religious piety. It is this claim that physicians labored to refute. It was important that they challenge the assumption that medicine and religion could not coexist in the person of the physician, even if their tracts were not widely read by the lay public, because their professional authority depended upon their good judgment and character. By writing for each other, they helped form their own self-image, one that they wished to present to the public: the godly physician who possessed sound morals and good judgment. These two essential qualities were the product of their university education and physicians argued were the key elements that enabled them to properly advise and care for their patients.

Notes

1   B. Franklin, *Poor Richard's Almanac* (1744).

2   T. Dekker, *The Gull's Hornbook* (1609). Cited in Paul Brewster, 'Physician and Surgeon as Depicted in 16th and 17th Century English Literature,' *Osiris* 14 (1962), 20.

3   F.P. Wilson (ed.), *The Plague Pamphlets of Thomas Dekker* (Oxford: Clarendon Press, 1925), 188-9.

4   L. Beier, *Sufferers and Healers: The Experience of Illness in Seventeenth-Century England* (New York: Routledge, 1987); D. Nagy, *Popular Medicine in Seventeenth-Century England* (Bowling Green: Bowling Green State University Popular Press, 1988); R. Porter, 'The Patient's View: Doing Medical History from Below,' *Theory and Society* 14, no. 2 (1985); R. Porter, 'The Patient in England, C. 1660-C.1800,' in A. Wear (ed.), *Medicine in Society* (New York: Cambridge University Press, 1992); and R. Porter and D. Porter, *In Sickness and in Health: The British Experience 1650-1850* (London: Fourth Estate, 1988).

5   The phrase 'hierarchy of resort' was coined by anthropologist Lola Romanucci-Ross and is described in M. Pelling, *Medical Conflicts in Early Modern London: Patronage, Physicians, and Irregular Practitioners, 1550-1640* (Oxford: Clarendon Press, 2003), 230. See also M. MacDonald, *Mystical Bedlam: Madness, Anxiety, and Healing in Seventeenth-Century England* (Cambridge: Cambridge University Press, 1981) and D. Nagy, *Popular Medicine in Seventeenth-Century England*. Lucinda Beier has also argued that educated lay people read medical books and did not hesitate to treat themselves when ill. See L. Beier, *Sufferers and Healers: The Experience of Illness in Seventeenth-Century England*.

6   R. Porter, 'The Patient in England, C. 1660-C. 1800,' 98-99.

7   A. MacFarlane, ed., *Diary of Ralph Josselin 1616-1683* (London: Oxford University Press, New Series, 1976), 584, 595, 634, 642, 392.

8   A. Wear, 'Religious Beliefs and Medicine in Early Modern England,' in H. Marland and M. Pelling (eds), *The Task of Healing: Medicine, Religion and Gender in England and the Netherlands, 1450-1800* (Rotterdam: Erasmus Publishing, 1996).

9   J. Earle, *Microcosmographie, or a Piece of the Worlds Discovered in Essays and Characters* (1529).

10   T. Middleton, *A Fair Quarrel* (1613), IV, ii.

11   B. Jonson, *The Poetaster* (1616), V.i.

12   T. Dekker, *The Pleasant Comedie of Old Fortunatus* (1600), II, ii and V, ii.

13   B. Jonson, *Volpone* (1606), I, iv.

14   W. Shakespeare, *Timon of Athens* (1623 (first folio publication)), IV, iii.

15   P. Massinger and T. Dekker, *Virgin Martyr* (1622), IV, i.

16   J. Ford, *Perkin Warbeck* (1634), V, iii.

17   B. Jonson, *Volpone*. I.i., B. Jonson, "The Silent Woman," (1610), Iv.i, Thomas Lyle, *Campaspe* (1632), V.iv.

18   J. Ford, *The Lover's Melancholy* (1629), I, ii.

19   W. Birken, 'The Social Problem of the English Physician in the Early Seventeenth Century,' *Medical History* 31 (April 1987), 215.

20   T. Pollard, '"No Faith in Physic": Masquerades of Medicine Onstage and Off,' in S. Moss and K.L. Peterson (eds), *Disease, Diagnosis, and Cure on the Early Modern Stage (Literary and Scientific Cultures of Early Modernity)* (Aldershot: Ashgate Publishing, August 2004), 29-30.

21   J. Webster, *Duchess of Malfi* (1613), II, i.

22   P. Kocher, *Science and Religion in Elizabethan England* (New York: Octogon Books, 1969), 41. The 'odour of impiety' is further discussed in A. Cunningham, 'Sir Thomas Browne and His *Religio Medici*: Reason, Nature and Religion,' in O.P. Grell and A. Cunningham (eds), *Religio Medici: Medicine and Religion in Seventeenth-Century England* (Aldershot: Scolar Press, 1996).

23   Excerpt from *The Diary of the Rev. John Ward,* 100. Cited in J. Axtell, 'Education and Status in Stuart England: The London Physicians,' *History of Education Quarterly* 10, no. 2 (Summer 1970), 159.

24   J. Axtell, 'Education and Status in Stuart England," 88-9. This same point is made in P. Kocher, *Science and Religion in Elizabethan England*, 258-321.

25 A. Wear, 'Religious Beliefs and Medicine in Early Modern England,' 148.

26 Taken as a whole, the contributors to *Religio Medici* agree on this con-clusion. O.P. Grell and A. Cunningham (eds), *Religio Medici: Medicine and Religion in Seventeenth-Century England* (Aldershot: Scolar Press, 1996), 2. See also Andrew Cunningham's Introduction 'Where there are three physicians, there are two atheists' in which he makes the point that 'religious sensitivity and sensibility were still everywhere around the eighteenth-century physician.' O.P. Grell and A. Cunningham (eds), *Medicine and Religion in Enlightenment Europe* (Aldershot: Ashgate, 2007), 1.

27 N. Sirasi, 'Oratory and Rhetoric in Renaissance Medicine,' *Journal of the History of Ideas* 65, 2 (April 2004), 201.

28 E. Gayton, *The Religion of a Physician: Or, Divine Meditations* (1663).

29 R. Burton, *The Anatomy of Melancholy, What It Is: With All the Kinds, Causes, Symptomes, Prognostickes, and Several Cures of It. In Three Maine Partitions with Their Several Sections, Members, and Subsections. Philosophically, Historically, Opened and Cut Up* (1621).

30 Sir T. Browne, *Religio Medici* (1642), 5. For secondary work on Browne's religious beliefs as they pertain to his medicine, see A. Cunningham, 'Sir Thomas Browne and His *Religio Medici*: Reason, Nature and Reli-gion' in O.P. Grell and A. Cunningham (eds), *Religio Medici: Medicine and Religion in Seventeenth-Century England;* P. Kocher, *Science and Religion in Elizabethan England;* and A. Debus, 'Chemists, Physicians, and Chang-ing Perspectives on the Scientific Revolution,' *Isis* 89 (1998).

31 Sir T. Browne, *Religio Medici*. Cited in A. Cunningham, 'Sir Thomas Browne and His *Religio Medici*: Reason, Nature and Religion,' 41-2.

32 C. Bartholin, *De Studio Medici* (1628). Discussed in O.P. Grell, 'Caspar Bartholin and the Education of the Pious Physician,' in O.P. Grell and A. Cunninham (eds), *Medicine and the Reformation* (London: Routledge, 1993), 78-9.

33 W. Schleiner, *Medical Ethics in the Renaissance* (Washington, D.C.: George-town University Press, 1995), 97-8.

34 W. Schleiner, *Medical Ethics in the Renaissance,* 97-8.

35 The sixteenth-century physician Alvise Luisini wrote that the Christian physician was the best for this reason, while in the eighteenth cen-tury the Methodist preacher John Wesley came to the conclusion that 'No man can be a thorough Physician without being an experienced Christian.' These writers, despite their varied backgrounds, believed the

combination of a morally upright physician and a penitent patient was the best way to insure a positive outcome. W. Schleiner, *Medical Ethics in the Renaissance*, 97-8.

36   O.P. Grell, 'Caspar Bartholin and the Education of the Pious Physician,' 78.

37   W. Schleiner, *Medical Ethics in the Renaissance*, 165.

38   B. a Castro, *Flagellum Calumniantium* (Amsterdam: 1631), 84.

39   W. Schleiner, *Medical Ethics in the Renaissance*, 86.

40   All from D. Harley, 'Spiritual Physic, Providence and English Medicine, 1560-1640,' in O.P. Grell and A. Cunningham (eds), *Medicine and the Reformation* (London: Routledge, 1993), 112.

41   R. Burton, *The Anatomy of Melancholy, What It Is: With All the Kinds, Causes, Symptomes, Prognostickes, and Several Cures of It. In Three Maine Partitions with Their Several Sections, Members, and Subsections. Philosophically, Historically, Opened and Cut Up* (1621). See Roy Porter, *Disease, Medicine, and Society in England, 1550-1860* (Basingstoke: Macmillan, 1987), 173.

42   S. Mercurio, *De Gli Errori [Popolari D'italia]* (Venice: 1603). Cited in R. Palmer, 'The Church, Leprosy and Plague in Medieval and Early Modern Europe,' in W.J. Sheils (ed.) *The Church and Healing* (Oxford: Basil Blackwell, 1982), 82-85.

43   N. Culpeper, *Compleat Method of Physick, Whereby a Man May Preserve His Body in Health; or Cure Himself, Being Sick, for Three Pence Charge, with Such Things Only as Grow in England, They Being Most Fit for English Bodies* (1652), A2.

44   See for example P. Leven, *A Right Profitable Booke for All Disseases* (1582) and C. Hueber, *A Riche Storehouse or Treasurie, for the Sicke* (1578).

45   R. Anselment, *The Realms of Apollo: Literature and Healing in Seventeenth-Century England,* (Newark: University of Delaware Press, 1995), 23, 216.

46   W. Vaughan, *Directions for Health* (1617). R. Anselment calls this the 'Christian variation of the Aristotelian relationship between the health of the soul and the health of the body.' R. Anselment, *The Realms of Apollo: Literature and Healing in Seventeenth-Century England*, 25.

47   D. Irish, *Levamen Infirmi: Or, Cordial Counsel to the Sick and Diseased Containing I. Advice Concerning Physick, and What a Physician Ought to Be; with an Account of the Author's Remedies, and How to Take Them. Ii. Concerning Melancholy, Frensie, and Madness; in Which, Amongst Other Things, Is Shew'd, How Far They Differ from a Conscience Opprest with the Sense of Sin, and Likewise How They Differ among Themselves. Iii. A Miscellany of Pious*

Discourses, Concerning the Attributes of God; with Ejaculations and Prayers, According to Scripture Rule. Likewise an Account of Many Things Which Have Happen'd since the Creation. To Which Are Added Several Predictions of What May Happen to the End of the World. The Whole Being Enrich'd with Physical, Pious, Moral & Historical Observations, Delightful to Read, & Necessary to Know (1700).

48 L. Riviere, *The Practice of Physick*, trans. N. Culpeper, A. Cole, and W. Rowland (1655).

49 D. Nagy, *Popular Medicine in Seventeenth-Century England*, 41.

50 J. Cotta, *A Short Discouerie of Seuerall Sorts of Ignorant and Vnconsiderate Practisers of Physicke in England with Direction for the Safest Election of a Physition in Necessitie* (1619), 36-7.

51 R. Burton, *The Anatomy of Melancholy, What It Is: With All the Kinds, Causes, Symptomes, Prognostickes, and Several Cures of It. In Three Maine Partitions with Their Several Sections, Members, and Subsections. Philosophically, Historically, Opened and Cut Up*. Such thinking could pose a problem in times of epidemic disease, such as plague. Doreen Nagy cites the physician Robert Bayfield, who in 1655 concluded there could be no 'general method of cure' for the plague, since it was a punishment meted out in godly 'rage.' However, he listed an assortment of readily obtained ingredients for those who wished to attempt a cure. D. Nagy, *Popular Medicine in Seventeenth-Century England*, 36.

52 Richard Bannister, *A Treatise of One Hundred and Thirteene Diseases of the Eye* (1622). Cited in R. Anselment, *The Realms of Apollo: Literature and Healing in Seventeenth-Century England*, 28.

53 A. Read, *The Manuall of the Anatomy or Dissection of the Body of Man Containing the Enumeration, and Description of the Parts of the Same, Which Usually Are Shewed in the Publike Anatomicall Exercises. Enlarged and More Methodically Digested into 6. Books* (1638). Cited in R. Anselment, *The Realms of Apollo: Literature and Healing in Seventeenth-Century England*, 28.

54 T. Brugis, *The Marrow of Physicke. Or, a Learned Discourse of the Severall Parts of Mans Body* (1640). Cited in R. Anselment, *The Realms of Apollo: Literature and Healing in Seventeenth-Century England*, 28.

55 P. Leven, *A Right Profitable Booke for All Diseases*. Cited in R. Anselment, *The Realms of Apollo: Literature and Healing in Seventeenth-Century England*, 28.

56 Cited in R. Anselment, *The Realms of Apollo: Literature and Healing in Seventeenth-Century England*, 28.

57 S. Mercurio, *De Gli Errori [Popolari D'italia]*.

58 W. Parke, *A Tractat of the Universal Panacaea of Soul and Body* (1665).

59 E. Gayton, *The Religion of a Physician: Or, Divine Meditations*.

60 S. Mercurio, *De Gli Errori [Popolari D'italia]*, B.

61 A. Read, *The Manuall of the Anatomy or Dissection of the Body of Man Containing the Enumeration, and Description of the Parts of the Same, Which Usually Are Shewed in the Publike Anatomicall Exercises. Enlarged and More Methodically Digested into 6. Bookes,* (1638).

62 P. Holland, *Cyrupaedia the Institution and Life of Cyrus, the First of That Name, King of Persians. Eight Bookes. Treating of Noble Education, of Princely Exercises, Military Discipline, Vvarlike Stratagems, Preparations and Expeditions: As Appeareth by the Contents before the Beginning of the First Booke. Written in Greeke by the Sage Xenophon. Translated out of Greeke into English, and Conferred with the Latine and French Translations* (Coventry: 1632), 208. See also W. Charlton, *Immortality of the Human Soul* (1657).

63 J. Ferrand, *Erotomania or a Treatise Discoursing of the Essence, Causes, Symptomes, Prognosticks, and Cure of Love, or Erotique Melancholy* (1640), 23-4.

64 J. Archer, *Every Man His Own Doctor, Compleated with an Herbal Shewing, First, How Every One May Know His Own Constitution and Complexion by Certain Signs : Also, the Nature and Faculties of All Food ...* (1673), 3-4.

65 W. Cole, *A Physico-Medical Essay Concerning the Late Frequency of Apoplexies Together with a General Method of Their Prevention and Cure: In a Letter to a Physician* (1689).

66 Anon., *Levinus Lemnius, the Secret Miracles of Nature in Four Books: Learnedly and Moderately Treating of Generation, and the Parts Thereof, the Soul, and Its Immortality, of Plants and Living Creatures, of Diseases, Their Symptoms and Cures, and Many Other Rarities...*(1658).

67 W. Cole, *A Physico-Medical Essay Concerning the Late Frequency of Apoplexies Together with a General Method of Their Prevention and Cure: In a Letter to a Physician*, 13.

68 T. Adams, *Diseases of the Soule a Discourse Diuine, Morall, and Physicall* (1616), 3.

69 S. Mercurio, *De Gli Errori [Popolari D'italia]*, B6. R. Palmer, 'The Church, Leprosy and Plague in Medieval and Early Modern Europe.' 85-86. Winfried Schleiner made a similar point during his discussion on Girolamo Bardi who noted that physicians should follow the lead of Galen in making 'the treatment of body and mind one.' This insistence that the habits of the mind and the condition of the body are inter-

dependent is a tenant basic to humoral medicine. W. Schleiner, *Medical Ethics in the Renaissance*, 96-97.

70 D. Irish, *Levamen Infirmi: Or, Cordial Counsel to the Sick and Diseased Containing I. Advice Concerning Physick, and What a Physician Ought to Be; with an Account of the Author's Remedies, and How to Take Them. Ii. Concerning Melancholy, Frensie, and Madness; in Which, Amongst Other Things, Is Shew'd, How Far They Differ from a Conscience Opprest with the Sense of Sin, and Likewise How They Differ among Themselves. Iii. A Miscellany of Pious Discourses, Concerning the Attributes of God; with Ejaculations and Prayers, According to Scripture Rule. Likewise an Account of Many Things Which Have Happen'd since the Creation. To Which Are Added Several Predictions of What May Happen to the End of the World. The Whole Being Enrich'd with Physical, Pious, Moral & Historical Observations, Delightful to Read, & Necessary to Know,* 48, 55-6.

71 On the subject of the secularization of medicine, see A. Blair and A. Graftton, 'Reassessing Humanism and Science,' *Journal of the History Of Ideas* 53, no. 4 (Oct- Dec 1992); B.C. Southgate, '"Forgotten and Lost": Some Reactions to Autonomous Science in the Seventeenth Century,' *Journal of the History Of Ideas* 50, no. 2 (Apr-Jun 1989); and B. Shapiro, *Probability and Certainty in Seventeenth-Century England: A Study of the Relations between Natural Science, Religion, History, Law, and Literature* (Princeton: Princeton University Press, 1983).

72 R. Anselment, *The Realms of Apollo: Literature and Healing in Seventeenth-Century England*, 23. Medical tracts are often so similar to sermons in incorporating religious material that they sometimes resemble religious writing more than medical writing. A typical example is J. Jonas, *The Arte and Science of Preserving Bodie and Soule in Healthe, Wisdome, and Catholike Religion: Physically, Philosophically, and Divinely Devised by John Jonas, Physitian* (1579), which begins with a passage from Proverbs: 'Hearken unto my wordes, encline your eares unto my sayings: for they are life unto those that find them, and health unto all their bodies,' The tract includes a prayer and acknowledgment of God's role in healing.

73 N. Sirasi, 'Oratory,' 204.

74 H. Cook, 'Good Advice and Little Medicine: The Professional Authority of Early Modern English Physicians,' *The Journal of British Studies* 33, no. 1 (January 1994), 4, 11-13.

75 N. Sirasi, *Medieval and Early Renaissance Medicine: An Introduction to Knowledge and Practice* (Chicago: University of Chicago Press 1990), 123.

76 H. Cook, 'Good Advice and Little Medicine,' 12-13, 28.

77 H. Cook, 'Good Advice and Little Medicine,' 112.

78 B.H. Traister, "'Note Her a Little Farther': Doctors and Healers in the Drama of Shakespeare," in S. Moss and K.L. Peterson (eds), *Disease, Diagnosis, and Cure on the Early Modern Stage (Literary and Scientific Cultures of Early Modernity)* (August 2004), 44-45. Traister notes that in several of Shakespeare's plays, doctors are not identified by their title or profession, so presumably their dress would have made them instantly recognizable, even if this required the anachronism of the character predating the actual dress code.

79 D. Harley 'Rhetoric,' 426-8

80 T. Dekker, *The Gull's Hornbook*. For examples of similar criticism in drama, see references to the character of Mr. Plaster in T. Nabbes, *The Bride* (1638), V, iv, who speaks in Latin gibberish to impress the patient, although he has no real understanding of the patient's condition, and T. Middleton, *A Fair Quarrel* (1613), IV, ii.

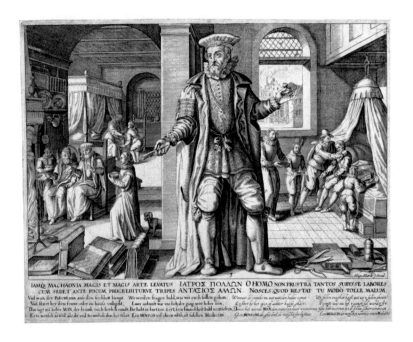

Figure 6: The medical practitioner appearing as a mere human when he
has succeeded in curing the sick
Courtesy Wellcome Library, London

2

'A Sacred Anatomy Both of Soul and Body'[1]:
Godly Physicians in Sermon Literature

The image of the physician as a poisoning, jargon-slinging, atheistic fop was a popular one in early Stuart drama. However, the stage provided only one perspective on the profession's multi-faceted reputation. There was another form of media, equally if not more popular, throughout the seventeenth century that depicted the physician in a much different light: religious sermons. Unlike the largely unflattering depictions of physicians on stage, sermons provided a fund of positive imagery.

Physicians were not alone in positing the idea that the health of the body was entwined with that of the soul, or that the physician possessed the moral authority to heal. Seventeenth-century sermons frequently employed medical metaphors that compared the physician to Christ. The metaphors were based upon Providential doctrine, which held that God sent disease to punish sin. Providential doctrine also stressed the connection of the body and the soul in terms of individual health, thereby ensuring that religion and medicine remained connected in an intimate and essential way.

Comparing God with a physician was an ancient analogy, developed by Church fathers, particularly Saint Augustine. In passage after passage, St. Augustine compared God to a physician. In the following passage, Augustine urged his listeners to trust in God as their physician, for His purpose was not to please the patient but only to heal him: 'For the sick person asks much of the physician, but the physician does not give it to him. He does not hear him for his will but, for his health. Therefore make God your physician.' The implication was a flattering one for the physician: that he knew what was best for his patients and remained steadfast in his treatment.[2] The writings of Augustine influenced seventeenth-century sermon writers who expounded upon the Christ-as-physician metaphor. John Donne frequently quoted Augustine in his sermons when he described Christ as the physician of man: 'He prepared and prescribed this physick for man, when he was upon earth...

then when he died, he became our physician.'[3]

Seventeenth-century writers were highly attuned to the philosophical and linguistic appeal of metaphors. Their use was sometimes prone to criticism because of metaphors' undue power over the collective imagination. John Locke warned that metaphors 'move the passions, and thereby mislead the judgment, and so indeed, are perfect cheats, and therefore, however laudable…or [however they] intend to perform or instruct, [are] wholly to be avoided.'[4] Metaphors are compelling rhetorical devices. Sara Covington has argued that metaphors possess the power of 'redescribing reality.' Metaphors can also 'mediate' social reality, as 'images which a social group forms of itself are interpretations which belong immediately to the constitution of the social bond.'[5] In the case of seventeenth-century England, the 'social bond' (or social body) was metaphorically perceived as diseased, and physician metaphors were popular methods of describing the necessary remedy.

Medical imagery was relied upon because it was familiar to people. Familiarity, in fact, is the key to an effective metaphor, which relies on an easily understood subject to shed light on something that is unfamiliar, intangible, or ineffable.[6] The prevalence of disease imagery in early modern writing illustrates that medical matters were within the grasp of the common people, or else they would not have been effective as metaphors.[7]

Early modern writing was rich with metaphors, and disease imagery proved an especially popular manner of illustrating conflict or corruption in early modern society. Whether the subject was the church, the state, or the family, the underlying notion was that all parts needed to be healthy in order for the whole to function harmoniously and effectively. In sermons, moral tracts, and even political treatises, images of disease in need of healing by a learned physician were common literary currency. For instance, authors expounding on the topic of corruption of the state routinely employed disease metaphors to demonstrate how infectious it could be.[8] Disease imagery proved a popular manner of conceptualizing the perceived problems afflicting the state, solved by a metaphorical physician who could restore health to the country. In one such tract, the entire nation was rendered 'very sick and weak' by corruption, causing the outcry: 'Is there no Balm for such wounds as ours? Is there no Physitian in the English Nation?' In order to restore the health of the nation, the author (a minister) suggested not only following the advice of the spiritual physician, but the earthly physician as well: 'I know not how to take a better course, then to imitate Physitians, who consult not mere reason, but likewise the experience of former times.'[9] Tracts such as this one compared the diseased kingdom with a diseased body, and the cure was reform, cloaked as physic, administered by a physician.[10] *A Vision: Wherein is manifested the disease and cure of the kingdome* and *A Medicine for Malignancy: Or, Parliament Pill, serving to purge out the Malignant humours of men dis-affected to the Republick* both employed such metaphors, and both suggested a learned physician administer a cure for the afflictions.[11] *The Parliament mended or ended; or, A Philter and halter for the two Houses. Prescribed by their Doctor Mercurius Elenticus* contained poems as well as a play in which the doctor prescribed the cure for the parliament as a recipe that mixed virtuous intangible attributes together as if they were tangible physic. The physician's goal was to cure 'the vulgar' who were 'generally infected, and desperately overrun with a disease [called Parliament].' He therefore ordered the recipe to be mixed together, 'with a hand not spotted with Rebellion, murthers, oppressions, cruelties, and Impieties,' and to be boiled in a caldron filled with their own 'teares of Contrition' so that a pristine and pure parliament might be restored.[12] These tracts provided a positive image of the physician as healer of the state. [13]

One reason why the image of disease running rampant and only to be cured by the physician was especially popular during the seventeenth century is that it provided a concrete way of describing a tumultuous and interrelated political and religious climate. The religious landscape of seventeenth-century England was intimately linked with political developments, from the Reformation Parliament of 1529, through the Elizabethan Settlement, to the challenges faced by the Anglican church as the Puritan movement flourished during the 1620s and 1630s, and right through the Civil War, Commonwealth, and the Glorious Revolution.[14] The conflict lent itself to images of a weak, sickened body that could benefit from the ministrations of a competent physician.

By setting up physicians as the healers of the metaphoric diseases of the state, political tracts were complimentary to them. However, even more helpful to physicians were the disease metaphors utilized by religious sermons that compared Christ with a physician. Alongside the lampooning and criticizing of physicians, sermons offered an alternative, idealized image of the profession in early modern culture.[15] Sermons also helped the image of the ideal physician by putting into metaphorical terms concepts of sin and physical disease, affliction and healing, and the interconnectedness of body and soul that were already prevalent among the godly, patients and practitioners alike.[16] The basic tenet of the Christ-as-physician metaphor, which equated God's healing power of the soul with the physician's healing of the

47

physical body, and which linked Christ with the physician, glorified the role of the earthly physician, validated his ability to care for the body as Christ's approved healer, and simultaneously linked body and soul together in the overall health of the individual.

Sermons proved powerful in disseminating the image of the godly physician throughout seventeenth-century culture. In addition to being heard by churchgoers, religious sermons also enjoyed considerable popularity and a wide readership. Religious writing dominated the published material available in the seventeenth century. In 1623, there were 327 publications in England. Of these, 120 were religious in nature, 84 dealt with current events, often oriented to a scriptural interpretation, and 60 were educational, most of which stressed piety and were morally instructive. Of 327 publications, therefore, 264 (eighty percent) could be said to be explicitly or implicitly religious in nature.[17] It is not surprising that in seventeenth-century England sermons were ubiquitous. Moral tracts and sermons were the most frequently published literature and as such constituted one of the main forms of mass media prior to the newspaper in the late seventeenth century.[18] In fact, the public appetite for printed sermons as well as preached sermons was phenomenal.[19] Everyone was required to attend church services, and although we cannot tell whether listeners were enrapt or napping, we know that the majority of people were exposed to sermons. We also know that all levels of society were strongly encouraged to read or hear sermons, and that even in the case of servants, sometimes derided as less than pious, it was not unusual for them to spend their leisure time on Sundays attending sermons.[20]

Published sermons were even more effective since they could be read on multiple occasions and referred back to, as noted in the following sermon: 'The Word preached is too soon forgotten, and reacheth but to few, but Printed may be seen by many, and perused at pleasure.'[21] Furthermore, writers marketed their sermons to less educated and less wealthy readers, not just to a small segment of the population. Title pages of sermons and moral tracts often stated that they were written in simple language so that all could read and readily comprehend their message. In *Christ the Physician of the Soul* predominantly positioned on the title page was the phrase: 'This sermon is preached in Market-Language, which [the author] thinks most likely to be understood and remembered by the common People.'[22] Sometimes such a statement was made directly in the title as exemplified in the following treatise: *A Caveat for Cold Christians Wherein the Common Disease of Christians, with the Remedie, Is Plainly and Excellently Set Downe for All That Will Use It.*[23] Edward

Lawrence's sermon provides a more blatant example: *Christ's Power Over Bodily Diseases Preached in several sermons…and published for the instruction especially of the more ignorant people in the great duty of preparation for sickness and death.*[24] Historians have found that even the poorest homes often possessed an array of such works, which makes printed sermons a useful tool to historians of medicine in the quest to uncover popular ideas in the collective world of seventeenth-century society.[25]

Historians have suggested that the carefully crafted rhetoric of sermons could enforce or even alter public perception, in this case as it pertains to the culture of medicine and illness.[26] Many seventeenth-century sermons directly addressed the culture of medicine and illness for their own purposes, yet these sermons had significant repercussions for the medical profession as well. Sermons purposefully constructed a link between spiritual and physical health, attributing bodily illness to sin while simultaneously stressing the importance of both in terms of one's overall health.

Part of the reason why sermons were effective was because they often employed metaphors as a rhetorical tool in preaching to people used to reasoning by analogy.[27] As was the case with political literature, one of the most enduring metaphors utilized in the sermons was that of disease, which frequently relied on the image of Christ as a physician, eradicating the disease of sin afflicting the bodies of mankind. When writers depicted Christ as a physician, He cured the soul, through redemption, and physic served as the linguistic bridge connecting the physical and spiritual worlds.[28] Medical metaphors enlisted in sermons, therefore, often consisted of Christ as the physician of the soul, who offered the 'certain cure for all diseases.'[29]

In seventeenth-century sermons, Christ was a divine physician, healing the soul the way a physician heals the body. In *Christ the Physician of the Soul*, the Reverend Whitefield promised his readers that the faithful could be made whole by Christ's grace if they were to partake in his righteousness, and would 'spend an eternity in praising this physician.'[30] Christ was a 'great physician' or a 'blessed physician.' By the end of the sermon, Christ was simply referred to as 'physician.' The degree of repetition emphasized the link between the two to the reader.

In F. Bamfield's tract, he delineated the physician as 'a wise comforter in the Word of God.' Healing was a virtue, and along with it, the physician could offer the patient 'his savoury, seasonable, suitable counsel.' The message was that his healing power and his sage counsel came from God.[31] Thomas Dekker forged a similar association by referring to the physician as 'God's second,' who 'in a duell or single fight (of this nature) will stand bravely to thee. A Good Physitian comes to thee in the shape of an Angell, and therefore let him boldly take thee by the hand, for he has been in Gods garden, gathering herbes: and soveraine rootes to cure thee.'[32] Dekker's allusion to the divine origin of the physician referred to a passage in Ecclesiasticus 12:6:

> From God the doctor has his wisdom. God makes the earth yield healing herbs which the prudent should not neglect...He endows humans with the knowledge to glory in his mighty works, Through which the doctor eases pain and the druggist prepares his medicines; Thus God's creative work continues without cease in its efficacy on the surface of the earth.

The verses seemed to offer proof of medicine's divine origin and the physician's ability to deliver them properly.

Thus, sermons helped bolster the authority of the physician by reiterating the link in people's minds between the learned physician and Christ. This gave the physician an advantage over the unlicensed healer, as the sermons were specific in their use of the word 'physician' rather than the more general term 'healer' when setting up the metaphor. The overriding message was a powerful and positive one for the physician: that he was God's ordained minister for healing on earth.

Ministers collected metaphors and analogical arguments to illustrate their sermons, and they found that the practice of medicine provided a fund of familiar metaphors. The flourishing of Calvinism during the second half of the seventeenth century contributed to the expansion and abundant reproduction of medical metaphors.[33] Calvinism's doctrine of Providential theory held that God used illness for a multitude of higher purposes, as an affliction against the ungodly, a trial, or even a mark of divine favor. The influence of Providentialism on sermons can be seen in their focus on the individual and God's purposes for him or her when it came to explaining sickness.[34] Providentialism encouraged a distinct attitude toward medicine that was favorable to physicians, as well as a fund of religious metaphors that reflected that attitude.

Most people in seventeenth-century England subscribed to the belief that God sent disease. Illness and suffering were incorporated into both Catholic and Protestant ideology as part of God's plan for mankind. God's interference in the health of His people could signify His displeasure with rampant human sinfulness or lukewarm religious faith. God sent specific diseases, most notably plague, as punishment or prodding to an individual sufferer or to an entire town. Pestilence, along with famine and war, was one of God's three arrows, which could at various times, for various purposes, be directed towards a populace. Sermons, therefore, worked on the assumption that people needed to repent in order to spare themselves God's wrath. M. Henry Burton's sermon demonstrated the 'necessity of Selfe-denyall and Humiliation, by Prayer and Fasting before the Lord, in regard of the present Plague we now lye under, which God, in his good time, remove from amongst us.'[35] This notion was ingrained in the *Book of Common Prayer* in assertions such as 'whatsoever your sickness is, know you certainly, that it is God's visitation.'[36] Clerics were fond of quoting biblical passages in their sermons that expressed this concept, such as Deuteronomy 28.20:

> The Lord shall smite them with a consumption,
> and with a feaver, and with an inflammation, and
> with an extreme burning. He shall smite them
> with the botch of Egypt, and with the Emerods,
> and with the scab, and with the itch (with a
> botch that cannot be healed, from the sole of the
> foot to the crown of the head.) …there shall be no
> health in their bodies, because of his displeasure;
> nor any rest in their bones by reason of their sin.[37]

As the passage indicates, the sinful nature of humanity was responsible for earthly suffering, and disease itself was a perpetual *memento mori*, with death constituting a release from the 'vale of tears' that signified earthly life.[38]

The disease metaphors in sermons illustrated this point. Christ was the physician who possessed the power not only to heal disease, but to afflict people with disease and suffering as well.[39] In *A Triple Antidote* the 'great physician' purged the body of mankind 'sometimes by fire, sometimes by water, & generally by many great, & common destructions'[40] *Christ's Power Over Bodily Diseases* reiterated that God could command illness, as 'all diseases are at the will of Jesus Christ.'[41] God was often compelled to do so because of an individual's sins, which sermons repeatedly insisted were 'the procuring cause of sickness.'[42] Sin resulted in physical sickness, a notion common in sermons: 'Our sins have brought us down under a great number of diseases, and laid us upon a bed of affliction.'[43] *The Plague of the Heart* put the matter succinctly: 'sin is against mans health: Hence come all diseases and sicknesses, till sin there were no such things.'[44]

Sermon writers took great care to describe meticulously the diseases of the soul that sickened their flock, often couching their description of spiritual diseases in terms of physical symptoms in order to make them more readily comprehensible to the reader. Daniel King described how the souls of sinners are 'burthened, and extreamly pressed' by sin, that 'Canker [that] eats out all their Comforts, and keeps their Souls under continuall fears and Distractions.'[45] In some sermons, the sins themselves became metaphorical diseases that 'waste the *body*, fill it with diseases; abate its strength, shorten its day, obstruct its lawful delights, and keep off the solid comforts of life.'[46] Other sermons anthropomorphized sin in order to highlight the physical, debilitating effects that it had on the body of the sinner.[47] In the most repetitive, if not obvious of these, sin was put on trial, charged with threatening 'mans present good in this life' including 'the good of his body' and 'the good of his soul…For on both it hath brought a curse and death.' Sin was further accused of having 'corrupted mans blood, and made his body mortal, and thereby render'd it a vile body.'[48]

The relationship whereby man sinned and God punished his body with disease was depicted as the natural state of affairs after the fall:

> The Godly, though they be the Sons of God by the grace of Adoption, yet they are the Sons of Adam by natural production: And as the Wood breeds a Worm that eats it, the Garment a Moth that frets it, and Fruit that which doth corrupt it, so natural bodies produce Diseases to destroy them.[49]

Since it was the sons of Adam's natural propensity to destroy their physical body through sin, there was not surprisingly an epidemic of diseased souls. In *The Diseases of the Soule*, Thomas Adams asserted, 'Soul-sick stomachs are so childishly weak, they know not how to refuse the evill, and choose the sound and good food for souls.'[50] Such people were doomed 'unlesse some speedie remedy be applied to this desperate disease, and the great God himselfe become our Phisitian and heale our distempers.'[51] Fortunately, the sermons offered a remedy. *Jewish Hypocrisie* advised those sick of soul to use all of 'Christ's prescriptions' (scripture) or else 'fall into a more dangerous distemper.' If people failed to make use of Christ's prescriptions the way they should make use of wholesome medicines, they would continue to suffer for their sins.[52]

The best way to remain healthy, then, was to avoid incurring the wrath of God, as stressed in the sermon *A Storehouse of Comfort for the Afflicted in Spirit*, which used Exodus 15.26 to illustrate the point:

> If thou wilt diligently hearken into the voice of the Lord thy God, and wilt doe that which is right in his sight, and wilt give eare unto his commandments, and keepe his ordinances, then I will put none of these diseases upon thee, which I brought upon the Egyptians: for I am the Lord that healeth thee.[53]

God was not eager to send diseases, according to the sermons. In fact, He was slow to anger: 'For he doth not afflict willingly.'[54] He did so only when prompted by mankind's sins, and in His mercy sent them remedies to counteract the diseases that sin wrought upon the physical body.

The metaphorical remedy was often scripture, as suggested in the title of the sermon *Physicke for body and soule...with a remedie against both, prescribed by our heauenly physitian Jesus Christ*.[55] Daniel King suggested the cure for the diseased soul was a 'compound' of scripture, which together with the blessing of God would prove medicinal.[56] In a similar vein, the sermon *Jewish Hypocrisie* depicted repentance as a remedy that 'expels and heals all such matters in the soule.' The tract extended the metaphor to compare consumption of the lungs with consumption of the soul:

> We see in nature euery part hath a faculty of expelling what is noxious and harmfull: the lungs haue their cough; the braine his sneezing, and other excretions; the stomacke will turne it selfe topsie turuie, but it will bring up (by vomit) that which offends...The souls of man in this condition wherein it contracts corruption, hath this faculty of repentance put into it, whereby it empties it selfe of all that is offensiue.[57]

Using the physical to describe the spiritual was an effective way of making the intangible more accessible, but it was more than a literary device. There was a real sense in these sermons that the health of the body and that of the soul were intimately connected and together made up the overall health of the individual.[58]

This stress on the symbiotic relationship of body and soul was a favorite metaphor in sermons, which asserted that 'The Spirit, Soul and Body in man have a mutual influence upon each other, and it is often well or ill with the one, as it is well or ill with the other.'[59] In another sermon, sin was described as 'the sicknesse of the soule,' and therefore 'the reall and radicall cause of all bodily sicknesse.'[60] A similar parallel was drawn between the health of the body and the health of the soul in John Donne's writing, which surmised that just as there was a bodily leprosy so there was a spiritual one, and just as the physician 'must consider excrements, so we must consider sin, the leprosie, the pestilence, and ordure of the soule.'[61] *A New Letter, to All Drunkards, Whoremongers, Thieves, Disobedience to Parents, Swearers, Lyers* cautioned against destroying the health of the body as well as the soul by partaking in such vices since sinful behavior would lead to the 'ruin both of soul and body in the world to come unless repented.'[62] Conversely, the sins of the body could likewise effect the soul, as illustrated in *The Christian Diary*, which warned that the sin of gluttony resulted not only in the 'infirmities of body' but also cast down the soul, leaving it in a 'miserable state…polluted & plunged in the flesh.'[63]

Henry King, Bishop of Chichester, was well known for the numerous Calvinist sermons he penned. His sermons might cover both the plague of the physical body and a metaphorical spiritual plague that infected the soul precisely because sermon writers typically described the physical and spiritual in interchangeable terminology.[64] Sermons such as King's, in which the health of the body and soul were interdependent, were supported by perceived reality, as physical illness and especially plague were seen as having both physical and spiritual causes and remedies. By similar token, the soul's cure could heal the body.[65] The upside of this interdependence for pious Christians was that they could learn from illness in one how to avoid illness in the other. *The Plague of the Heart* recommended using bodily illness as a spiritual warning: 'One Plague suggested another to the good mans thoughts: and indeed it is no unusuall thing with pious persons, to make even the diseases of their bodies, administer matter of devout meditation for the health of their souls.'[66] Such use of sickness was consistent with Calvin's teaching that Christ's healing was intended for the spiritual purpose of enlightening the sick and to prove His divinity, an idea that was propounded in the sermon *Christ the Physician of the Soul*: 'It is true God often is pleased to make use of the sickness of the body in order to make the soul sick, and in order to bring the soul home to Jesus Christ to get saving health…For, as there is a *bodily*, so there is a *spiritual* sickness.'[67]

As David Harley has pointed out, the medical metaphors in sermons that illustrate the link between sin and its negative effects on the body, along with depictions of God as a physician, helped emphasize the fluid lines between physical and spiritual healing. Writers of these sermons saw the practice of medicine as entirely compatible with true religion, both appointed by God for the welfare of humanity, both healing with the providence of God. This analogy between God and the medical practitioner was reinforced by the frequency of the comparisons made between the means of salvation and the means provided by God for recovery from sickness, which were seen as almost precisely homologous.[68]

It is difficult to assess the result of the positive images of physicians presented by sermons and in the writing of physicians themselves. However, evidence that the public internalized ideas about godly physicians can be found in a biased source: the sermons themselves. If we consider the warnings and admonitions of sermon writers that society was more concerned with the advice of the physician than with that of the minister, there is ample evidence to suggest that people were in fact viewing physicians as authority figures who had expertise and knowledge.

Sermons presented an epidemic of diseased souls, sickened by sin, and in desperate need of a cure. Yet to the dismay of ministers, people seemed far more concerned with the health of their bodies than their souls. Some took up the topic as the main subject of their sermons, such as *The Invaluable price of an immortal soul shewing the vanity of most people in taking care for the body, but neglect their duty as to the preservation of their never-dying souls.*[69] The writers of such tracts lamented that when people fell sick, they focused on bodily health: 'When therefore God summons thee, do not as the common course is, send first for the bodily physician, and when thou art past natural care, then for the divine; but contrarily let the divine begin.'[70] Such reproving of their readers was no doubt a response to a lapse in what ministers considered to be the proper chain of response to illness, laid out in a 1511 statute passed by the House of Commons concerning Ecclesiastical licensing. The statute stated that since the soul was far more precious than the body, no physician should prescribe for the health of the body anything that might prove perilous to the soul. Should the patient summon the physician first to the sickbed, the physician was obligated to persuade the patient 'to send for the physician of the soul; that after the sick person hath taken care of his spiritual medicament, he may with better effect proceed to the cure of his body.'[71] For all the rhetoric of the godly physician, there is a sense in some sermons that the writers were feeling dismayed by the public's impulse to consult a physician prior to a minister.

The fact that clergymen had to employ medical metaphors in the first place suggests that Christianity was remote from the experience of illness and suffering and that clerics knew that to make Christianity relevant they had to bring medicine and the bedside into religious discourse. Physicians were being called to sickbeds more frequently and earlier than ever before, and where previously a priest or minister might have been summoned, now a medical practitioner was first on the list. Seventeenth-century Christianity was attempting to counter this trend by bringing death, and even illness, more fully into the scope of religion as part of the attempt to govern all aspects and stages of life.[72]

This subtle friction between the minister and the physician concerning the proper protocol for calling them to duty speaks volumes about the inroads physicians were making in terms of public trust. Robert Bolton complained, 'They look no higher than to the hand of the Physitian, they depend onely on the power of physic for their deliverance and recovery.'[73] The author of the sermon *Jewish Hypocrisie* remonstrated that spiritual ailments should be attended to as speedily as physical ones: 'If a bodily disease breed on us, we loue to looke forth quickly. Thus it should be, when sin (an enemy, yea a sicknesse to the soul) doth so much as make entrance into us.'[74]

Urging people not to focus solely on their physical well-being reflected the concern that seventeenth-century people had with the health of their bodies. In *Physick to cure the most dangerous Disease, Desperation* the author remarked in his preface, 'It is a wonder of the world' how much care people took of their bodily health, while neglecting their spiritual care, which he deemed essential to 'euerlasting felicity both of soule and body.' He found it amazing that so many

either loathe and are afraide of bodily sicknesse…will send for and seeke…after bodily Physitions, and enquire after the best, the most expert & most skilfull of them, to learn by their direction, and to bee advised by their counsaile (though it cost their purse full deare) how to purge and auoide such corrupt humours as maybreede…noisome diseases, and sickness.

While on the other side, so few

> seeke after the spirituall Physition or prepare physicke to purge and
> expel those dangerous and peccant humours, of notorious and hay-
> nous sinnes, which in time will both breede & bring forth the most
> deadly disease of Desperation, the very Peste of soule and body for
> ever.[75]

The reprimands couched in such sermons imply that physicians were the first choice for many people when they fell ill.[76] They suggest a hierarchy of illness in which suffering individuals or their families summoned a physician prior to a cleric, an action which implies a much stronger reliance on and faith in the physician than might otherwise be assumed.

Medical metaphors and disease imagery contributed significantly to the cultural understanding of disease in the early modern era. The metaphors in these sermons illuminate the way people thought about the health of both body and soul, and the relationship of physical to spiritual wellness. Since their effectiveness rested on their familiarity to the intended audience, the metaphors can be viewed as a reflection of the way people conceptualized the causes of disease. By linking Christ's redemption of the soul with a physician's healing of the body, clergymen presented a positive view of the medical profession at a time when physicians were struggling to advance their profession in the face of burgeoning competition.

The messages emanating from sermons, and echoed in physicians' writing, also appear in lay comments and diaries. Lay attitudes about Providence and affliction were in line with those of both the minister and the physician, resulting in a common conception of illness in seventeenth-century England that would ultimately aid the physician's argument that the best healer was a pious physician, responsible for the whole health of the individual. The majority of the lay public interpreted illness in providential terms: disease was God's mode of instruction, and He had the power to punish humanity with disease.[77] People were accustomed to the idea that 'God hath his Quiver full of arrows, full of the Pestilence, of Fevers, and Dropsies, and consumptions, and all manner of diseases; and he shoots these arrows into our families, friends, and children.'[78] The diaries of individuals as diverse as Ralph Josselin and Samuel Pepys offer evidence that contemporaries internalized this idea. Lucinda Beier noted that Josselin considered the health of his family and friends 'hostages for his good behaviour.'[79] Samuel Pepys also saw his illness as a punishment meted out by God. When he suffered with a debilitating cold, he recorded in his diary 'it is a cold which God Almighty in justice did give me while I sat lewdly sporting with Mrs. Lane the other day with the broken window in my neck.'[80] The draft from the window no doubt played a part in the cold, according to Pepys, but equally damaging was his sinful conduct in precipitating his illness. Such ideas seem to have extended up the social ladder, as evidenced when Sir John Reresby noted that 'it hath pleased God to visit me with a rhumatisme,' while Lady Brilliana Harley commented to her son, 'It hath pleased God that I have been ill…but yet I rejoice in Gods mercy to me, that you enjoy your health.' She also attributed her miscarriages to the will of God. When studying lay perceptions of illness, historians have suggested that Providence was a familiar trope in the diaries of the godly. It was therefore logical that they should see God at work in their illnesses and cures.[81]

While it is difficult to determine the origination of ideas about Providence, sin, and illness, it is clear that ideas about illness were consistent in sermons, medical tracts, and among lay diary writers and served to reinforce one another. Together they contributed to the culture of illness in the seventeenth century: one that viewed sickness as an affliction that warranted careful notice by the godly sufferer in order to help determine God's plan for him or her. In *The Universal Medicine* affliction was defined as 'the bearing or enduring any injuries whatever; so that it may be said to be any trouble, grief, or evil that happeneth to Soul, Body, Name, or Estate, and that either for trial or punishment.'[82] This focus on affliction and the personal, spiritual lessons to be learned from the bearing of affliction meshed nicely with the significance Calvinists placed on their individual experiences and its relationship to Divine Providence. As John Beadle asserted, 'It is good to set down every affliction we have met within our time, and to observe Gods carriage toward us.'[83] There is evidence that the godly did just this. The diary of the Nonconformist Joseph Lister included his account of 'some of the most remarkable passages of Providence towards myself.' Lister singled out his sickness in order to emphasize the drama of his deliverance: 'Yet at last God was pleased to step in with light, and love, and clear satisfaction; and I could not hold, but cried out aloud, "He is come! He is come!" Which made the affliction on my body the more light and easy, the remainder of the time I was under it.'[84] John Lowther described his wife's death in childbirth in terms of her patient endurance of affliction: 'shee was hourely afflicted which [with?] extremitie of sickness,…yet in all her sickness was singularly patient penitent and full of ejaculation and prayers that god would be merciful to hir that he [would] pardon her sinnes and receive hir soule.'[85]

Sermons depicted affliction as useful to the sufferer, often as a form of spiritual physic to purge and cleanse the soul. John Donne stated, 'Affliction is my Physick; that purges, that cleanses me,' while Thomas Adams described affliction as a bitter pill administered by the Divine Physician that would ultimately help the penitent in the next world.[86] The godly lay population similarly tended to embrace affliction as a sign of grace. Joseph Hall declared, 'Not to be afflicted is a sign of weakness…when I am stronger, I will look for more.'[87] Lady Margaret Hoby saw her ailments as useful. When she described the pain in her shoulder in 1605, she declared that it did her good, as 'afflictions draw one nearer to god.'[88] As these examples illustrate, affliction did not always signify divine punishment for sinful behavior but could be construed as a sign of God's grace and was sometimes welcomed by the godly as such. Jane Turner, a Newcastle Baptist, wrote 'Being under a bodily affliction, the Lord was pleased to visit me with his loving kindness, that I can truly say, it was a time of great joy to my soul.'[89] These diarists were reflecting the idea of the spiritual significance of sickness, one of the favorite topics of ministers employing the Christ-as-physician metaphors, that because sickness was God's will, those who were ill should be calm under their afflictions, or even welcome them as a means of spiritual and physical purification.[90]

Bearing affliction, however, did not mean forgoing the means of a cure, but quite the opposite. David Harley has found that even insistence that only divine will determined the course of healing did not imply fatalism: although God may have appointed the length of each individual's life, the obligation to preserve it was widely recognized.[91] Most people seemed to accept the thinking that 'Physicke is good, if we intreat God by Prayer to giue a blessing to it.'[92] Although Calvinist theology did make a strong connection between sin and illness, it did not lead to fatalistic acceptance of sickness but instead to active searching for cures and treatment.[93] Patients typically desired to keep both body and soul in good order, using a combination of natural and spiritual remedies to do so.[94] For the godly, therefore, the means employed by the physician were to be respected but not solely relied upon: 'The more we depend on a wise Physitian, the more wee will observe his *directions*, and be carefull to use what hee prescribes; yet wee must use the meanes as meanes, and not set them in Gods roome, for that is the way to blast our hopes.'[95] In this sense, active, daily monitoring of one's health could be viewed as tantamount to fulfilling one's religious duty, taken so seriously that Margaret Pelling has described it as the 'health-related activity most characteristic of early modern people.'[96]

This interest in monitoring one's health with vigor was often extended to self-cure, as the sick typically treated themselves when they fell ill.[97] This does not necessarily indicate that people saw no value in employing a physician or that they did not respect his expertise. Physicians actually endorsed the idea of taking care of oneself for most ailments. As Roy Porter has noted, textbooks and case notes reveal just how commonly learned Humanist physicians recommended relatively non-medical remedies to their patients: riding, a change of air or diet, a trip to the waters, a holiday. Within that framework, which required a patient to be active, self-treatment could complement rather than countermand the recommendations of orthodox physic.[98] In this respect, physicians' advice was in agreement with lay common sense in believing that health was a measure of the proper workings of the individual constitution, and sickness was a sign of its malfunctioning. To maintain good health, one needed to ensure proper diet, monitor both exercise and evacuations, get an adequate amount of sleep, reside in as healthy an environment as possible, and regulate one's passions. The different qualities vital for life must be well balanced. The body should not be allowed to become too hot or cold, too wet or dry (fevers or colds would result). These ideas about health stemmed from traditional Hippocratic teaching about regulating one's lifestyle through a combination of the aforementioned factors. Such early modern medical theories about health and disease allowed anyone to take rational measures to maintain an appropriate balance of all bodily functions, either alone or with the help of medical professionals. All an individual needed was a good knowledge of his or her own unique constitution and reaction to the non-naturals before charting a desirable lifestyle that would preserve the state of health.[99] As the French physician Arnulfe d'Aumont declared, 'There does not exist a definition of health applicable to everyone, each has his own state of well-being.'[100] This preventative view made good sense at a time when curative medicine was little advanced, a point that has led Roy Porter to conclude that one way in which people in traditional society coped with the fact that doctors were not miracle workers was to view their health as ultimately their personal responsibility.[101]

In Porter's view, illness for the lay population was typically not seen as a random accident striking from the outside, but as a deeply significant life event, integral to the sufferer's whole being—spiritual, moral, and physical. This may account for why patients took to heart the Galenic notion that the mind and body were connected, which ministers and physicians expanded to include spiritual aspects as well. It was their responsibility to keep their spirits up, whether through resisting sinful actions that could lead to bodily illness or through maintaining a positive attitude. Sir Ralph Verney's comments on his daughter-in-law's illness illustrate this point. When Mary Verney's physician, Dr. Denton, reported her low-spirited and in deteriorating health in 1663, Sir Ralph Verney responded, 'All the Phisick in the world will not cure her, unless she strive against her Malancholly, & in a good measure prove her owne Doctor.'[102] Sir Walter Scott endorsed this view of low spirits adversely influencing the body: 'My bile is quite gone. I really believe it arose from mere anxiety. What a wonderful connexion between the mind and body.'[103] John Locke commented upon the necessity of good spirits for good health in a letter to his friend Philip Van Limborch:

> Since nothing so promotes and restores the health of the body as does tranquility of the mind, you cannot doubt that your most enjoyable letters, evidence of your affection and good will, have been the greatest comfort to me in my protracted condition of poor and variable health.[104]

According to lay and medical thinking alike, the sick person's duty lay in mustering good spirits to drive away the disease.[105] They did this best by avoiding sin and excessive passion, both of which inevitably caused an ill mind, an idea summed up in the writing of Robert Boyle, a leading philosopher and scientist of his day. When people subdued their lusts and passions, he reasoned, they helped preserve their bodies by

> exempting them from those vices…which are not enemies to man's life and health barely upon a physical account, but upon a moral one, as they provoke God to punish them with temporal as well as spiritual judgment; such as plagues, wars, famines…besides those personal afflictions of bodily sickness and disquiet of conscience, that do both shorten men's lives and imbitter them.[106]

His view is representative of educated contemporary thinking wherein mind and body were factors in health, and both fell under the domain of Divine

Providence.

For both the physician and the patient, it was important to bear in mind that remedies could be expected to work only if they had God's blessing. Both the physician and the patient should do all that they could to ensure health, including keeping spiritually healthy, but ultimately a person's fate was in God's hands. Physicians could not be expected to understand God's plan for a patient. They could only do their best to help him or her. The concept of Divine Providence, therefore, had some positive attributes for physicians. Providentialism provided a convenient excuse for ineffective medical treatment since God's assistance was required to make medical intervention successful. Ultimately, no physician's expertise could preserve a life that was divinely preordained to end at a certain time.[107] David Harley has argued that Providentialism actually led to a greater confidence in the ministrations of physicians since their remedies were not expected to have automatic efficacy.[108] A funeral sermon for the High Sheriff of Suffolk insisted that the physician was not to be blamed for the man's demise, as nothing could be done 'if God shooteth his arrow.' Since healing was a gift from God, He might choose to cloud the physicians' judgment: 'If a skilfull Phisician doth us no good, it is because it pleaseth God to hide the right way of curing at that time from him.' God could also suspend the action of medicine, no matter how skillful the physician administering it. If sin was being punished, and the patient was still meant to suffer affliction, then despite the best efforts of physicians, 'Physicke ministred doth often lose its working.'[109] Physicians, then, could fall back upon the belief that even the most competent and expert efforts could be overridden if God had another plan for the afflicted, a concept that proved instrumental in shaping patient expectations during the period.

Over time, medical science would change significantly, thus altering the relationship between religion and medicine. The spiritual and physical duality would not be as implicit as the secularization of medicine gained ground. However, in the seventeenth century, there remained present a conceptual framework wherein Christianity and medicine interacted on a regular basis. The relationship between the physician's job of healing did not contrast with commonly held beliefs about Providence. The two actually complemented one another, to the benefit of the seventeenth-century physician and his limited efficacy.

By the end of the seventeenth century, physicians had come a long way in gaining personal trust. In 1464 Margaret Paston warned her husband, 'For

Goddys sake be war what medesyns ye take of any fysissyans of London.'[110]
In the 1747 publication of his *Primitive Physick*, the Methodist preacher John
Wesley, who was at best leery of the medical trade, had this to say on the subject of physicians: 'In uncommon or uncomplicated cases…I again advise
every man without delay to apply to a Physician that fears God.'[111] Wesley's
comments illustrate what has been the objective of this chapter: to demonstrate that physicians were not at odds with religion, but that religion and morality formed an important part of physicians' conception of their offerings.

In his work on Calvinist diaries and autobiographies, Harley demonstrated that the Calvinist minority was in fact convinced that pious medical
men were the best choice. As leaders among their communities, the godly
were influential in establishing the authority of regularly educated medical
practitioners.[112] Perhaps it was enough to aid physicians' struggle for more
authority and respect in society for them to be viewed by the godly as a reasonable option for ensuring health. Their job was ordained by Christ, and
they incorporated the physical and spiritual aspects of healing and thereby
assured the best chance for a blessing of the means and outcome of the healing process. This certainly was not a ringing endorsement for the fledgling
profession, but it may have been just enough to disentangle them from the
crowd of empirics offering healing without the spiritual components.

Given the expense and the dubious efficacy of their treatments, Roy
Porter, Doreen Nagy, Margaret Pelling, and Lucinda Beier have argued that
most people would have been better off without the intervention of physicians, and they are no doubt correct.[113] We owe much of our understanding of the lay culture of illness and healing to these studies. They have offered invaluable insight into the thinking and beliefs of seventeenth-century
people. These studies convincingly demonstrate the divergence between lay
and medical beliefs, but it is also helpful to appreciate the commonalities. In
this culture, the value of physical and spiritual health as contributing equally
to one's overall wellbeing was more than a figurative trope—it possessed
literal and practical importance in the maintenance of health and was of essential importance to the way in which illness was culturally constructed in
seventeenth-century England.

Counteracting the negative depiction of physicians on stage were religious
sermons, published throughout the century, many of which employed the
Christ-as-physician metaphor. Along with disease imagery, sermons offered

an example of the 'All-wise Physician' who 'graciously at once provided both for the health of Mens bodies, and for the salvation of their Souls.'[114] The pious physician described in these sermons offers an alternative, idealized version of what the perfect medical practitioner should be, and they demonstrated what such a practitioner *could* be. Since the metaphors are specific in comparing the physician with Christ, and because we know that the metaphors were repeated often enough to become part of the mental landscape, we can use these sermons to glean a better understanding of what seventeenth-century people thought about physicians. These sermons suggest to us that physicians were generally respected and had the reputation of being competent healers.

Raymond Anselment has concluded that by the end of the century, people were less dependent upon religious consolation and more reliant upon medical care.[115] This is the time period when historians generally acknowledge the rise in prominence of the physician. Advances in scientific thinking and an increasing secularization of society changed the way people viewed their ill health and the options available to restore and maintain health. Eighteenth-century disease theory would come to be less tied to the spiritual qualities of the individual and less dependent on the will of God. However, physicians laid the groundwork for the rise of the medical profession in the seventeenth century, and its base was just as spiritual and moral as it was scientific.

As the next chapter will demonstrate, once physicians made inroads in establishing an image of their profession as learned and godly, it was necessary to capitalize on these gains in status. They would do so in part by attacking their competitors for the same flaws their critics saw in them. Perhaps most ironically, they would push to separate themselves from the clergy, whose metaphors had proven so instrumental in developing the image of the godly physician.

Notes

1   J. Smith, *Gerochomia vasilike King Solomons portraiture of old age : wherein is contained a sacred anatomy both of soul and body, and a perfect account of the infirmities of age, incident to them both : and all those mystical and aenigmatical symptomes expressed in the six former verses of the 12th chapter of Ecclesiastes, are here paraphrased upon and made plain and easie to a mean capacity* (1666), title page.

2   W. Schleiner, *The Imagery of John Donne's Sermons* (Providence: Brown University Press, 1970), 71. See also G.B. Ferngren, 'Early Christianity as a Religion of Healing,' *Bulletin of the History of Medicine* 66 (1992). For additional information on St. Augustine's use of the image of Christ as medicine, see R. Walker, *A Learned and Profitable Treatise of Gods Providence* (1608).

3   [1:313, 9:458], 68 cited in R. Anselment, *The Realms of Apollo: Literature and Healing in Seventeenth-Century England* (Newark: University of Delaware Press, 1995), 23. Donne calls God's grace 'physicke of the soul.' The image of a healer of body and soul harkens back before even biblical references to Apollo, who, for Plato and the Western tradition was a physician of the body and the soul. Andrew Wear studies the similarities between Catholic and Protestant depictions of Christ as the good physician. A. Wear, 'Religious Beliefs and Medicine in Early Modern England,' in H. Marland and M. Pelling (eds), *The Task of Healing: Medicine, Religion and Gender in England and the Netherlands, 1450-1800* (Rotterdam: Erasmus Publishing, 1996) 147-8, 150, 152.

4   S. Covington, *Wounds, Flesh, and Metaphor in Seventeenth-Century England* (New York: Palgrave Macmillan, 2009), 4.

5   S. Covington, *Wounds, Flesh, and Metaphor in Seventeenth-Century England,* 5.

6   Other helpful sources covering metaphors and disease include A. Weinstein, *Contagion and Infection* (Baltimore: Johns Hopkins University Press, 2003); A. Mack, ed., *In Time of Plague: The History and Social Consequences of Lethal Epidemic Disease* (New York: New School for Social Research, 1988); and H. Skulsky, *Language Recreated: Seventeenth-Century Metaphorists and the Act of Metaphor* (Athens: University of Georgia Press, 1992).

7   The diseased state of the kingdom could be extended to include the church as well. See for example John Taylor's 1642 tract, in which he

suggests *Rare Physick for the Church Sick of an Ague*, to be prescribed by the parliament, 'those admirable physicians of the church and state.' J. Taylor, *Rare Physick for the Church Sick of an Ague with the Names of Every Particular Disease, and the Manner How She Contracted Them, and by What Means, as Also Prescripts to Remedy the Same. Humbly Commended to the Parliament, Those Admirable Physicians of the Church and State* (1642). Disease metaphors were also applied to nonconformists, as illustrated by Francis Bugg's tract, *The Pilgrim's Progress, from Quakerism to Christianity* (1700), in which the doctrine and politics of Quakerism is likened to an epidemic disease. The tract offers 'a remedy proposed for this malady, and the cure of Quakerism,' in the preface.

8   These tracts often take for granted the idea of the body politic. For more on body politic theory, see R. Braverman, *Plots and Counterplot: Sexual Politics and the Body Politic in English Literature, 1660-1730* (New York: Cambridge University Press, 1993); J.G. Harris, *Foreign Bodies and the Body Politic: Discourses of Social Pathology in Early Modern England* (New York Cambridge University Press, 1998); and S. Melzer and K. Norberg (eds), *From the Royal to the Republican Body: Incorporating the Political in Seventeenth- and Eighteenth-Century France* (Berkeley: University of California Press, 1998).

9   S. Patrick, *Jewish Hypocrisie, a Caveat to the Present Generation* (1660). The author states that he knows not how 'to take a better course, then to imitate Physitians, who consult not inner reason, but likewise the experience of former times.'

10   Anon., *The Disease of the House: Or, the State Mountebanck: Administering Physick to a Sick Parliament* (1649). In this satire, the French quack has come over to cure the sick nation and turn a quick profit. He soon flees the land when he realizes how corrupt and diseased it is. A learned English physician draws the same conclusion as the mountebank about the hopelessness of the case: the land that murdered the king is now the realm of the devil, who wishes disease on them, and curses them with no cures: 'Let no Physition, or learned Doctor spend / A Pill, but what may send them to their end.'

11   E. Pool, *A Vision: Wherein Is Manifested the Disease and Cure of the Kingdome* (1648). W.L., *A Medicine for Malignancy: Or, Parliament Pill, Serving to Purge out the Malignant Humours of Men Dis-Affected to the Republick* (1644). See G. Burnet, *The Plague at Westminster. Or, an Order for the Visitation of a Sick Parliament, Grievously Troubled with a New Disease, Called the Consump-*

tion of Their Members (1609). The tract describes hostility at home as a disease that 'consumes the Vitals,' leaving only a 'wasted and exhausted Carcasse.' See also J. Tichborne, *A Triple Antidote against Certaine Very Common Scandals of This Time, Which, Like Infections and Epidemicall Diseases, Have Generally Annoyed Most Sorts of People Amongst Us, Poisoned Also Not a Few, and Divers Waies Plagued and Afflicted the Whole State* (1609).

12 Anon., ———, *the Parliament Mended or Ended; or, a Philter and Halter for the Two Houses. Prescribed by Their Doctor Mercurius Elenticus* (1648). The recipe is comprised of 'twelve ounces of Loyaltie, a Vegitable to be found in each corner of the pleasant Garden, called the word of God, with a good quantity of Order and Discipline, with as much of Law and Justice; a pound of Penitence, with Competency, of the ancient Religious practices.' For a similar message, see Anon., *A Cure for the State. Or, an Excellent Remedy against the Apostacy of the Times* (1659). The author recommends a remedy 'approved by the College of Physicians' and 'made publick for the good of the Common-wealth.' It includes a satirical recipe that, when taken every morning with fasting, 'will preserve you from the like Apostacy, that the Army and other Saints have of late fallen into, and make you stick close to the Parliament.'

13 It can be difficult to differentiate the political tract from the sermon, such as in W. Stampe, *A Treatise of Spiritual Infatuation, Being the Resent Visible Disease of the English Nation. Delivered in Severall Sermons* (1650). In this tract the subject matter is political, yet it is crafted to resemble a strictly religious sermon, from the title to the inclusion of biblical passages on the title page. See also Anon., *The Sad State of the Kingdom, Being an Account of the First Years Charge of Our Reformation*, in which the author lists the 'debts' and 'credits' of England, so that by knowing the 'disease' of the kingdom, those that love it may find the cure.

14 R. Hutton, *The Restoration: A Political and Religious History of England and Wales 1658-1667* (Oxford: Clarendon Press, 1985), introduction.

15 H. Cook, 'Good Advice and Little Medicine: The Professional Authority of Early Modern English Physicians,' *The Journal of British Studies* 33, no. 1 (January 1994), 24.

16 Michael MacDonald has argued that the idea of combining spiritual and physical means of healing were images and themes 'familiar to every Christian and deeply embedded in popular culture. They were the central devices in medieval drama, and they lingered on in plays, sermons, and devotional works into the eighteenth century.' M. Mac-

Donald, 'Psychological Healing in England, 1600-1800' in *The Church and Healing*, ed. W. J. Sheils (Oxford: Basil Blackwell, 1982), 116.

17 J. Simmons, 'Publications of 1623,' in *The Library* (1966). Cited in D. Nagy, *Popular Medicine in Seventeenth-Century England* (Bowling Green: Bowling Green State University Popular Press, 1988), 35.

18 A. Wear, 'Puritan Perceptions of Illness in Seventeenth Century England,' in R. Porter (ed.), *Patients and Practitioners: Lay Perceptions of Medicine in Pre-Industrial Society* (Cambridge: Cambridge University Press, 1985), 67-8; D. Harley, 'Medical Metaphors in English Moral Theology, 1560-1660,' *Journal of the History of Medicine and Allied Sciences* 48, no. 4 (1993), 396; and D. Harley, 'Spiritual Physic, Providence and English Medicine, 1560-1640,' in O.P. Grell and A. Cunningham (eds), *Medicine and the Reformation* (London: Routledge, 1993).

19 L.A. Ferrell, *Government by Polemic: James I, the King's Preachers, and the Rhetorics of Conformity, 1603-1625* (Stanford: Stanford University Press, 1998), 10-11.

20 M. Spufford, *Small Books and Pleasant Histories: Popular Fiction and Its Readership in Seventeenth-Century England* (London: Methuen and Company, 1981).

21 T. Allefree, *Epaphroditus's Sickness and Recovery, in Three Sermons* (1671), A2.

22 G. Whitefield, *Christ the Physician of the Soul* (1750).

23 P. Bayne, *A Caveat for Cold Christians Wherein the Common Disease of Christians, with the Remedie, Is Plainly and Excellently Set Downe for All That Will Use It* (1618).

24 E. Lawrence, *Christ's Power over Bodily Diseases Preached in Several Sermons* (1662).

25 This idea forms the basis of David Harley's argument in 'Medical Metaphors in English Moral Theology, 1560-1660,' 396-7.

26 See L.A. Ferrell, *Government by Polemic: James I, the King's Preachers, and the Rhetorics of Conformity, 1603-1625* and D. Harley, 'Spiritual Physic, Providence and English Medicine, 1560-1640,' 110-112.

27 This point is argued in W. Schleiner, *The Imagery of John Donne's Sermons* (Providence: Brown University Press, 1970).

28 Ferrell and Harley both work in the linguistic aspects of sermons and metaphors. See L.A. Ferrell, *Government by Polemic: James I, the King's Preachers, and the Rhetorics of Conformity, 1603-1625* and D. Harley, 'Medical Metaphors in English Moral Theology, 1560-1660.'

29 W. Parke, *A Tractat of the Universal Panacaea of Soul and Body* (1665).

30 G. Whitefield, *Christ the Physician of the Soul,* 21-22.

31 F. Bampfield, *All in One, All Useful Sciences and Profitable Arts in One Book of Jehovah Aelohim, Copied out and Commented Upon in Created Beings, Comprehended and Discovered in the Fulness and Perfection of Scr[i]pture-Knowledges* (1677).

32 F. Wilson, ed., *Plague Pamphlets of Thomas Dekker* (Oxford: Clarendon Press, 1925), 188-9.

33 D. Harley, 'Spiritual Physic, Providence and English Medicine, 1560-1640,' 101.

34 R. Porter, 'The Patient in England, C. 1660-C.1800,' in A. Wear (ed.), *Medicine in Society,* (New York: Cambridge University Press, 1992), 96. Porter asserts that Divine Providence proved a fundamental tenet of popular works, and that books on spiritual and practical physic similarly explained God's punishing hand. This focus was reiterated in medical writings of the period, as the next chapter will demonstrate.

35 M. Henry Burton, *A Most Godly Sermon: Preached at St. Albons in Woodstreet on Sunday Last, Being the 10 of October, 1641* (1641). Burton's sermon demonstrated the 'necessity of Selfe-denyall and Humiliation, by Prayer and Fasting before the Lord, in regard of the present Plague we now lye under, which God, in his good time, remove from amongst us.' See also W. Gouge, *God's Three Arrowes: Plague, Famine, Sword* (1636) and M.H. Burton, *A Most Godly Sermon: Preached at St. Albons in Woodstreet on Sunday Last, Being the 10 of October, 1641* (1641).

36 R. Anselment, *The Realms of Apollo: Literature and Healing in Seventeenth-Century England.* 25.

37 Anon., 'A Sermon, Containing the Strangeness, Frequency, and Desperate Consequence of Impenitency,' in *Six Semons Preached by the Right Reverend Father in God, Seth Lord Bishop of Sarum* (1672). Sermons at times discussed why God would send disease for sin, see W. Bridge, *Two Sermons: I. The Diseases That Make a Stoppage to Englands Mercies Discovered, and Attended with Their Remedies Ii. A Preparation for Suffering in These Plundering Times* (1642) and H. Gosson, *Christs Teares over Jerusalem. Or, a Caveat for England, to Call to God for Mercy, Lest We Be Plagued for Our Contempt and Wickedness* (1624).

38 This idea is expressed in K. Thomas, *Religion and the Decline of Magic* (New York: Scribner, 1971) and W. Shiels, ed., *The Church and Healing.*

39 Diseases inflicted by God were often referred to in sermons as 'the

rod of the lord.' T. Allefree, *Epaphroditus's Sickness and Recovery, in Three Sermons*, 12-14.

40   For an example of this in sermons, see T. Burroughs, *A Soveraign Remedy for All Kinds of Grief* (1662); G. Lesly, *The Universal Medicine: A Sermon* (1678); J. Edwards, *The Plague of the Heart* (1665); R. Venning, *Sin, the Plague of Plagues; or, Sinful Sin the Worst of Evils.* (1669); and W. Bridge, *The Diseases That Make a Stoppage to Englands Mercies Discovered, and Attended with Their Remedies* (1642).

41   E Lawrence, *Christ's Power over Bodily Diseases Preached in Several Sermons*, 18. The logic is usually that God sends sickness as a reminder to a sinful people to repent now, so that their souls can be saved before it is too late. For additional examples, see T. Vincent, *God's Terrible Voice in the City* (1667); W. Gouge, *God's Three Arrowes: Plague, Famine, Sword;* and Gosson, *Christs Teares over Jerusalem. Or, a Caveat for England, to Call to God for Mercy, Lest We Be Plagued for Our Contempt and Wickedness.*

42   T. Allefree, *Epaphroditus's Sickness and Recovery, in Three Sermons*, 12-14 and N. Bownd, *A Storehouse of Comfort for the Afflicted in Spirit* (1604).

43   S. Patrick, *Jewish Hypocrisie, a Caveat to the Present Generation* (1660).

44   J. Edwards, *The Plague of the Heart* (1665), 26-27.

45   D. King, *A Discovery of Some Troublesome Thoughts Wherewith Many Godly Precious Souls Are Burthened, and Extreamly Pressed: That Like a Canker Eats out All Their Comforts, and Keeps Their Souls under Continuall Fears and Distractions. Together with a Compound of Some Scripture and Experimentall Cordials, for the Refreshing of Those Who Are Sick of Such a Disease; and through the Blessing of God, May Prove Medicinall, to the Cure of Some, and the Comforting of Others* (1651).

46   D.D. Perrinchief, *A Sermon Preached before the Honourable House of Commons, at St. Margarets Westminster, Nov. 7 Being the Fast-Day Appointed for the Plague of Pestilence* (1666), 31-2.

47   R. Venning, *Sin, the Plague of Plagues; or, Sinful Sin the Worst of Evils* (1669).

48   R. Venning, *Sin, the Plague of Plagues; or, Sinful Sin the Worst of Evils*, 21.

49   T.   Allefree, *Epaphroditus's Sickness and Recovery, in Three Sermons*, 11-12.

50   T. Adams, *Diseases of the Soule a Discourse Diuine, Morall, and Physicall* (1616). See also J.B., *The Journal or Diary of a Thankful Christian* (1656).

51   T.   Burroughs, *A Soveraign Remedy for All Kinds of Grief* (1662), A2. This same notion is expressed in W. Bridge, *Two Sermons: I. The Diseases That Make a Stoppage to Englands Mercies Discovered, and Attended with Their*

Remedies Ii. *A Preparation for Suffering in These Plundering Times* (1642).

52 S. Patrick, *Jewish Hypocrisie, a Caveat to the Present Generation*, 77 and T. Adams, *Physicke from Heaven* and Cawdry, *Treasurie of Similies* both mention a spiritual panacea.

53 N. Bownd, *A Storehouse of Comfort for the Afflicted in Spirit.*

54 W. Gouge, *God's Three Arrowes: Plague, Famine, Sword*, 11. See a similar message in E. Lawrence, *Christ's Power over Bodily Diseases Preached in Several Sermons.*

55 E. Heron, *Physicke for Body and Soule Shevving That the Maladies of the One, Proceede from the Sinnes of the Other: With a Remedie against Both, Prescribed by Our Heauenly Physitian Iesus Christ* (1621).

56 D. King, *Self the Grand Enemy of Jesus Christ, and Mortall Disease of Man. Or, a Treatise Discovering What a Heart-Plague Self Is with Its Mischief and Danger: Also, Special Remedies for Its Cure* (1660).

57 S. Patrick, *Jewish Hypocrisie, a Caveat to the Present Generation*, 19.

58 See J. Flavel, *Pneumatologia, a Treatise of the Soul of Man Wherein the Divine Original, Excellent and Immortal Nature of the Soul Are Opened, Its Love and Inclination to the Body, with the Necessity of Its Separation from It, Considered and Improved, the Existence, Operations, and States of Separated Souls, Both in Heaven and Hell, Immediately after Death, Asserted, Discussed, and Variously Applyed...*(1685); K. Digby, *Two Treatises in the One of Which, the Nature of Bodies: In the Other, the Nature of Mans Soul Is Looked into in Way of Discovery of the Immortality of Reasonable Souls* (1658); J. Dunton, *The Visions of the Soule, before It Comes into the Body in Several Dialogues* (1692); and T. Manlove, *The Immortality of the Soul Asserted, and Practically Improved Shewing by Scripture, Reason, and the Testimony of the Ancient Philosophers, That the Soul of Man Is Capable of Subsisting and Acting in a State of Separation from the Body, and How Much It Concerns Us All to Prepare for That State...*(1697). See also J. Howell, *The Vision or a Dialog between the Soul and the Bodie, Fancid in a Morning-Dream* (1651); Anon., *Saint Bernard's Vision (a Brief Discourse Dialogue-Wise) between the Soul and Body Of a Damned Man Newly Deceased, Laying the Faults One Upon Other: With a Speech of the Devils in Hell* (1640); Anon., *A Moral Essay Upon the Soul of Man in Three Parts: I. The Preference Due to the Soul above the Body...Ii. Of Our Duties of Religion and Morality...Iii. Concerning Our Duties of Time and Eternity;* E. Carrey, *A Serious Meditation for Sinners Which Is Set Forth in Several Discourses, Which Passed between a Soul at Her Departure, and the Members of the Body* (1688); and J. Davies and T. Jenner, *A Work for None but Angels...A Book Shew-*

ing What the Soule Is, Subsisting and Having Its Operations without the Body (1658).

59   F. Bampfield, *All in One, All Useful Sciences and Profitable Arts in One Book of Jehovah Aelohim, Copied out and Commented Upon in Created Beings, Comprehended and Discovered in the Fulness and Perfection of Scr[i]pture-Knowledges*. Winfried Schleiner has described illness, with its connotations of bodily corruption, as a 'ready metaphor' for depictions of sin and the soul's corruption. W. Schleiner, *The Imagery of John Donne's Sermons*, 69.

60   W. Schleiner, *The Imagery of John Donne's Sermons*, 72.

61   (9:208, 8:708), (10:123, 5:160) cited in W. Schleiner, *The Imagery of John Donne's Sermons*, 71.

62   J.F., *A New Letter, to All Drunkards, Whoremongers, Thieves, Disobedience to Parents, Swearers, Lyers* (1696). For additional examples, see S. Haworth, *Anthropologia, or, a Philosophic Discourse Concernng Man Being the Anatomy of Both His Soul and Body: Wherein the Natue, Origin, Union, Immaterality, Immortality, Extension, and Faculties of the One and Parts, Temperament, Complexions, Functions, Sexes, and Ages Respecting the Other Are Concisely Delineated* (1680), which takes into account the wholeness of a person's health, including that of body and soul, and R. Overton, *Man Wholly Mortal, or, a Treatise Wherein 'Tis Proved Both Theologically and Philosophically, That as Whole Man Sinned, So Whole Man Died Contrary to That Common Distinction of Soul and Body* (1655), in which sin is shown to effect the whole man, both body and soul. See also J. Smith, *The Pourtract of Old Age Wherein Is Contained a Sacred Anatomy Both of Soul and Body, and a Perfect Account of the Infirmities of Age Incident to Them Both: Being a Paraphrase Upon the Six Former Verses of the 12. Chapter of Ecclesiastes,* and J. Harris, *The Divine Physician, Prescribing Rules for the Prevention, and Cure of Most Diseases, as Well of the Body, as the Soul Demonstrating by Natural Reason, and Also Divine and Humane Testimony, That, as Vicious and Irregular Actions and Affections Prove Often Occasions of Most Bodily Diseases, and Shortness of Life, So the Contrary Do Conduce to the Preservation of Health, and Prolongation of Life: In Two Parts* (1676), wherein the author sermonizes on the need for both the body and soul to be healthy in order for happiness to be enjoyed.

63   N. Caussin, *The Christian Diary* (1648), 87.

64   See 'The Literall Plague of Disease and Noysome Pestilence or the Metaphoricall Plague of Sinne; Dangers of the Body or of the Soule,' cited in A. Wear, 'Religious Beliefs and Medicine in Early Modern

England,' 151. On body/soul duality in early modern England see P. Boitani and A. Torti, eds., *The Body and the Soul in Medieval Literature: The J.A.W. Bennett Memorial Lectures, Tenth Series, Perugia, 1998* (Rochester: D.S. Brewer, 1999).

65   A. Wear, 'Religious Beliefs and Medicine in Early Modern England,' 151 and M. Hobbs (ed.), *The Sermons of Henry King (1592-1669), Bishop of Chichester* (Cranbury, New Jersey: Associated University Press, 1992), 209. See for example T. Vincent, *God's Terrible Voice in the City*, 31-2. The tract chronicles the Lord's infliction of plague and fire on the city. A parallel is drawn between disease's wasting of the body and sin's wasting of the soul.

66   Edwards, *The Plague of the Heart*, 2-3.

67   Cited in A. Wear, 'Religious Beliefs and Medicine in Early Modern England,' 152, 155. See also T. Becon, *Prayer for Them That Are Sick*. Becon asks God to be a physician to those who are diseased either in body or soul, and after He gives His loving correction, 'restore unto them the bounty of health, both corporally and spiritually.' For additional primary examples, see Bishop E. Stillingfleet, *The Works of Dr. Edward Stillingfleet*, 6 vols., vol. 1 (London: 1704), 544; J. Pearson, *An Exposition of the Creed* (1659), 39; G. Rust, *Funeral Sermon Preached at the Obsequies Of...Jeremy, Lord Bishop of Down* (1668), 6; T. Woolnough, *The Dust Returning to Earth* (1669), 2; W. Bates, *A Funeral Sermon Preached Upon the Death of Mr. Thomas Gouge* (1681), 4; and R. Allen, *A Gainful Death at the End of a Truly Christian Life* (1700), 22.

68   D. Harley, 'Medical Metaphors in English Moral Theology, 1560-1660,' 401.

69   R. Baxter, *The Invaluable Price of an Immortal Soul Shewing the Vanity of Most People in Taking Care for the Body, but Neglect Their Duty as to the Preservation of Their Never-Dying Souls* (1681).

70   D. Harley, 'Spiritual Physic, Providence and English Medicine, 1560-1640,' 106.

71   J.R. Guy, 'The Episcopal Licensing of Physicians, Surgeons, and Midwives,' *Bulletin of the History of Medicine* 56 (1982), 530.

72   A. Wear, 'Religious Beliefs and Medicine in Early Modern England,' 165,151. A similar sentiment is expressed in M. MacDonald, 'Psychological Healing in England, 1600-1800,' 118.

73   R. Bolton, *Instructions for a Right Comforting Afflicted Consciences with Speciall Antidotes against Some Grievous Temptations: Delivered for the Most Part in the*

Lecture at Kettering in North-Hampton-Shire (1631).

74 S. Patrick, *Jewish Hypocrisie, a Caveat to the Present Generation,* B1, 17.

75 W.W., *Physick to Cure the Most Dangerous Disease, Desperation* (1607). See also the same author's preface in W.W., *The Anchor of Faith. Upon Which, a Christian May Repose in All Manner of Temptations* (1628). This tract includes the biblical quotation, 'The Body will beare his infirmitie; but a Broken and Wounded Spirit who can beare,' Prov. 18. 14, A2-A3.

76 This was still was not a possibility for many, due to financial and geographical reasons.

77 K. Thomas, *Religion and the Decline of Magic.* and MacFarlane, ed., *Diary of Ralph Josselin 1616-1683.* See also Wear, 'Puritan Perceptions of Illness in Seventeenth Century England,' 115, in which he makes the point that Ralph Josselin frequently saw the workings of God's Providence in everyday encounters.

78 R. Anselment, *The Realms of Apollo: Literature and Healing in Seventeenth-Century England,* 26-7.

79 L. Beier, 'In Sickness and in Health: A Seventeenth Century Family's Experience,' in R. Porter (ed.), *Patients and Practitioners: Lay Perceptions of Medicine in Pre-Industrial Society* (Cambridge: Cambridge University Press, 1985), 122. Keith Thomas makes a similar point in *Religion and the Decline of Magic* (New York: Scribner, 1971), 96.

80 R. Latham and W. Matthews (eds.), *The Diary of Samuel Pepys,* 11 vols. (London: Bell & Hyman, 1970-83), III, 318.

81 R. Anselment, *The Realms of Apollo: Literature and Healing in Seventeenth-Century England,* 16-17. A similar argument is presented in A.Wear, 'Religious Beliefs and Medicine in Early Modern England,' 152-3. Wear notes that at the individual level, there was similarity between connection between illness, sin and God.

82 G. Lesly, *The Universal Medicine: A Sermon,* 4.

83 J. Beadle, *The Journal or Diary of a Thankful Christian* (1656), 55.

84 T. Wright (ed.), *The Autobiography of Joseph Lister, of Bradford in Yorkshire* (London: John Russell Smith, 1842), 29.

85 J. Lowther, *Lowther Family Estate Books, 1617-1675,* vol. 191. C.B. Philips (ed.) (Gateshead: Northumberland Press, 1979), 62. The above cited in R. Anselment, *The Realms of Apollo: Literature and Healing in Seventeenth-Century England,* 16-17.

86 C8 (6:237, 11:538) cited in W. Schleiner, *The Imagery of John Donne's Sermons,* 75. See also L. Andrews, *A Sermon of Pestlience, Preached at Chis-*

wick, 1603 (1636). English ministers stressed the spiritual significance of sickness. See for example T. Becon, *Prayer for Them That Are Sick* in which the author points out that those who are most sinful often are not visited with sickness, but in the end receive the eternal pains of hell. Cited in A. Wear, 'Religious Beliefs and Medicine in Early Modern England,' 151-152.

87 S. Clarke, 'The Marrow of Ecclesiastical Historie,' (1650), 239.

88 D.M. Meads (ed.), *The Diary of Lady Margaret Hoby, 1599-1605* (1930), 220.

89 J. Turner, *Choice Experiences of the Kind Dealings of God* (1653), I. Similar attitudes regarding patients' bearing of and usefulness of affliction are found in E. Calamy, *The Art of Divine Meditation, or, a Discourse of the Nature, Necessity, and Excellency Thereof with Motives to, and Rules for the Better Performance of That Most Important Christian Duty: In Several Sermons on Gen. 24:63* (1680) and N. Bisbie, *Prosecution No Persecution: Or, the Difference Between Suffering for Disobedience and Faction, and Suffering for Righteousness and Christ's Sake* (1682).

90 P. Slack, 'Mirrors of Health and Treasures of Poor Men: The Uses of the Vernacular Medical Literature of Tudor England,' In C. Webster (ed.), *Health, Medicine, and Mortality in the Sixteenth Century* (New York: Cambridge University Press, 1979), 270.

91 See D. Harley, 'Spiritual Physic, Providence and English Medicine, 1560-1640.' 101-4. Harley reiterates this point in 'From Providence to Nature: The Moral Theology and Godly Practice of Maternal Breast-Feeding in Stuart England,' *Bulletin of the History of Medicine* 69 (1995).

92 R. Sibbes, *The Soules Conflict with It Selfe* (1665).

93 D. Harley, 'The Theology of Affliction and the Experience of Sickness in the Godly Family, 1650-1714: The Henrys and the Newcomes,' in A. Cunningham and O.P. Grell (eds), *Religio Medici: Medicine and Religion in Seventeenth-Century England* (Aldershot: Scolar Press, 1996).

94 See P. Slack, *The Impact of Plague in Tudor and Stuart England* (London: Routledge & K. Paul, 1985), 270.

95 See F. Bunny, *A Guide Unto Godliness* (1617); R. Walker, *A Learned and Profitable Treatise of God's Providence* (1608), 46-7, 55; and R. Sibbes, *The Soules Conflict with It Selfe*.

96 M. Pelling, *The Common Lot: Sickness, Medical Occupations and the Urban Poor in Early Modern England* (New York: Longman, 1998), 229.

97 R. Porter, 'The Patient in England, C. 1660-C. 1800,' 98-99. See also

L. Beier, 'In Sickness and in Health: A Seventeenth Century Family's Experience,' and D. Nagy, *Popular Medicine in Seventeenth-Century England.*

98   R. Porter, 'The Patient in England, C. 1660-C.1800,' 98.

99   G. Risse, 'Medicine in the Age of Enlightenment,' in A. Wear (ed.), *Medicine in Society: Historical Essays* (Cambridge: Cambridge University Press, 1992), 150. See also L.J. Rather, 'The Six Things "Non-Natural": A Note on the Origins and the Fate of a Doctrine and a Phrase,' *Clio Medica* 3 (1968); R.C. Burns, 'The Non-Naturals: A Paradox in the Western Concept of Health,' *Journal of Medicine and Philosophy* 3 (1976); and P. H. Niebyl, 'The Non-Naturals,' *Bulletin of the History of Medicine* 454 (1971).

100   In G. Risse, 'Medicine in the Age of Enlightenment,' 151.

101   R. Porter, 'The Patient in England, C. 1660-C. 1800,' 95.

102   Cited in R. Porter and D. Porter, *In Sickness and in Health: The British Experience 1650-1850*, 72-4

103   Cited in R. Porter and D. Porter, *In Sickness and in Health: The British Experience 1650-1850*, 72-4

104   Cited in R. Porter and D. Porter, *In Sickness and in Health: The British Experience 1650-1850*, 72-4.

105   R. Porter and D. Porter, *In Sickness and in Health: The British Experience 1650-1850*, 73.

106   T. Birch (ed.), *Robert Boyle, the Works*, vol. 4 (Hildesheim: George Olms Verlagsbuchhandlung, 1965), 39.

107   R. Anselment, *The Realms of Apollo: Literature and Healing in Seventeenth-Century England*, 26. Doreen Nagy has argued that Providentialism was a hindrance to the medical profession: 'In a climate where an all-powerful and righteous God held sway, the costly treatments of licensed practitioners were unnecessary if God willed recovery and a needless waste if the patient died.' D. Nagy, *Popular Medicine in Seventeenth-Century England*, 42. Nagy cited support for her opinion in P. Seaver, *Wallington's World* (Stanford: Stanford University Press, 1985), 228.

108   D. Harley, 'The Theology of Affliction and the Experience of Sickness in the Godly Family, 1650-1714: The Henrys and the Newcomes,' 274-5. For discussions of the interplay between the spiritual and physical, see K. Thomas, *Religion and the Decline of Magic* (London: Weidenfeld and Nicolson, 1971); D. Amundsen, 'Medicine and Faith in Early Christianity,' *Bulletin of the History of Medicine*, 56 (1982), 326-50; and G.Ferngren, 'Early Christianity as a Religion of Healing,' *Bulletin of the*

History of Medicine, 66 (1992), 1-15.

109 T. Oldman, *Gods Rubuke in Taking from Us That Worthy and Honourable Gentleman Sir Edward Lewkenor Knight* (1619), 43-4 and R. Sibbes, *The Soules Conflict with It Selfe*, 355. Above examples cited in D. Harley, 'Spiritual Physic, Providence and English Medicine, 1560-1640,' 107.

110 R. Porter, 'The Patient in England, C. 1660-C.1800,' 98.

111 J. Wesley, *Primitive Physick: Or, an Essay and Natural Method of Curing Most Diseases* (1747). Cited in G.S. Rousseau, 'John Wesley's *Primitive Physic* (1747),' *Harvard Library Bulletin* 16 (1968), 242-56.

112 D. Harley, 'Medical Metaphors in English Moral Theology, 1560-1660,' 433-35.

113 D. Nagy, *Popular Medicine in Seventeenth-Century England;* R. Porter, *Disease, Medicine, and Society in England, 1550-1860;* M. Pelling, *Medical Conflicts in Early Modern London: Patronage, Physicians, and Irregular Practitioners, 1550-1640* (Oxford: Clarendon Press, 2003); and L. Beier, *Sufferers and Healers: The Experience of Illness in Seventeenth-Century England.*

114 A. Wear, 'Religious Beliefs and Medicine in Early Modern England,' 157.

115 R. Anselment, *The Realms of Apollo: Literature and Healing in Seventeenth-Century England*, 48. Roy Porter came to the same conclusion in 'The Patient in England, C. 1660-C.1800,' 96.

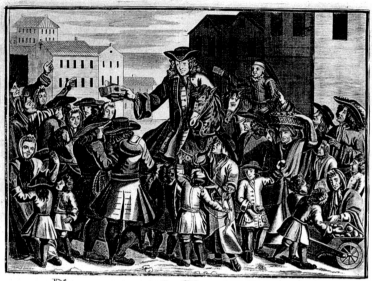

Pharmacopola Circumforaneus, OR
The Horse Doctor's Harangue to y Credulous Mob

GENTLEMEN, I Waltho Van Claturbank, High German Doctor, Chymist & Dentifricator, Native of Arabia Deserta, Citizen and Burgomaster of the City of Brandipolis, Seventh Son of a Seventh Son, Unborn Doctor, of above 60 Years Experience; having Studied over Galen, Hypocrates, Albumazor & Paracelsus, am now become the Æsculapius of this Age: Having been Educated at 12 Universities, and Travell'd through 52 Kingdoms, and born Counsellor to the Counsellors of several Monarchs, Natural Son of the Wonder working Chymical Doctor Signior Hanesio, lately arriv'd from the farthest Part of Utopia, Famous throughout all Asia, Africa, Europe and America, from the Sun's Oriental Exaltation to his Occidental Declination: Out of meer Pity to my own Dear Self, and languishing Mortals, have by the earnest Prayers and Intreaties of several Lords, Earls, Dukes and Honourable Personages, been at last prevail'd upon to oblige the World with this Notice.

That all Persons, Young & Old, Blind or Lame, Deaf or Dumb, Curable or Incurable, may Know where to repair for Cure, in all Cephalalgia's, Paralytick Paroxysms, Palpitations of the Pericardium, Empyema's, Syncopes & Nausea's, arising either from a Plethory or a Cacochymy, Vertiginous Vapours, Hydrocephalous Dysentery's, Odontalgic or Podagrical Inflammations, Iliac Passions, Ilierical Effusions, Exanthemata, the Hen Pox, the Hog Pox, the Whores Pox, and the Small Pox, the Alcites, Tympanites, Anasarca, and the entire Legion of Lethiferous Distempers.

Imprimis, Gentlemen, I have a never failing Styptic, Corroborating, Odoriferous, Anodinous, Balsamic Balsam of Balsams, made of dead Mens Fat, Rosin, and Goose Grease; which infallibly Restores Lost Maidenheads, Raises Demolish'd Noses, and by its Abstersive, Cosmetic Quality, preserves Superannuated Bawds from Wrinkles.

Item. I have the True Carthamophera of the Tripple Kingdom, my never failing Heliogenes, being the Tincture of the Sun, deriving Vigor, Influence, and Dominion from the same Light: It causes all Complexions to laugh or smile, at the very Time of Taking it: Is 7 Years in preparing, and being compleated, secundum Artem, by

by Fermentation, Cohobation, Calcination, Sublimation, Fixation, Philtration, Circulation and Quidlibitification, in Balneo Mariæ, Crucible and Fixatory; the Athanor, Cucurbita and Reverberatory; is the only Sovereign Medicine in the World. This is Nature's Palladium, Healths Magazine, it Works 7 manner of Ways, in order as Nature her self, requires, for it seems to be confin'd to any particular way of Operation: so that it effecteth the Cure, either Hypnotically, Hydrotically, Cathartically, Poppilmatically, Hydrogogically, Pneumatically, or Synecdochically: it Mundifies the Hypogastrium, wipes off abstersively, those tenacious conglomerated sedimental Sordes, adhere to y Œsophagus & Viscera: Extinguishes all Supernatural Fermentations & Ebullitions, & in fine Annihilates all Nosporophical Morbific ideas of the whole Corporal Compages.

A Dram of it is worth a Bushel of March Dust: For if a Man chance to have his Brains beat out or his Head chopd off, 2 Drops (I say) 2 Drops Gentlemen, seasonably apply'd, will recall y fleeting Spirits, reinthrone y depopd Archeus, Cement y discontinuity of y Parts & in 6 Minutes restore y lifeless Trunk to all its pristine Functions, Vital, Natural & Animal: So y this believe me Gentlemen, is the only Sovereign Remedy in the World.

I have y chiefest Antepuckenda Gangran Specific in Venus's Regalia, which infallibly Cures y French Pox, with all its train of Gonorrhea's, Bubo's and Shankers, Carnosity's, Phymosis, Paraphymosis, Christalline, Priapismus, Caudalomata & Ragades, without Baths & Stoves, & that with as much Pleasure as y same was contracted: so that its worth any Persons while to get y modish Distemper once a Fortnight, if it be to be had for Love or Money, to enjoy the Benefit of so diverting a Remedy.

I have the Panchymagogon of Hermes Trismegistus, an Incomparable Spagyric Tincture of the Moons Horns, which is the only infallible Antidote against the contagion of Cuckoldom.

Besides my Vermifugo Pulvis, or Antivermatical Worm conquering Powder, so famous for destroying all y sorts of 'em, incident to humane Bodies, breaking their complicated Knots in y Duodenum, & dissolving y Phlegmatick Crudities that produce their Anthropolagous Vermine: it hath brought

away Worms by Urine, as long as the May-Pole in the Strand, when it flourish'd in its Primitive Prolixity, tho' I confess not altogether so thick.

Look ye GENTLEMEN, I have it under the Hands and Seals of all the Greatest Sultans, Sophys, Bashaw's, Viziers, Chams, Seraskiers, and Muftis, &c. in Christendom, to verificate the Truth of my Operations, that I have actually perform'd such Cures as are really beyond human Abilities.

I Cur'd Prestor John's Godmother, to the great Admiration of all the Court, of a stupendous Dolor about the Os Sacrum, so that the good Old Lady really feared the Perdition of her Huckle Bone; I did it by fomenting her Posteriors, with a Mummy of Nature, alias call'd Pilgrims Salve, mixt up with the Spirit of Mugwort, tartaragraphated throw an Alembick of Christalline Transfluency.

Thence was I sent for to Sultan Gilgon, Despote of Bosnia, who was violently afflicted with the Spasmus, He came to meet me 300 Leagues in a Go Cart: But I gave him to speedy an Acquittance of his Dolor, that the next Night I caused him to dance a Saraband, with Flipflaps and Somersets.

I Restor'd Virility and the Comforts of Generation, to above 150 Eunuchs in the Grand Seignior's Seraglio, and by a Pair of Prolific Pills lately caus'd a Vintner's Widow, who had been barren all her Days, to conceive of a Man-Child in the Twelfth Lustre of her Age, without the Help of her Husband.

I Cur'd likewise the Dutchess of Boromolpho of a Cramp in her Tongue, and the Count de Rodomontado Corrept with an Iliac Passion, contracted by eating butter'd Parsnips.

I also Cured an Alderman of Grand Cairo, who had been sick 7 Years of the Plague, in 4 Minutes: And by the like Empyrical Remedie I lately Cur'd Duke Phlioris, of a Dropsy, of which he Dy'd.

Venienti occurrite Morbo, Down with your Dust. Prœuniquiobsia. No Cure, no Money. Quæ omnia Pecunia primum. Be not sick too late.

Figure 7: A quack and his assistant arriving on horseback in a crowded town square, and text containing a parody of a quack's harangue
Courtesy Wellcome Library, London

3

'Medling Fops' with their 'Gagling Goose-quils'[1]:
The Competition

Every one striveth to be a physitian in the Country, no sooner can any one be pricked with a pin, or stung with a Bee, but every one gives his counsel and presenteth himself to be a phisitian for the patient. [2]

Dr. J.D. Alsop

I n spite of the advantages that sermons yielded to physicians in their effort to be viewed as professionals, they still faced a series of hurdles if they were to establish themselves as expert authorities whose services were routinely employed. One of the most pressing problems was competition from other medical practitioners who treated the vast majority of individuals who fell ill, especially outside of the Royal College of Physicians' seven-mile radius of jurisdiction.[3] Making matters worse, the lay public had their own ideas about health, illness, and medicine.[4] Physicians faced the difficult task of convincing the public that they offered a unique service that justified the expense. This service consisted of advice tailored to each patient's individual lifestyle and constitution, a practice grounded in their university education and the sound judgment it imparted.[5]

Medicine was one of the three learned professions surviving from the middle ages, along with the Church and law.[6] However, unlike lawyers and clerics, physicians faced challenges from competitors that were unique to the field of medicine, particularly by those who practiced medicine on a part-time basis and those who offered medical services gratis to the poor.[7] Margaret Pelling has argued against even referring to medicine as a profession, opting instead for the term 'medical occupations,' as early modern medicine was a combination of craft and trade.[8] Her description stems from the fact that although large numbers of practitioners existed, many, if not most, engaged in other activities of economic significance. In rural areas, where multiple means of employment and seasonal working were the rule rather than the exception, medicine was equally likely to be a part-time occupation. Pelling has therefore concluded that the economic framework of medicine as an occupation during this period makes it inappropriate to conceive of the modern ideal of the full-time dedicated member of the professional classes. However, within the varied medical occupations, as early as the sixteenth century physicians began evolving an ideology closely related to modern professional ideals.[9]

Harold Cook has argued that among all the number and variety of medical practitioners in early modern England, one small group self-consciously considered itself professional: physicians. Physicians purposely used the word 'profession' with regard to themselves and to no other medical practitioners, clearly identifying their profession as something other than a mere occupation.[10] Cook has maintained that physicians' struggle to define themselves as a profession has been a crucial test case for various definitions of what a profession is or was.[11] Because of the challenges posed by their varied and numerous competitors, studying how physicians garnered authority within the medical ambit and eventually secured a monopoly in terms of licensing can help shed light on how professions form. One key component was the development of a clear sense of what it meant to be a physician. This chapter will argue that this development evolved as physicians defined themselves in contrast to what they were not: uneducated or part-time practitioners.

Physicians distinguished themselves in part through their education and the sense of morality and wisdom that such an education wrought. They claimed a professional authority based on two key concepts: judgment and advice, in similar fashion to lawyers and clerics. Sound judgment and advice were considered to be related to sound morality at least as much as to knowledge and were attributed to a university education, which shaped their characters as much as their minds.[12]

Physicians attempted to differentiate themselves from other healers, calling attention to the shortcomings of their competitors while highlighting their own virtues. Indeed, the very forming of the occupation as we would characterize it today began in the seventeenth century when physicians defined themselves as a profession, separate and superior to other types of healers, at least in their opinion. The way in which physicians struggled to remain differentiated in the public's mind from their competition would set the tone for their approach to medicine and public health and would have greater ramifications for the profession for the remainder of the seventeenth century and beyond.

There has been much work done on the aggressive stance of the Royal College of Physicians in relation to irregular healers who practiced within the RCP's jurisdiction.[13] These studies have generally pointed to the futility of such actions, given that licensed physicians were a miniscule group in the seventeenth century. Margaret Pelling has estimated that in 1600 the population of London was approximately 200,000, while the average membership of the college between 1580 and 1640 was thirty-one. Although it was not possible for such a small group of physicians to attend to all the healthcare needs in London, not to mention the outlying areas, Pelling has made the point that the college was just as concerned with illicit practice as it was with malpractice.[14] This chapter attempts to explain the stance of the college, and of university-educated physicians in general, as one in which anxieties over part-time healers went deeper than simply guarding their turf against encroachers. The RCP, like the majority of formally educated physicians, viewed their offering as truly unique, and they were interested in distinguishing themselves from their competition in order to convince the public that they could provide them with a valuable service.

This chapter is interested primarily in the self-fashioning of physicians, as defined in the Introduction as university educated, although not necessarily licensed by the RCP. They considered themselves different from and in many ways superior to other members of the tripartite system of medicine: the surgeons and apothecaries. They were concerned with surgeons and apothecaries encroaching on their professional turf, but the quarrels they had with these two groups were somewhat different from the ones they had with part-time healers, women healers, and quacks. Surgeons and apothecaries had their own charters. They were regulated. There existed internal organization to their professions. They occupied a distinct place in the medical hierarchy, at least in theory, as in reality there was a considerable degree of overlap. In short, the relationship between the three professions was at least defined, if not always practiced. Therefore, although physicians may have been keen to differentiate themselves from surgeons and apothecaries, they fell into a different category of competition than those who practiced medicine part-time or without formal training for a particular medical occupation.

The field of competition within seventeenth-century medicine is a vast one in terms of historiography, and coverage of all aspects encompasses more than can be included in a single chapter. This chapter will *not* chronicle the quarrels between surgeons or apothecaries but instead focuses on part-time healers, women healers, and quacks. Furthermore, the chapter does not delve into the exact nature of a medical education and the changes that took place. Instead, the focus is on education as conceived of by physicians, in terms of instilling in them not just more knowledge than their competitors, but the fundamentals of advice and judgment that went along with a university degree. No detailed history of the Royal College of Physicians and its struggles, either internally or with its competition, is provided. Perhaps most significantly, the chapter does not consider competition in the medical marketplace from the irregular healers' point of view. There has been excellent work done on this subject, most notably by Roy Porter, Lucinda Beier, and Margaret Pelling, from whose work this chapter draws. They have established that the skill levels of other healers and their motivations varied and that they were an integral part of seventeenth-century health care.[15] The emphasis here will be on the physicians' reaction to competition by 'unlearned' healers, as this was ultimately helpful to the establishing of professional authority for physicians in that it forced them to hone their image of a godly physician: one that combined education and morality to offer a unique service.

Physicians faced difficulties professionalizing in part due to the manner in which early modern society viewed medicine. As has been discussed previously, there was an entrenched culture of self-treatment for ailments. Many people treated themselves when they became ill, and even if they enlisted professional help, they tended to be very opinionated about treatment options. Unlike lawyers and clergymen, physicians had to convince people to trust in (and pay for) a professional rather than rely on themselves or family members. They also had to compete with people who offered their services gratis to the poor and who treated the ill on a part-time basis. The challenge for physicians was to make the public (and other practitioners) see that medicine was best practiced by full-time, university-educated professionals, and to convince the public that this type of medical professional could offer them the best outcome. Therefore, the seventeenth century witnessed an attempt by physicians to close ranks against those who practiced medicine without the proper credentials, particularly empirics, clergymen practicing medicine, and women healers, both lay and professional.

The term 'empiric' covers a broad range of practitioners, from respected healers whose services formed a vital part of health care in seventeenth-century society to itinerant quacks whose nostrums promised to cure any ailment imaginable. Their most obvious characteristic was the lack of a formal university education in medicine. They were not licensed, and consequently those who practiced within the RCP's jurisdiction did so illegally. Henry VIII attempted to address the issue of irregular practitioners with an act that reflected the concern that:

> [Physic and Surgery] is daily within this Realm exercised by a great multitude of ignorant persons as common artificers, smiths, weavers and women who boldly and customably take upon them great cures and things of great difficulty in the which they partly use sorcery and witchcraft to the grievous hurt, damage, and destruction of many of the King's liege people.[16]

The act ordered that only graduates of the universities or persons licensed by the bishops, after careful examination by experts, would be permitted to practice physic or surgery. Although this act might have seemed to establish a monopoly, it proved one impossible to maintain. Legislation such as the Quack's Charter of 1542 recognized the dearth of licensed practitioners and allowed those with medical knowledge to alleviate the suffering of the multitude.[17] Consequently, there existed a tradition of supporting the idea of a medical monopoly, but of not actually enforcing one.

There has been much attention focused on the RCP's reaction to empirics. Yet for all the attempts to curtail the illicit practicing of medicine and selling of remedies, empirics flourished. The College simply lacked the power to force them out of existence or even to drive them underground.[18] Empirics proliferated in the rapidly growing commercial economy of the period. Frequently, the medicines they offered were commodities, sometimes even pre-packaged, brand-labeled, and sold throughout the realm for a set price.[19] Selling a single remedy to anyone went against the tenets of Galenic medicine espoused by the majority of physicians. One seventeenth-century physician argued that empirics were dangerous because their remedies were so popular with the public. He complained that empirics 'steal away the affections of the inconstant multitude, from the Learned Professors of that Faculty.'[20] By leading the populace away from the physician's remedies, empirics made the public suffer for their ignorance, as they 'stab to the heart their poor and silly patients, ere they be aware or once suspect such uncouth treachery.'[21] Warning against all-too popular empirics was a means by which physicians sought to protect naive patients.

Physicians used the threat to the public's health to object to non-for-mally educated healers who lacked the wisdom necessary to provide proper care and the morality to be trusted with the gullible and capricious public. Physicians had scant faith in the wisdom and the integrity of irregular healers: 'But our Empirics and Imposters, as they are too ignorant either to teach or to practice Physic…and too insolent, and too arrogant…to be reduced into order: so are they the most dangerous and pernicious unto the Weale public.'[22] In the eyes of physicians, the public was perhaps the only group more ignorant than empirics, as they were depicted in physicians' writing as easily duped by lofty promises and incapable of differentiating between solid medical advice and outright quackery. As the physician and author of *The Tomb of Venus* lamented, the public all too often believed the 'usual practice of boasting Empiricks' who attempted to 'ruin the Reputation of others, to endeavour the building up of their own.' It was exceedingly difficult for the public to discern between 'the real Physician and the Pretender' when 'even the most ignorant of Quacks' claimed skill in healing.[23] It was therefore imperative that empirics not be allowed to practice medicine, as the public could not be trusted to know better than to succumb to their promises, thereby risking great damage to their 'Purse' and 'Persons.'[24]

Perhaps the most thorough description of the way physicians viewed empirics was encapsulated in the anonymous 1676 publication, *The Character of a quack doctor*, which described in great detail a quack's unsavory characteristics:

> To trace his *Pedigree*, is to rake a *Dunghil*, and write the *Genealogy* of *Mushrooms* for his *Birth* is (commonly) as wretched as his *Breeding*, both being below *Mechanick*, not to be found, but amongst the *Feeces* of the *Bedraggled Rabble*; yet he might have Liv'd well at his *Primitive Handicraft*, but Extravagance put him upon shifts, & *Idleness* made him Abandon his *Anvil* or his *Loom*, his *Aul* or his *Thimble*, & pitch upon this safe and *Thriveing* course of *Pocket-Picking*, no *Jiltor, Legerdemain*, being now a days so Effectual as a *Catholick Pill* or *Universal* Potion…His prime care, and greatest trouble, is to get the *Names* of Diseases *Without Book*, & a Beadrole of Ratling *Terms* of Art, which he desires only to *Remember*, not *Understand*, so that he has more *Hard words* than a *Juggler*, and uses them to the same Purpose, to *amuse* and beguile the Ignorant or unwary, first of their *Wit*, and next of their *Mony*.[25]

The main objections to unlearned healers were all accounted for in *The Character of a quack doctor*. They were ill-bred (a preoccupation with status-anxious physicians that will be discussed later in this chapter), they were lazy and therefore looking to make quick money the easy way, and they preferred to feign knowledge rather than acquire it, which due to their ignorant nature would have no doubt proved a futile undertaking regardless.

The above tract was subtitled 'The Abusive practices of *impudent* illiterate pretenders to physick exposed,' a telling choice in that impudence was a trait frequently associated with quacks and thought to be a sign of their lack of knowledge of the art of physic. The journalist New Ward included impudence when delineating the character of a quack. Such people were 'A Shame to Art, to Learning, and to Sense / A Foe to Virtue, Friend to Impudence, / Wanting in Nature's Gift and Heaven's Grace, / An Object Scandalous to the Human Race.'[26] Impudence reflected not only a lack of judgment, but of morality as well, a point lamented by John Cotta:

> This scum and off-scouring of people, without conscience and honesty…being withal conscious to themselves of their own insufficiency, and ignorant of the signs, causes, and consequently of the right cure of disease, to the attaining of which the most learned Physicians bestow no small labour and pains.[27]

Quacks represented for Galenic physicians everything they were not.[28] Empirics of all kinds therefore became essential negative examples for physicians, helping orthodox physicians develop a strong sense of professional ethics and a clearer idea of how their offering diverged from that of their competitors. It was against empirics that physicians would define who they were, a definition of contrasts that physicians hoped would cement in the public's mind the difference between the wisdom and integrity of the learned physician versus the fraudulent antics and ignorance of empirics.

Clergymen aided physicians in denouncing the dangers of irregular healers. Ministers appreciated the potential danger of unlearned and unskillful pretenders to the practice of medicine because it related to similar threats they faced from unqualified clerics in religion. In 1667, the minister George Castle lamented that quackery was rampant in medicine and religion, and that ignorance 'is become as necessary a qualification for the profession of *Physick*, as it us'd to be for *Preaching*.'[29] Both the physician and minister had to be ever vigilant of intruding quacks who might distract people from the true professionals, ordained by God to perform either physical or spiritual healing. Such people would 'pretend at a two-penny charge to give professional balsams for all wounds; and for as much more to cure I know not how many desperate diseases.' Yet their unfortunate customers would soon come to realize that they could receive no help from such people, so they 'begin to ask after the method of the great Physitian, and to enquire what God would have them do, that they may be healed.'[30] There was sympathy between the two professions, as both practitioners were educated and saw themselves performing both a religious duty and a public service in their vocations. Further adding to the connection was the mixing of the two professions that had traditionally taken place. The correlation between the clergyman and the physician was logical and long-standing, as pastoral care and physic were complementary activities that clergymen had combined for centuries.[31] Historians have noted that clergymen frequently slipped into the role of healer, either to supplement their income or as an act of charity when no alternative was available.[32]

Clergymen-physicians were not rarities in the seventeenth century.[33] In a sermon in 1608, George Downame described the ideal pastor as one meant 'to instruct the ignorant, to reduce the erroneous, to heal the diseased, [and] to admonish the disorderly.'[34] For some, the decision to preach and practice medicine was a voluntary one. Others claimed it arose from necessity. The dissenting minister Richard Baxter noted in the late seventeenth century that he had been 'forced by the Peoples Necessity to practice Physick…no Physician being near,'[35] a notion seconded by Edmund Gayton who argued that a physician and a Divine were 'not inconsistent,' as 'the late times made many Preachers Physicians.'[36] The preacher Hugh Smythson justified his publication of *The Compleat Family Physician* on the grounds that 'in the remoter provinces of the kingdom of Great Britain (and indeed, in every part of it, except the metropolis and its environs) medical assistance is placed at such a distance from the major part of the inhabitants, and the expense of obtaining it is so considerable' that self-medication was the only preservative of health.[37] His publication was therefore filling a gap in medical care that physicians were not able or willing to fill.

Many seventeenth-century physicians did not approve of clerics like Smythson dipping into the medicinal arts. As early as 1612, the practice of combining professions in the church and in medicine drew criticism from members of the medical profession. John Cotta denounced 'beneficed practicers' in his treatise *Ignorant Practisers of Physicke*. Cotta adopted the argument of 'one calling,' which he claimed was taken from the Christian view propounded by St. Paul. He repeatedly used religious arguments to support his charges: 'it is manifest, that this fluctuation of these men between two callings is offensive to God, scandalous unto religion and good men, and injurous unto commonweales, and but presumption borrowing the face of Divinitie.'[38] Physicians were interested in establishing clear lines of demarcation between the two professions. This issue was taken up by the Royal College of Physicians in 1623, when that group complained to the upper house of convocation about clergy practicing medicine. The archbishop's response was that clergy would be prohibited from practicing physic except in their own parishes and for charitable purposes only.[39] However, the practice continued. Enforcement was an issue, as was a dearth of qualified medical practitioners, particularly those interested in caring for the rural poor.

One major motivation for separating the two professions was for physicians to protect themselves from competition for fee-paying patients, as the issue seemed to turn on whether 'beneficed practitioners' accepted payment for their healing. For example, Cotta had no objection to divines who gave medical assistance to the sick poor out of charity. He was concerned with those who charged for their services, thereby depriving 'the more worthy of his fee.'[40] Physicians' concern with their fees was acknowledged by the Anglican priest George Herbert, when he advised parsons to be familiar with at least one book of physic and one herbal, but then explicitly warned them to be careful not to divest others of their profession.[41]

However, as the seventeenth century progressed, physicians increasingly objected to the mixing of professions under any circumstances, even treating the poor gratis. If medicine was to be a respectable profession, it had to be a distinct profession, as argued by the physician James Hart in *Arraignment of Urines*:

> Is it not apparent that many of our Parsons and Vicars…have like usurpers intruded upon other mens right? Now that the preaching of the word…and practising of Physicke are in the word of God two seuerall distinct callings I thinke cannot be denied. And in the second place…whosoever will consciensably performe the worke of the ministry as he ought, shall therein finde worke enough without meddling in the health of the body.[42]

Hart delineates several points in support of his argument, accusing clergy-men of usurping the rights of physicians, claiming biblical reference to the distinction of the two professions, and suggesting that if clerics looked prop-erly after their flocks, they would have no time to meddle in medical matters.

Physicians even used Christian doctrine to bolster their argument against clergymen practicing medicine. Calvin taught that the age of miracles lay in the past, and learned physicians interpreted this to mean that lay healers could no longer claim to have divinely given powers. In addition, clergymen should not practice medicine since the age of miraculous curing had passed. John Cotta asserted: 'I know the gift of healing in the Apostles as the gift of God in his grace and speciall favour and allowance unto them for those times; but it was in them a miraculous and divine power consecrated unto a holy end: but in these times it is an acquired faculty.'[43] Cotta's point was that while the two professions may have mixed in the past, such intermingling was no longer permissible.[44]

Attempts by the Royal College of Physicians to disengage clerics from the practice of medicine began in the mid-sixteenth century when the College denied anyone in holy orders admission to its Fellowships.[45] In 1601, this ban was extended to licentiates as well, and it was under this pretext that the College prosecuted two well-known Puritan ministers, Dr. John Burgess and Dr. Alexander Leighton, for practicing medicine within the confines of London. Another Puritan physician, Dr. Edmund Wilson, was forced to forego ordination as a canon of Windsor for a similar reason, in order to become a Fellow of the College.[46] The RCP deemed a disassociation from the clergy necessary in order to gain ground in their struggle for respectability, accep-tance, and social status.[47] It is somewhat ironic, however, that measures to shed their 'clerical odour' coincided with physicians' embracing of the link between physical and spiritual healing so articulately and frequently demar-cated in religious sermons, which they hoped might convince the public of their moral respectability and thereby help shed the profession's 'odour of impiety.'

Attempts by physicians to close ranks become clearer when viewed against the backdrop of anxieties about the status of the medical profes-sion. Depicting the Royal College of Physicians as a small, aggressive group, jealously guarding its privileges from all competitors is not an inaccurate portrayal, yet such a representation yields little understanding of the deeper motives, aside from jealousy and greed, at work. In fact, there were underly-ing reasons for the College to force physicians to choose medicine as their sole profession or to abandon it altogether. While this principle of exclusivity or total dedication to one's career is assumed in our modern conception of professionalism, William Birken has pointed out that it was not assumed in the seventeenth century, and by taking such a stand, the College was quite consciously innovating.[48] They were motivated to agitate for exclusivity to one career by the struggle to gain in status and professionalism that stemmed from acute issues of low social standing.[49]

Past historiography has assumed the physician was drawn from the upper echelons of society, as illustrated in 1951 by Bernice Hamilton's observation that 'In 1660 a physician was a gentleman, while apothecaries and surgeons were mere craftsmen.'[50] Wallace Notestein similarly observed that 'The long training required meant that recruits to medicine came largely from the well-to-do classes.'[51] James Axtell suggested that the physician in Stuart England was 'a gentleman by education, by profession, and usually by birth.'[52] Yet recent research has called into question the gentlemanly status of the early modern physician. William Birken has conducted extensive research of the ledgers of medical schools to determine the social standing of seventeenth-century physicians. He has concluded that the medical profession drew its members primarily from the middle ranks of English society, adding that if there was a 'gentleman's profession' in the seventeenth century, a true offshoot of the gentry, it was law, rather than medicine. He has noted that the average Fellow of the College of Physicians in the early seventeenth century was not likely to be the younger son of a gentleman but rather the eldest son of a plebian or clerical family, eager to advance the family fortune and social status through the vehicle of the medical profession.[53]

Birken has asserted that throughout the seventeenth century the social acceptance and status of the physician was lower than previously assumed by historians.[54] The following letter convincingly illustrates the depth of this status issue. In 1656 John Stuteville advised Sir Justinian Isham not to allow a marriage to take place between his daughter and the son of one of the most prominent and wealthiest physicians in England, Dr. Lawrence Wright:

> In these degenerating times, the gentry had need to close nearer together, and make a banke and bulwarke against that Sea of Democracy which is over running them: and to keep their descents pure and untainted from that mungrill breed, which would faigne mixe with them.

The 'mungrill breed' to which Stuteville referred was the physician. Stuteville was clear in his view of the low status of the mid-seventeenth-century physician:

> I know a Gentleman related to your Selfe, but a younger Brother and every way farre your inferior, who was offred a very considerable fortune with a wife, beyond either his desert or expectation: yet because it was with a Physitian's daughter, the very thought of ye Blister-pipes did Nauseate his Stomacke. And great is the discourse at this very time about a Norfolk Baronets matching with a Doctor of Divinities daughter in Cambridge, and yet we know Divinitie is the highest, as Physicke is the lowest of Professions.[55]

What could account for such a negative perception of the physician? Why might medicine compare so unfavorably with the other two learned professions, divinity and law?

One of the main differences between the status of a lawyer or a cleric and a physician arose from the gender associations of both the work carried out by medical practitioners and their social relationships. Issues of gender intensified the anxiety physicians felt about their social status, in particular, their intimacy with bodily functions and their healing work that was associated in the mind of the public with labour traditionally carried out by women.[56] The form of competition in which issues of gender and status became the most acute was undoubtedly that of the female healer, particularly the midwife.

While all seventeenth-century physicians had reason to feel insecure about their professional status, this was particularly true for those who worked, and sought to work, in obstetrics. As early as the seventeenth century, physicians became interested in assuming an increasingly significant role in the lucrative field of childbirth.[57] Yet obstetrics was a field fraught with challenges to a fledgling profession already struggling with issues of professionalism and status. They faced an uphill battle in gaining the acceptance of women, as the ceremony of childbirth had traditionally been a social construct developed and maintained by women.[58] Midwives had typically handled all normal births. Male practitioners were summoned only when there was a difficulty with the birth, for example to perform a craniotomy in the case of obstructed births by the head, in order to extract a dead child and save the life of the mother.[59] When male practitioners became interested in delivering babies, they found themselves in the unenviable position of being in direct competition with a group of women, and a group who were firmly entrenched at that. Making matters worse, the midwife's role was linked to more traditional female healing and often included performing household tasks during labor and sometimes after delivery.[60] Physicians who wished to deliver babies were loath to have their expertise compared to women who cooked and cleaned as part of their usual services.

In light of such unfortunate associations, physicians found it impossible to envision entering the field of childbirth as peers of midwives. This attitude accounts for their refusal to regulate midwives. In the early seventeenth century, the Church subjected midwives to a system of licensing in order to assure that they were properly skilled in their craft. However, enforcement of licensing varied greatly from one community to the next, so the Church's efforts were not very successful in establishing uniform standards for the profession.[61] Such a disparity in skill level was detrimental to the profession of midwifery. In 1616 several midwives, with the help of Peter Chamberlen, petitioned the king and Parliament for the incorporation of a midwives' company that would be responsible for the training and licensing of midwives. The Royal College of Physicians blocked the effort, giving the following reason: '[the RCP] think it neither necessary nor convenient that they [the midwives] should be made a Corporation to govern within themselves, a thing not exampled in any Commonwealth.'[62] Two more schemes for licensing and training midwives were attempted during the seventeenth century; neither was successful. Lucinda Beier has contended that rather than offering them training, the physicians and surgeons attempted to drive midwives and other unlearned healers from medical practice altogether.[63] Regulation would have yielded midwives a certain legitimacy that physicians did not wish to see in any healers but themselves. Physicians were much more interested in distancing themselves from uneducated women. While the Royal College of Physicians sought to control the activities of midwives, they had no intention of enhancing their status by regulating them in any sort of formal manner.[64]

Women who cared for the sick out of charity proved an equally difficult issue for physicians. Like midwives, they were performing duties that women had always assumed. As much as physicians would have preferred to ban all unlicensed competitors from practicing medicine, this was not practical. What they settled upon, albeit uneasily, was deriding female healers in general while simultaneously acknowledging their necessity to a pool of patients whose needs could never be served by the tiny minority of learned physi-

91

cians. When Richard Banister wrote his treatise on diseases of the eye, he criticized women healers in general but made an exception for gentlewomen who treated the poor 'not for gain,' as their charitable relief of the poor was a necessity. He singled out one woman in particular, Lady Grace Mildmay, because 'her cures were attended with due care, and ended with true charity.' Curing gratis helped win approval from Dr. Banister, as did her good judgment to know her limitations: 'In cases of physic, she would use the approbations of a physician; in surgery, the aid of a surgeon and for the eyes, the assistance of myself.'[65] As Dr. Banister's compliment toward Lady Mildmay demonstrates, women who cared for the poor out of charity were permissible, provided they were aware of their limitations and deferred to physicians whenever possible. Good judgment in this case was not the result of a university education but instead was reflected in Lady Mildmay's understanding of her limitations and her willingness to consult a more learned healer.

A similar logic was outlined in the 1697 book *The Character of a Good Woman*. A good woman 'distributes among the indigent, money and books, and clothes and physick, as their several circumstances may require.' She should help 'her poor neighbor in sudden distress, when a doctor is not around, or when they have no money to buy what may be necessary for them.' The actions of good women were approved by God who 'gives a *peculiar blessing* to the practice of those women,' but the text was specific in stressing that the women's motives must be pure and their ministrations limited to physician-approved remedies. They must

> have no other design in this matter, but the doing good: that neither prescribe where they may have the advice of the learned, nor at any time give or recommend any thing to try experiments, but what they are assured from former trials is safe and innocent; and if they do not help cannot hurt.[66]

The author is adamant that women should not innovate or in any way presume to perform the higher functions of a physician. Once again, the line of demarcation is clearly drawn between charity and work that could compete with livelihood of the physician. John Tanner professed to write in order 'To help Ladies and gentlewomen who are [able] to help their poor sick neighbours' with their ailments, so that 'all women may the better understand the Physitians Directions and with more prudence govern the sick.'[67] Even when healing was an act of charity, women still required the guidance and tutelage of physicians.[68]

Due to the risk involved in relying on the care of female healers, their patient pool should be restricted to the poor who had no other healthcare options. Furthermore, women should never be so bold as to offer their services in competition with male medical practitioners, thereby claiming them to be of equivalent skill, a point made in verse in James Primrose's *Popular Errours*: 'Loe here a *woman* comes in *charitie* / To see the *sicke*, and brings her *remedie*.' She boasted that her remedies, 'Will doe more good, and is of more desert, / Then all *Hippocrates*, or *Galens* Art.' But her audacity was soon checked by a higher power:

> But Loe, an *Angell* gently puts her backe,
> Lest such *erroneous* course the sicke doe wracke,
> Leads the *Physitian*, and guides his hand,
> Approves his *Art*, and what he doth must stand.
> Tis *Art* that God allowes, by him 'tis blest
> To cure diseases, leave then all the rest.[69]

The poem appeared opposite the title page in Primrose's book, a work whose expressed purpose was to correct the 'errours of the people in physick,' in this case the near hubris of a female healer to claim expertise in a field divinely ordained for physicians alone. As these examples suggest, physicians generally accepted the traditional charitable role of women in health care, as long as women's ministrations did not impact physicians' pocket books, and as long as physicians reserved the right to condemn women as uneducated, inferior, and dangerous, despite their best intentions.[70]

In spite of their efforts, physicians were not particularly successful in discouraging competition from women practicing the healing arts. Female healers remained a staple of healthcare in seventeenth-century England, causing the male practitioner Samual Purchas to lament, 'How many old Women preferred before their greatest Doctor?'[71] The clergy proved equally recalcitrant. William Birken concluded that keeping the two professions separate in the seventeenth century must have been a very real and constant problem for the Fellows of the College of Physicians of London, as there was not much the College could do to discourage the simultaneous practice of medicine and ministry beyond its borders in London. As a result, dual practice flourished in the rest of country.[72] Empirics were similarly ubiquitous, as noted by the frustrated physician James Young: 'I believe there are more strowling Quacks in this Nation than in all Europe besides, who have nothing to recommend them but their Impudence.'[73] The variety and disparate skill level of those offering medical services illustrates that the practice of medicine as a sole profession was anything but a forgone conclusion in the seventeenth century.

While it is clear that physicians were not particularly successful in keeping others from practicing medicine, too much emphasis should not be placed on the lack of progress physicians made in the seventeenth century. Physicians were pitting themselves against groups who were firmly entrenched in the culture of healing and who would not be displaced easily, in part because they were filling a necessary void in health care due to the dearth of licensed healers, particularly outside of London. Although physicians would have liked to be viewed as the preeminent medical practitioner, it is quite possible that even they realized this vision of medicine as practiced exclusively by university-educated physicians was not particularly practical in the seventeenth century. By objecting to other healers, physicians were more clearly defining their own offerings as unique and valuable, a not altogether fruitless enterprise. Despite the uphill battles of circumscribing competing groups who had long established themselves in the practice of healing, the College of Physicians remained dedicated to the exclusive advancement of their own profession. They felt the need to differentiate themselves from these groups because allowing clergy members (or anyone else) to engage in medicine as a secondary undertaking devalued medicine as a full-time profession. Being forced to compete with uneducated women similarly threatened the sense of professionalism that physicians were aiming to capture, as did competition with empirics who had no formal education yet professed to be able to cure almost any ailment. Their objection to these groups ultimately aided the profession in that it prompted them to articulate their vision of a professional physician. The superior medical practitioner healed both body and soul. The ability to do so was predicated upon a consideration of learning and morality. The acquisition of these traits lay far beyond the reach of amateurs.

Historians studying the history of medicine have often cited the eighteenth century as a watershed in the rise of medicine as a profession. They have gone so far as to argue that there really was no organized medical profession prior to the eighteenth century. Rather, pre-eighteenth century medicine was defined by traditional healing, which included a hodge-podge of healers, some licensed, some not, some competent, some quacks.[74] There is much truth in these statements, yet the complexity of seventeenth-century healing and the inroads made by medical men to organize and define their profession should also be considered. The attempts to professionalize were there, however inchoate they may appear to modern observers. Physicians considered their medical treatment to be dramatically different from their competition, in spite of the fact that their remedies were not necessarily drastically different from those of lay healers or empirics. They marketed their learning, which provided them not only with skill, but also with sound moral judgment necessary to provide a life regimen crucial for a patient's overall health. This they contrasted with their competitors, whom they presented as lacking in both learning and judgment.

The need to distinguish themselves from their competition stemmed from physicians' motivation to carve a niche for themselves in a crowded field. Additionally, issues of status and gender made it unacceptable for them to be compared to those who did not receive the same education, a necessary step in order to elevate their status and authority. Particularly in the realm of childbirth, where midwives were associated with domestic duties, such issues became critical, as lamented by one seventeenth-century physician: 'For in all times, in the opinion of the multitude, witches and old women and impostors have had a competition with physicians.'[75] Competition, particularly by women, forced physicians to make a pedigree for themselves that involved their education and morality.

It was crucial that physicians honed their self-image in the seventeenth century. As the next chapter will demonstrate, the way in which medicine was marketed and delivered was beginning to change, and the profession of medicine would have to change as well. The struggle against their competition would prove to be a critical one in their development of authority and status in that it spurred the medical profession to construct new images of medical authority: not just as purveying remedies, but as creating the realm of reputable knowledge.

Notes

1   J. Young, *Medicaster Medicatus, or a Remedy for the Itch of Scribling* (1685), 2.
2   Cited in D. Nagy, *Popular Medicine in Seventeenth-Century England* (Bowling Green: Bowling Green State University Popular Press, 1988), 42.

3   See M. Pelling, 'Irregular Practitioners: A Wilderness of Mirrors,' in M. Pelling (ed.), *Medical Conflicts in Early Modern London: Patronage, Physicians, and Irregular Practitioners, 1550-1640* (Oxford: Clarendon Press, 2003), 68.

4   On lay perceptions of medicine, see R. Porter, 'The Patient's View: Doing Medical History from Below,' *Theory and Society* 14, no. 2 (1985); M. Pelling, 'Medical Practice in Early Modern England: Trade or Profession?' in W. Prest (ed.), *The Professions in Early Modern England* (London: Croom Helm, 1987); and L. Beier, 'In Sickness and in Health: A Seventeenth Century Family's Experience,' in R. Porter (ed.), *Patients and Practitioners: Lay Perceptions of Medicine in Pre-Industrial Society* (Cambridge: Cambridge University Press, 1985).

5   H. Cook, 'Good Advice and Little Medicine: The Professional Authority of Early Modern English Physicians,' *The Journal of British Studies* 33, no. 1 (January 1994), 4-5.

6   H. Cook, 'Good Advice and Little Medicine: The Professional Authority of Early Modern English Physicians,' 1-2.

7   See for example H. Vollmer and D. Mills (eds.), *Professionalization* (Englewood Cliffs, New Jersey: Prentice Hall, 1966); T.J. Johnson, *Profession and Power* (London: Macmillan, 1972); and E. Freidson, *Professional Powers: A Study of the Institutionalization of Formal Knowledge* (Chicago: University of Chicago Press, 1986).

8   M. Pelling, *Medical Conflicts in Early Modern London: Patronage, Physicians, and Irregular Practitioners, 1550-1640* (Oxford: Clarendon Press, 2003),7

9   M. Pelling, *Medical Conflicts in Early Modern London: Patronage, Physicians, and Irregular Practitioners,* 23-24, 7.

10 H. Cook, 'Good Advice and Little Medicine: The Professional Authority of Early Modern English Physicians,' 2, 4.

11 Other significant studies focusing on the professionalization of medicine include E. Freidson, *Profession of Medicine: A Study of the Sociology of Applied Knowledge* (New York: Dodd, Mead & Co., 1974); J. Berlant, *Profession and Monopoly: A Study of Medicine in the United States and Great Britain* (Berkeley: University of California Press, 1975); and N. Parry and J. Parry, *The Rise of the Medical Profession: A Study of Collective Social Mobility* (London: Croom Helm, 1976).

12 H. Cook, 'Good Advice and Little Medicine: The Professional Authority of Early Modern English Physicians,' 4-5.

13 For some examples see W.J. Birkin, 'The Royal College of Physicians of London and Its Support of the Parliamentary Cause in the English

Civil War,' *The Journal of British Studies* 23, no. 1 (1983); M. Pelling, 'Irregular Practitioners: A Wilderness of Mirrors'; and R. Porter, *Health for Sale: Quackery in England 1660-1850* (Manchester: Manchester University Press, 1989). Even historians who paint the RCP in a favourable light allude to this. See R.S. Roberts, 'The Royal College of Physicians of London in the Sixteenth and Seventeenth Centuries,' *History of Science* 5 (1966) and Sir G. Clark, *History of the Royal College of Physicians of London* (Oxford: Clarendon Press, 1964).

14 M. Pelling, 'Thoroughly Resented? Older Women and the Medical Role in Early Modern London,' in L. Hunter and S. Hutton (eds), *Women, Science and Medicine 1500-1700* (Gloucestershire: Sutton Publishing, 1997), 68.

15 R. Porter, 'The Patient's View: Doing Medical History from Below,' R. Porter, *Health for Sale: Quackery in England 1660-1850*, R. Porter, 'The Patient in England, C. 1660-C.1800,' in A. Wear (ed.), *Medicine in Society* (New York: Cambridge University Press, 1992); L. Beier, *Sufferers and Healers: The Experience of Illness in Seventeenth-Century England* (New York: Routledge, 1987); M. Pelling, 'Irregular Practitioners: A Wilderness of Mirrors'; and M. Pelling, *Medical Conflicts in Early Modern London: Patronage, Physicians, and Irregular Practitioners, 1550-1640*.

16 Statutes of the Realm, 3 Henry VIII, Ch. 11. Cited in R. O'Day, *The Professions in Early Modern England, 1450-1800* (New York: Pearson, 2000), 192.

17 R. O'Day, *The Professions in Early Modern England*, 193, 196. The Quack's Charter, 34 & 35 Henry VIII, c. 8.

18 R. Porter, *Health for Sale: Quackery in England 1660-1850* (Manchester: Manchester University Press, 1989), 187.

19 H. Cook, 'Good Advice and Little Medicine: The Professional Authority of Early Modern English Physicians,' 5.

20 J. Oberndoerffer, *The Anatomies of the True Physician and Counterfeit Mountebank,* trans. Francis Herring (1602), preface. See also Joseph Cam's similar complaint in the eighteenth century that empirics endear themselves to the public, who 'pass Judgment by the Force of their Affections, and not their Judging Faculty,' J. Cam, *A Rational and Useful Account of the Venereal Disease: With Observations on the Nature, Symptoms, and Cure, and the Bad Consequences That Attend by Ill Management* (1740), 16.

21 J. Cam, *A Rational and Useful Account of the Venereal Disease: With Observations on the Nature, Symptoms, and Cure, and the Bad Consequences That*

Attend by Ill Management (1740), 16.

22 J. Oberndoerffer, *The Anatomies of the True Physician and Counterfeit Moun-tebank*, trans. Francis Herring (1602), preface.

23 Anon., *The Tomb of Venus* (1710), preface.

24 J. Archer, *Secrets Disclosed, or, a Treatise of Consumptions; Their Various Causes and Cure* (1693), 26.

25 Anon., *The Character of a Quack Doctor, or, the Abusive Practices of Impudent Illiterate Pretenders to Physick Exposed* (1676), 1-2.

26 R.Porter, *Health for Sale: Quackery in England 1660-1850*, 5.

27 J. Cotta, *A Short Discouerie of Seuerall Sorts of Ignorant and Vnconsiderate Practisers of Physicke in England with Direction for the Safest Election of a Physition in Necessitie* (1619), 45-6.

28 A.K. Lingo, 'Empirics and Charlatans in Early Modern France: The Genesis of the Classification of the "Other" in Medical Practice,' *Jour-nal of Social History,* Vol. 19, No. 4 (Summer 1986), 591-2.

29 Cited in M. Jenner, 'Quackery and Enthusiasm, or Why Drinking Water Cured the Plague,' in A. Cunningham and O.P. Grell (eds), *Religio Medici: Medicine and Religion in Seventeenth-Century England* (Aldershot: Scolar Press, 1996), 329.

30 S. Patrick, *Jewish Hypocrisie, a Caveat to the Present Generation* (1660), 5.

31 M. MacDonald, 'Psychological Healing in England, 1600-1800' in W.J. Sheils (ed.), *The Church and Healing* (Oxford: Basil Blackwell, 1982).

32 D. Amundsen and R.L. Numbers (eds), *Caring and Curing: Health and Medicine in the Western Religious Traditions* (New York: Macmillan, 1986), 531 and D. Nagy, *Popular Medicine in Seventeenth-Century England*, 38-9. See also the study of the Quaker George Fox's fascination with medicine and how his understanding of disease was clearly related to the 'spiritual' character of his religion in P. Elmer, 'Medicine, Science and the Quakers; the "Puritanism-Science" Debate Reconsidered,' *The Journal of the Friends' Historical Society* 54, no. 6 (1981), especially 266-7, 268-9.

33 R. Anselment, *The Realms of Apollo: Literature and Healing in Seventeenth-Century England* (Newark: University of Delaware Press, 1995), 29. Anselment uses the examples of John Ward, Richard Baxter, and John Allin.

34 G. Downame, *Two Sermons, the One Commending the Ministrie in General: The Other Defending to Office of Bishops in Particular* (1608), 15-16 cited in N. Enssle, 'Patterns of Godly Life: The Ideal Parish Minister in

Sixteenth- and Seventeenth-Century English Thought,' *Sixteenth Century Journal* 28 (1997), 3.

35   Cited in A. Wear, 'Religious Beliefs and Medicine in Early Modern England,' in H. Marland and M. Pelling (eds), *The Task of Healing: Medicine, Religion and Gender in England and the Netherlands, 1450-1800* (Rotterdam: Erasmus Publishing, 1996), 98.

36   E. Gayton, *The Religion of a Physician: Or, Divine Meditations* (1663).

37   A. Wear, 'Religious Beliefs and Medicine in Early Modern England,' 98. See also L. Gatford, *Logos Alexipharmakos, or, Hyperphysicall Directions in Time of Plague. Collected out of the Sole-Authentick Dispensatory of the Chief Physitian Both of Soule and Body, and Disposed More Particularly (Though Not without Some Alteration and Addition) According to the Method of Those Physicall Directions Printed by Command of the Lords of the Councell at Oxford 1644. And Very Requisite to Be Used with Them. Also, Certain Aphorismes, Premised, and Conclusions from Them Deduced, Concerning the Plague, Necessary to Be Knovvn and Observed of All, That Would Either Prevent It, or Get It Cured* (1644).

38   J. Cotta, *A Short Discouerie of Seuerall Sorts of Ignorant and Vnconsiderate Practisers of Physicke in England with Direction for the Safest Election of a Physition in Necessitie* (1619).

39   R. O'Day, *The Professions in Early modern England*, 218.

40   J. Cotta, *A Short Discouerie of Seuerall Sorts of Ignorant and Vnconsiderate Practisers of Physicke in England with Direction for the Safest Election of a Physition in Necessitie*, 88, 89, 84, 87.

41   R. Anselment, *The Realms of Apollo: Literature and Healing in Seventeenth-Century England*, 39.

42   J. Hart, *Arraignment of Urines* (1623), A3-A4.

43   J. Cotta, *A Short Discouerie of Seuerall Sorts of Ignorant and Vnconsiderate Practisers of Physicke in England with Direction for the Safest Election of a Physition in Necessitie*, 88. Learned physicians also argued that the Christian doctrine on charitable care of the sick poor did not justify unlearned medical practice. See A. Wear, 'Religious Beliefs and Medicine in Early Modern England,' 141, 161.

44   For more primary source examples, see D. Nagy, *Popular Medicine in Seventeenth-Century England*, 39, 41 and A. Wear, 'Religious Beliefs and Medicine in Early Modern England,' 163-5.

45   W. Birken, 'The Social Problem of the English Physician in the Early Seventeenth Century,' *Medical History* 31 (April 1987), 207.

46 Sir G. Clark, *History of the Royal College of Physicians of London*, 97.

47 W. Birken, 'The Social Problem of the English Physician in the Early Seventeenth Century,' 208, 204.

48 W. Birkin, 'The Royal College of Physicians of London and Its Support of the Parliamentary Cause in the English Civil War,' 53.

49 For discussions on the status of medical men, see Sir G. Clark, *History of the Royal College of Physicians of London;* M. Pelling, 'Medical Practice in Early Modern England: Trade or Profession?'; and W. Birken, 'The Social Problem of the English Physician in the Early Seventeenth Century.'

50 B. Hamilton, 'The Medical Professions in the Eighteenth Century,' *The Economic History Review* IV, no. 2 (1951), 141.

51 W. Notestein, *The English People on the Eve of Colonization 1603-1630* (New York: Harper, 1954), 103. Cited in W. Birken, 'The Social Problem of the English Physician in the Early Seventeenth Century,' 202.

52 J. Axtell, 'Education and Status in Stuart England: The London Physicians,' *History of Education Quarterly* 10, no. 2 (Summer 1970), 148.

53 W. Birken, 'The Social Problem of the English Physician in the Early Seventeenth Century,' 206, 209. Birken found that of 71 civil lawyers admitted to the Doctors Commons between 1590 and 1641 who died after 1603, fully 35 were the sons of either gentlemen, esquires, or knights. Keith Wrightson uncovered similar findings relating to the status of lawyers: of all the entrants to the Inns of Court in the period 1610-39, some 90 per cent were sons of the aristocracy and gentry, with most of the rest being drawn from the highest ranks of trade and the professions. K. Wrightson, *English Society, 1580-1680* (London: Hutchinson, 1982), 189. Virtually non-existent among lawyers were the sons of clergymen, an element that Birken has found 'bulked so large in the composition of the Fellows of the College of Physicians, and physicians generally.' Of these 67 physicians who were Fellows of the College of Physicians, Birken uncovered the social origins of 57. Only 16 could have made any claims at all to gentle blood (and most of these minor gentry). Forty-one were of non-gentle, plebeian, or clerical origin. Within this group of 41, eldest sons predominated. (No less than 17 of those 41 came from clerical families). W. Birken, 'The Social Problem of the English Physician in the Early Seventeenth Century,' 204.

54 W. Birken, 'The Social Problem of the English Physician in the Early Seventeenth Century,' 210. There is also debate about how physicians' association with the clergy affected their status. James Axtell sees it

as positive for the profession, claiming that even before the medical profession had any sort of organization (prior to the seventeenth century) its members still had a substantial place in the social hierarchy due to its close association with the Church, which stood at the apex of society. J. Axtell, 'Education and Status in Stuart England: The London Physicians,' 141. However, William Birken views the association as negative for the profession, claiming that 'lower-class and clerical associations,' among other numerous factors, 'conspired to make the profession unattractive to the gentry and their sons.' W. Birken, 'The Social Problem of the English Physician in the Early Seventeenth Century,' 204.

55 Cited in W. Birken, 'The Social Problem of the English Physician in the Early Seventeenth Century.' In addition to William Birken, see M. Ashley, *Life in Stuart England* (London: Batsford, 1964), 50; C. Bridenbaugh, *Vexed and Troubled Englishmen 1590-1642* (London: Oxford University Press, 1976), 107; and R. Grassby, 'Social Mobility and Business Enterprise in Seventeenth-Century England,' in *Puritans and Revolutionaries*, ed. Donald Pennington (Oxford: Clarendon Press, 1982), 377.

56 M. Pelling, *Medical Conflicts in Early Modern London: Patronage, Physicians, and Irregular Practitioners, 1550-1640*, 14 and M. Pelling,'Compromised by Gender: The Role of the Male Medical Practitioner in Early Modern England' in H. Marland and M. Pelling (eds), *The Task of Healing: Medicine, Religion and Gender in England and the Netherlands 1450-1800* (Rotterdam: Erasmus Publishing, 1996).

57 For more on the traditions of childbearing and their effect on women's relationships with one another, see L. Pollock, 'Childbearing and Female Bonding in Early Modern England,' *Social History* 22, no. 3 (1997) and P. Crawford, 'The Construction and Experience of Maternity in Seventeenth-Century England,' in V. Fildes (ed.), *Women as Mothers in Pre-Industrial England. Essays in Memory of Dorothy Mclaren* (London: 1990).

58 For background on the traditional role of the midwife, see Linda Pollock, 'Embarking on a Rough Passage: The Experience of Pregnancy in Early-Modern Society,' in V. Fildes (ed.), *Women as Mothers in Pre-Industrial England. Essays in Memory of Dorothy Mclaren* (London: 1987); A. Clark, *The Working Life of Women in the Seventeenth Century* (London: Routledge and Paul, 1991); C. Bicks, 'Midwiving Virility in Early Modern England,' in N. Miller and N. Yavneh (eds), *Maternal Measures:*

Figuring Caregiving in the Early Modern Period (Burlington: Ashgate, 2000); and D. Evenden, 'Gender Differences in the Licensing and Practice of Female and Male Surgeons in Early Modern England,' *Medical History* 42 (1998).

59 See J. Towler and J. Bramall, *Midwives in History and Society* (London: Croom Helm, 1986) and H. Marland, *The Art of Midwifery. Early Modern Midwives in Europe* (London: Routledge, 1993).

60 L. Beier, *Sufferers and Healers: The Experience of Illness in Seventeenth-Century England*, 16.

61 This would only worsen in the next century. Despite increasing involvement of male practitioners in childbirth, the medical community refused to regulate the profession of midwifery throughout the eighteenth century, causing it to appear less and less reputable a profession to physicians and many members of the general public. See L. Beier, *Sufferers and Healers: The Experience of Illness in Seventeenth-Century England*, 16-8.

62 L. Beier, *Sufferers and Healers: The Experience of Illness in Seventeenth-Century England*, 17.

63 It was not until 1902 that midwives finally attained their own corporation. L. Beier, *Sufferers and Healers: The Experience of Illness in Seventeenth-Century England*, 19.

64 For examples of women specifically targeted by the college for practicing medicine without a license, see M. Pelling, 'Thoroughly Resented? Older Women and the Medical Role in Early Modern London,' and M. Pelling and C. Webster, 'Medical Practitioners,' in C. Webster (ed.), *Health, Medicine, and Mortality in the Sixteenth Century* (New York: Cambridge University Press, 1979).

65 R. Banister, *A Treatise of One Hundred and Thirteene Diseases of the Eye* (1622) cited in L. Pollock, *With Faith and Physic: The Life of a Tudor Gentlewoman, Lady Grace Mildmay, 1552-1620* (London: Collins and Brown, 1993), 109.

66 Anon., *Character of a Good Woman* (1697), 42-3.

67 J. Tanner, *The Hidden Treasures of the Art of Physicke: Fully Discovered in Four Books* (1658), To the Reader page.

68 See also the following, which discuss educating women as either healers or sufferers or both: L. Sowerby, *The Ladies Dispensatory Containing the Natures, Vertues and Qualities of All Herbs and Simples Usefull in Physick* (1651); *The Woman's Counsellor; or the Feminine Physitian*, trans. A. Massaria

(1657), 78; and R. Bunworth, *The Doctresse: A Plain and Easie Method of Curing Those Diseases Which Are Peculiar to Women* (1656).

69 J. Primrose, *Popular Errours. Or the Errours of the People in Physick* (1651).

70 D. Nagy, *Popular Medicine in Seventeenth-Century England*, 71.

71 P. Crawford, 'Attitudes to Menstruation in Seventeenth-Century England,' *Past and Present* 91 (1981), 69.

72 W. Birken, 'The Social Problem of the English Physician in the Early Seventeenth Century,' 204.

73 J. Young, *Medicaster Medicatus, or a Remedy for the Itch of Scribling* (1685), 94. This also accounts for physicians' criticism of quacks who boasted they could heal every ailment, as lampooned in the following ballad wherein a quack claimed he could cure anything—even poverty: 'All Sickness flies at his Approach, / Here, take his Pills—You'll keep your Coach…Come, here, who takes this little Box? / They'll cure both Poverty and Pox.' Anon., *The Quack Triumphant: Or, the N-R--Ch Cavalcade. A New Ballad* (1733).

74 See for example L. Beier, *Sufferers and Healers: The Experience of Illness in Seventeenth-Century England*, R. Porter and D. Porter, *In Sickness and in Health: The British Experience 1650-1850* (London: Fourth Estate, 1988) and D. Nagy, *Popular Medicine in Seventeenth-Century England*.

75 F. Bacon, *The Advancement of Learning* G.W. Kitchin.(ed.) (London: Everyman, 1965) in M. Pelling (ed.), 'Compromised by Gender: The Role of the Male Medical Practitioner in Early Modern England,' 101.

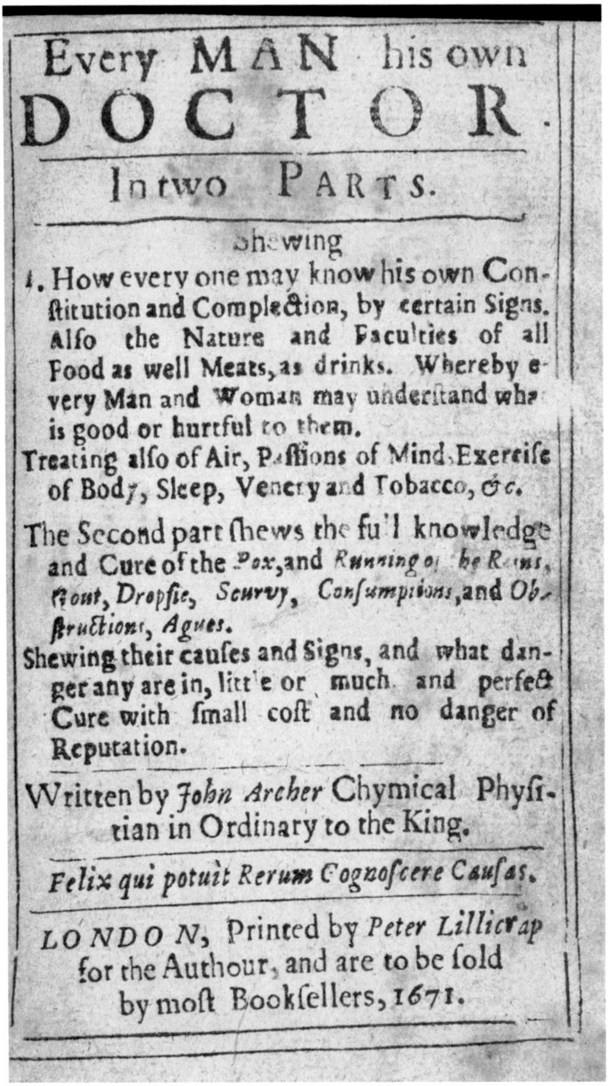

Every MAN his own

DOCTOR.

In two PARTS.

Shewing

1. How every one may know his own Constitution and Complection, by certain Signs.
Also the Nature and Faculties of all
Food as well Meats, as drinks. Whereby e-
very Man and Woman may underftand wha
is good or hurtful to them.

Treating also of Air, Paffions of Mind, Exercife
of Body, Sleep, Venery and Tobacco, &c.

The Second part fhews the full knowledge
and Cure of the Pox, and Running of he Reins,
Gout, Dropfie, Scurvy, Confumptions, and Ob-
ftructions, Agues.

Shewing their caufes and Signs, and what dan-
ger any are in, little or much and perfect
Cure with fmall coft and no danger of
Reputation.

Written by *John Archer* Chymical Phyfi-
tian in Ordinary to the King.

Felix qui potuit Rerum Cognofcere Caufas.

LONDON, Printed by *Peter Lillicrap*
for the Authour, and are to be fold
by moft Bookfellers, 1671.

Figure 8: Titlepage: Every man his own doctor
Courtesy Wellcome Library, London

4

'Every man his own doctor'[1]:
Physicians and the Printing Boom

Physicians' emphasis on the importance of their specialized knowledge, so crucial in differentiating themselves from their competition, was threatened by the increasing availability of printed medical works in English. Such works were often written by non-physicians whose aim was to disseminate basic medical knowledge to all readers. Worse still for physicians was the fact that the audience for such vernacular works was growing along with literacy, and writers were responding by using simple language so that everyone from an upper-class audience to the commonest reader had access to medical information.[2]

The increasing availability of medical publications in English was a potential problem for physicians, as these threatened both the value and mystique of the formal education upon which physicians differentiated themselves. Physicians were divided in their opinion about the appropriateness of publishing in the vernacular, particularly in the beginning of the century. Eventually, many physicians came to capitalize on the opportunities provided by the printing press and used it as a means of highlighting the deficiencies of their competitors and articulating their unique vision of health care.

The publications penned by physicians have been described by Lucinda Beier as a physician-led advertising campaign against irregular healers. Beier has argued that the medical profession launched a concerted and conscious effort to bolster their status through a campaign with a twofold aim: to create a favorable image for licensed healers and to destroy the reputation and practices of unlicensed healers.[3] William Eamon has made a similar suggestion but pointed out that physicians only learned the value of impugning their competition after being forced to defend themselves in print from the onslaught of empirics who attacked physicians first.[4] The antagonistic nature of physicians' writing, often defensive in tone and just as frequently offensively aggressive against their critics, needs to be placed in the context of a growing sense of professional calling and pride, one that Eamon has noted was felt not just in England, but throughout Europe.[5] This chapter draws upon these theories to demonstrate that publications in the vernacular by physicians were a crucial component in differentiating themselves in the public mind from other types of healers in order to bolster their status and to assume greater authority in public-health issues.

Physicians had reason to be wary of their place in a society in which medical knowledge was becoming more readily available to healers and patients alike, and in which learned counsel was being valued less in the emerging commercial world than empirical experience.[6] How then did the profession survive, and in the eighteenth century thrive? By publishing medical works in the vernacular, a practice to which many physicians were vehemently opposed earlier in the century, they were able to attack other types of healers while simultaneously establishing their credentials in the field of healthcare.

The flood of books that streamed from the presses began in the sixteenth century and by the seventeenth century had opened up a burgeoning market for self-help manuals in medicine, the crafts, and the domestic arts.[7] Competition now took on an entirely new dimension with the flourishing of the market for printed medical texts in English.[8] For centuries, anatomy had been the province of surgeons and physicians, trained to read and write in Latin, but publications in the vernacular threatened to change this.

The printing press provided a great opportunity for empirics to advertise their cures and to write health guides and medical treatises on any imaginable subject. In contrast with learned medical theory, works by empirics were accessible and practical. Rarely were the medical-theoretical underpinnings spelled out or disputed, because unlike physicians, empirics lacked motivation to establish intellectual authority over their patients or their competition.[9] Vernacular works also challenged the very type of care regimen advocated by physicians by giving remedies for specific ailments. Empirical publications generally did not concern themselves with the spiritual aspects of healing or with preventative medicine. They were focused on remedies for specific ailments. This was in stark opposition to what physicians envisioned as proper health care: instead of advocating sound advice on the ideal way to organize one's life and habits, such publications attempted to alter the conditions under which people lived through bad advice and powerful remedies.[10]

Vernacular works also challenged the exclusivity of medical knowledge by claiming the public had a right to medical information that learned practitioners were deliberately keeping from them:

106

How long would they [physicians] have people ignorant? Why grudge them physic to come forth in English? Would they have no man to know but only they? Or what made they themselves Merchants of our lives and deaths, that we should buy our health only of them, and at their prices?[11]

Such an argument was made repeatedly by empirics in their medical publications, of varying credibility, that purported to provide the reader with the information necessary to turn anyone into a physician.[12] The works are similar in that they were often written by non-physicians and were mainly comprised of 'kitchen physick.'[13] Their stated intention was usually to ease the afflictions of the poor and needy although their target audience was often gentlewomen and 'other such Persons, whose Stations requires their taking care of the House.'[14] Some overtly bypassed the physician, but most were more subtle, and instead attempted to sidestep physicians' objections by claiming to be of use when an 'able and honest Physician is not near at Hand' either because he was geographically out of reach or because the reader lacked the financial means to 'entertain a learned Physician.'[15] The authors of such tracts could legitimately make the argument that their publications were practical and provided a service for the public health by providing their information to those who could not employ a physician or for educational purposes intended for 'such Ladies and Gentlewomen, who of charity labour to doe good.'[16] Such arguments would prove difficult for physicians to refute.

In *Castel of Helthe*, Sir Thomas Elyot preemptively defended against criticism of publishing his work in the vernacular, citing historical precedent: 'But if Phisitions be angrye, that I have written phisicke in English, let them remember that the Greekes wrate in Greeke, ye Romanes in Latin…which were their owne proper and maternall tongues.'[17] He went on to charge that those who would restrain vernacular medical publications were greedier even than heathens of ancient times:

If they had bene as muche attached with envye and covetise, as somme nowe seeme to be, they would have devised some particular language, with a strange cipher or forme of letters, wherein they would have written their science…But those, although they were Paynims and Jewes, yet in this part of charity, they far surmounted us Christians, that they woulde not have so necessarye a knowledge as Physicke is, to be his from them."[18]

Providing medical information for the poor and those who charitably cared for them proved a popular justification for publishing in the vernacular, even by physicians. However, such publications also enabled anyone who had access to them to act as his or her own healer and thereby posed a threat to physicians.

Making matters worse, publications in the vernacular directly attacked traditional medicine and the manner in which physicians practiced it. Lucinda Beier has identified at least forty books published during the period 1500-1700 penned by medical empirics. She has argued that these texts comprised a legitimate cause for alarm for the medical establishment, as such writers maintained that classical medical education was virtually useless.[19] By claiming experience mattered more than formal education, the writers of vernacular medical works threatened to devalue Latin and thereby endangered the mystique of the physician along with it.[20] For instance, some writers were empirics who made a strong case against formal medical education. They maintained that in medical practice experience was more important than theory; consequently, extensive book learning was unnecessary. Some followed the lead of the popular sixteenth-century empirical writer, Leonardo Fioravanti, who claimed 'there is no science in the world wherewith a man may do good if therewith be no practice or experience, as a man may say. The which experience is master of all things, as it is plainly seen.'[21] The devaluing of Latin, and thereby of university education, constituted a key reason why physicians were so resistant to medical works published in the vernacular.

Vernacular publications were increasing at a time when medicine was already being accused of 'empty scholarship,' and empirical methods were gaining support. There was even debate within the profession regarding the value of a university education in the field of medicine. The leading promoter of the clinical method, Thomas Sydenham, was an outspoken advocate of apprenticeship for physicians, an idea that horrified university-educated physicians but made sense in light of new chemical remedies. Sydenham asserted that medicine was not to be learned by going to the universities, as 'one had as good send a man to Oxford to learn shoemaking as practicing physick.'[22]

The argument so often made in vernacular medical works that experience mattered more than formal education was used by a variety of competitors. Publications by seventeenth-century midwives used the premise that experience mattered more than formal learning to challenge directly the notion that male practitioners were better able to deliver babies than midwives. One such example is Jane Sharp's *The Midwives Book*, intended as a vernacular reference for midwives. She argued that although women could not hope to achieve the same level of learning as men (primarily because they did not have access to a formal education), they had 'natural propriety' on their side to practice the art, and they could further their knowledge through 'long and diligent practice' that might then be 'communicated to others of our own sex.' Sharp was critical of the notion that women who could not read Latin were therefore ignorant: 'It is not hard words that perform the work, as if none understood the Art that cannot understand Greek.' She derisively added:

> It is commendable for men to employ their spare time in some things of deeper speculation than is required of the female sex: but the art of midwifery chiefly concerns us, which even the best learned man will grant, yielding something of their own to us when they are forced to borrow from us the very name they practice by, and to call themselves man-midwives.[23]

For Sharp and many other midwives, the 'deeper speculation' of 'learned men' was not paramount to the art of midwifery. Women created the craft and indeed the name that male medical professionals were attempting to usurp.

A similar defense of the female midwife's skill in relation to the learned physician was echoed in the writing of the outspoken midwife Elizabeth Cellier. In her *A Letter to Dr.---*, Cellier stated that her purpose in writing the letter was to 'Deter any of you [physicians] from pretending to teach us the art of Midwifery, especially such as confess they never delivered Women in their lives.' She implied that men who would teach women midwifery yet lack practical experience in the field were going against the example set by Hippocrates, who swore, 'he will not cut those who have the Stone, but will leave it to the skilful in that Practice. But you, tho you understand nothing of it, pretend to teach us an Act much more difficult.'[24] Midwives, along with many other empirics, clearly valued experience and the expertise it afforded over the formal education that physicians were so fond of touting.

Printing in the vernacular posed a serious threat to learned medicine and the way it was practiced by physicians. Their formal learning was being devalued in favor of empirical methods. Physicians had reason to feel that their struggles to assume preeminence in the medical profession were threatened by this new way of disseminating medical knowledge to the public, which by making 'every man his own doctor,' (as at least one publication promised to do) threatened the entire manner in which medicine was practiced.[25] The dissemination of medical knowledge to the reading public arguably would pose the greatest challenge to the image of the godly physician and his conception of proper health care.

Early in the century, many physicians were at first vehemently opposed to printing in the vernacular. However, attitudes would slowly change, in part because many physicians came to realize they had no choice but to join in the wave of printing medical works in English. As they increasingly relied on the printing press to defend themselves against their critics, physicians discovered that they could also use the printing press as a propaganda weapon to demarcate the boundary between themselves and unlearned popular healers.[26] Physicians were therefore able to highlight the faults of unlearned healers and contrast their shortcomings with the qualities of the idealized, learned physician possessing good judgment and superior moral character, thereby dispersing the image of the godly physician to a wide and diverse audience.

The debate over publishing in English was a bitter one for physicians, as most were highly wary of eschewing their Latin for the vernacular, and by doing so making their medical knowledge more accessible to the public. For Dr. James Hart, the issue was clear cut: 'It may plainly appear that there can be no right use of such Bookes' as these 'might give the least encouragement to ignorant Droanes and Dunces, wherewith this Kingdome doth so abound.'[27] However, some physicians did advocate publishing medical works in the vernacular. One of the most boisterous supporters of the endeavor was the physician Nicholas Culpeper. Culpeper wrote numerous books aimed at disseminating medical knowledge to those who might be in a position to help the needy. In one of his tracts he outlined a method of physic in which 'a man may preserve his Body in Health; or cure himself, being sick, for three pence charge, with such things only as grow in England, they being most fit for English Bodies.'[28] He reasoned that books published in the mother tongue helped the poor and therefore did not hurt the medical professional, since 'the poor are but a trouble to him.' Books published in English, argued Culpeper, were actually beneficial to the public health because they provided medical knowledge to those other than physicians who might be of some assistance to the needy, as there were 'Industrious men that know no more Languages than their Native one, who may in a rational way contribute to the Necessities of the poor.' Furthermore, vernacular medical books led the rich to 'crave the Advice and Assistance of the Learned Physitian,' after seeing 'what a world of Considerations Cautions do belong to the knowledge and orderly cure of every Disease.' They therefore aided the physician by prompting the potential patient to 'be more fearful than ever he was before to commit himself to the Cure of any but a learned Physitian.'[29] Since Culpeper argued that there was no harm to the rich patient base through which the learned physician made his living, there should be no objection to disseminating medical knowledge to the public. Yet he lamented the opposition he encountered to such radical notions, as 'some men are so damnable proud and envious withal, that they would have no body know any thing but themselves.'[30] Hoarding medical knowledge, according to Culpeper, went against the nature of the art of physic, through which physicians were meant to glorify God (and themselves) through their medical knowledge and do good to their neighbors by alleviating their infirmities.[31]

Culpeper's ideas were not well received within the medical community. James Axtell has noted that the tenacity with which physicians clung to their Latin was evidenced by the vehemence directed towards physicians such as Nicholas Culpeper who translated Latin medical texts into English. Culpeper was accused of being a 'foul-mouth'd impudent scribler,' and the backlash against him was tremendous.[32] The backlash, however, was mostly published in English, an irony that suggests the issue was for the most part already decided. The debate was then recast by physicians as a struggle between learned, approved English works such as their own and the regrettable scribblings of unqualified and dangerous quacks.[33] Physicians justified their joining in the publication of medical works in English on the grounds that they were obligated to do so in order to combat the incorrect and dangerous information so readily available to a naïve public who were too eager to believe all that they read. In the physician J.S.'s tract on children's diseases, he warranted his decision to publish in the vernacular by lamenting, 'The true use of Physick is as difficult, as the abuse is dangerous,...the mistake whereof by the Vulgar, is often mortal...To prevent which, I present this Manual to you, pointing and holding forth what ought to be done, and what not, for the procuring & preserving the health.'[34] The physician Christopher Wirtzung declared that since there was 'no arte more falsified nor abused in these dayes…by the presumptuous intermeddling of audacious and unskill persons,' he was compelled to make up for the 'lack of good and wholesome writings in English for the instruction and safe direction of all those that have not always a good and learned Physition at hand.'[35] By publishing such works, physicians claimed to be acting as guardians of the public health.

What was particularly alarming to physicians was that anyone could publish a medical tract, including any information on remedies or health that he or she wished. The quality of information being circulated could not be assured. After reading a medical work written by a person with dubious credentials, the practitioner James Young commented: 'as we seldom see a wiseman gain knowledge from a Fool, so is it as rare to gain a wise Medicine from an ignorant Block. I would also know his Education, what esteem his Person, and Books have among the worthy Brotherhood in the Town.'[36] To the author, it was clear that only those properly educated had the right to advise others on matters of health, yet anyone could now publish a medical text.

The Royal College of Physicians was perpetually wary of medical information it could not control.[37] This, in fact, remained one of their justifications for regulating medical activity, at least within London, throughout the seventeenth century. In the eyes of the College, nothing was more dangerous to public health than the empiric who arrogantly treated the populace without the slightest knowledge of Latin.[38] Such men 'throw dirt in the face of the *Orthodox,* fill the world with much noise to no purpose,' and strive to 'outvie one another in *Ignorance,* as strenuously as if the prize of an Olympick Game were at stake, for the most obstreperous *Blockhead,* or *clamorous Fool* in print.'[39] Not only was the health of the populace at stake, argued physicians, but such vernacular publications cast a shadow on respectable medicine, that 'noble and very useful Art,' so that while

> Ingenious, and Inquisitive men, are labouring to improve and advance [the profession of medicine] and its esteem in the world…so many medling Fops busily interpose, and not only amuse, disturb, and discourage them by the gagling of their Goose-quils, but disparage the growing credit of the faculty, by their follys and falshoods.[40]

While physicians couched their objections to the dissemination of medical knowledge in terms of public health, just beneath the surface loomed the less civic-minded concern that such publications would negatively affect the physician's livelihood. As early as 1566 John Securis lamented that if medical books in English were allowed,

> every man, woman, and child that lyst, may use phisike…as well as we? And so, many tymes not only hinder and defraud us of our law-full stipende & [gains]: but (which is worst of all and to much to be lamented) shall put many in hasarde of their lyfe, yea & be the destruction of many.[41]

Securius's mention of the health risks to the public seem tacked on as an afterthought to what was truly riling him: the hindrance of the physician's gains.

However, for all the drawbacks of the increase in vernacular publications, there were some positives for the medical profession. By publishing their own works in the vernacular, physicians created an opportunity to publically tout what they considered to be their superior learning and moral character. The increasing dissemination of medical knowledge arguably had a positive effect on the medical profession in that the trend afforded them a valuable opportunity to reiterate to the public the difference, as they envisioned it, between themselves and their competition. In essence, they turned their competition into a medical 'other,' suggesting that the morals and skills of the competition were both sub-par to their own.[42]

It was therefore of prime importance when publishing in the vernacular that the learned physician set his work apart from the rest. Johannes Dryander, physician and professor of medicine, wasted no time in stressing the point that his medical work was not an imitation of other vernacular works, but was grounded upon established academic principles. He used this claim as an opportunity to expound upon the difference between 'inexperienced mountebanks, uneducated monks, Jews, and foolish old women' versus 'experienced physicians.' While the former were nothing more than 'bums and cheats' who had 'a drug, potion, salve, plaster, or some other absurd thing for every ailment,' the latter were 'pious, God-fearing, experienced, learned' and were 'certified by the community.' It was extremely important to choose healers wisely, as decisions to hire non-physicians often resulted in a life 'squandered away by them.' In contrast, a godly physician could be fully trusted to treat any illness and afforded the patient 'God's means in a physician and in medicine.'[43] The distinction between a learned physician and an imposter, Dryander implied, could not be greater or of more importance to the consumer of medical services.

Physicians viewed the lack of character of their competition as one of the main distinctions between 'learned' and 'unlearned' medicine. For instance, when John Cotta railed against the multitude of non-physicians, whom he termed 'illiterates' due to their ignorance of Latin, he not only condemned the lack of education and bad practices of such people, but above all their undisciplined characters and their lack of virtue.[44] As Harold Cook has noted, when physicians wrote against their competitors, it was not as much the treatments they used but their inner character and outward behavior that separated the physician from the rest, as they considered wisdom and prudence necessary attributes of a good physician. Because learning and character were so closely related, when Eleaza Dunk wrote that the difference between physicians and empirics was that empirics were 'ignorant,' he was referring to much more than their lack of formal knowledge. Dunk also pointed to their loquaciousness, their haste in judging diseases and promising cures before the cause had been ascertained, their forwardness in condemning and slandering proper physicians, and their boastfulness regarding their own skills. This type of behavior was not simply a reflection of their lack of knowledge, but a demonstration of their lack of discipline, which Cook has asserted symbolized for physicians outward signs of inward character.[45] Such people could not be trusted with the health care of the public.

Physicians became quite adept at warning the public against the lack of knowledge and virtue inherent in unlearned healers. In fact, physicians created an entire genre dedicated to exposing medical frauds and the 'popular errors' contained in their empirical publications and echoed in beliefs of the common people. This series of works on 'popular errors' was published in the late sixteenth and early seventeenth centuries in several European countries. In these works, physicians lashed out against popular superstitions, folklore, and the 'errors of the people' in medicine and health.[46] The first of the genre appeared in 1578 by Laurent Joubert, the chancellor of the Faculty of Medicine at Montpellier. He justified publishing on the grounds that popular culture was shot through with error, ignorance, and superstition. Empirics used faulty logic and failed to understand rational causes. The lay population dosed themselves with whatever medicines some midwife or empiric recommended, so that 'their poor bodies are altered and mixed up by a chaos of remedies, and their minds tossed about by hope and despair.' The main problem, he concluded, was that 'everybody makes medicine his business.' There were too many 'meddlers' who tried to 'cut in on a portion of the profession' with their quack remedies and panaceas. Joubert asked physicians everywhere to record popular errors in medicine and health and add them to his catalogue. They responded from cities throughout Europe. [47]

In England, the physician James Primrose railed against empirics who claimed to have mysterious secret remedies for which they overcharged the ignorant rabble. That was to be expected, given the gullible nature of the general public, reasoned Primrose. However, he also described a case in which a gentleman paid twenty pounds for one such secret that he could have purchased for far less from an apothecary, demonstrating the necessity of trusting only in a godly physician, as even the quality could be duped. Primrose took great pains to expose the trickery of unscrupulous empirics who often represented common remedies as 'great secrets, which they will reveale to no man.' This they did for good reason, because in reality 'they have nothing that is worthy the name of a secret.' The irony, as pointed out by Primrose, was that the empirics' secrets were often remedies that originally came from physicians, yet physicians would not keep such things secret but would prescribe the best medicines from experience. If only people would learn to avoid these quacks, there would be no need to lament, 'how many, both men and women here in England, are beguiled.'[48] Primrose's *Popular Errours* took the form of a warning against dangerous practices by the competition, yet devoted at least equal time to convincing the public what it was about the character of a good physician that made his services valuable.

Arguably the most comprehensive attack on common dangerous mistakes and fallacies in medicine was written by Sir Thomas Browne, whose *Religio Medico* so eloquently linked the piety of the physician to his duty in medicine and which also discussed in painstaking detail the causes of errors. Foremost was original sin, which made people naturally credulous and easily deceived. As did other physicians, Browne posited a decidedly negative view of the common people, whom he described as 'the most deceptable part of Mankind and ready with open arms to receive the encroachments of Error.' In Browne's view, the situation only worsened when the common people congregated in large groups:

> Their individual imperfections being great, they are moreover enlarged by their aggregation; and being erroneous in their single numbers, once huddled together, they will be a farraginous concurrence of all conditions, tempers, sexes, and ages; it is but natural if their determinations be monstrous, and many waies inconsistent with Truth.[49]

Browne's contribution therefore justified the importance of a wise physician to guide the common people in matters of health.

Publishing works that focused on the dangerous practices and commonly believed myths associated with medicine proved useful in uniting physicians throughout Europe in a common campaign against incorrect medical information circulating as a result of ignorant, unlearned writers. Doing so simultaneously discredited non-physicians offering medical advice and provided another reason for physicians' entry into the field of vernacular publishing. As the above examples indicate, empirics were widely criticized in physicians' publications. However, there was a sub-group of empirics who bore the brunt of the physicians' ire, namely midwives.

In his original *Popular Errours,* Laurent Joubert reserved special contempt for midwives who claimed to know secret arts. He expressed his disgust at what he saw as the common practice of midwives to hoard a few small remedies that they claimed were their own invention, but that Joubert asserted were actually taken from physicians and later passed around among themselves: 'For women have never invented a single remedy; they all come from our domain.' He furthermore scoffed at their attempt to dupe learned physicians by their tricks: 'They are very ignorant to think we do not know about these remedies and to think they know more about them than we do.'[50] William Eamon has suggested that Joubert's diatribe is indicative of the fact that in the struggle between orthodox medicine and empirical practice, women healers and midwives became symbolic of the ignorant intruder into the domain of official medicine. The hierarchy of medicine demanded that midwives, like surgeons and apothecaries, be instructed and overseen by physicians, as 'all illnesses are within his knowledge and under his jurisdiction.' Yet too often this was not the case. The problem, as Joubert saw it, was that women healers were ignoring their position in the medical hierarchy, forgetting that 'All those who meddle in treating any illness are underlings with respect to physicians, such as surgeons, who have middling jurisdiction, and midwives, who have the lowest.'[51] Women healers exhibited impudence in assuming that they had the right to practice medicine apart from the authority of the physician, an audacity that was exacerbated by those who dared to compete with men in healing. This point was made by Scipion Mercurio in his Italian contribution to popular errors publishing, in which he declared that 'most errors are committed by women, who intrude too much in medical matters.[52]

Physicians proved exceedingly boisterous in their disparagement of women healers. John Cotta devoted an entire chapter to women in his *Ignorant Practisers of Physicke*. Cotta pointed out women's deficiency in 'learned reasoning and understanding' in matters of life and death, as these were bestowed by 'God and Nature' to men, rather than women.[53] Because they lacked both the education and natural reasoning that men possessed, women healers, even the best intentioned, tended to be depicted by physicians as dangerous to their patients. The physician Richard Whitlock attacked 'she-physitians' in his 1654 *Zootomia*. He accused them of killing rather than curing patients, and added that 'all that falsely usurp the title of physitian, and practice it,' did so 'to the sad cost of many.' He included in this group 'Toothless women, fuddling gossips, and Chare-women, [and] talkative midwives,' which he referred to as 'the scum of mankind.'[54] Dr. Whitlock's work is representative of the views of the College of Physicians regarding female healers in general.[55] An underlying theme in Whitlock's work is that, similar to all uneducated practitioners of physic, women were dangerous. Richard Banister, whose favorable opinion of Lady Grace Mildmay was previously mentioned, nevertheless felt that women as medical practitioners posed a danger to their patients, claiming that their lack of formal education led to malpractice.[56]

Physicians used the belief that midwives in particular were uneducated as a further justification of printing medical works to educate them, again having the added bonus of allowing physicians to subtly undermine both the capacity and character of midwives. The works were clear in the message that physicians were providing a watered-down version of their knowledge in order to accommodate the inferior intellect of the midwives who would read them. *The Compleat Midwifes Practice* condescendingly assured midwives that in order to aid them to the fullest, the writing would be 'so plain, that the weakest capacity may easily attain the knowledge of the whole art.'[57] Even the physician Nicholas Culpeper, in many ways a champion of midwives, was quick to acknowledge their inferior intellect. In the preface of his directory for midwives, he assured his readers that he would provide them with information that was 'very plaine and easie enough' and would not 'burden [their] brain.' He professed to loathe a system that excluded so many from a medical education and lamented the subsequent ignorance of uneducated healers: 'What an insufferable injury is it, That Man and Woman should be trained up in such ignorance.'[58] Culpeper was unique in considering the underlying reasons for the lack of knowledge in healers who received no formal education. Most writing by physicians instead focused on the hazards to patients that an

117

uneducated midwife, or healer in general, posed.

Physicians used this supposed lack of knowledge and inability to grasp all but the simplest of language to question the fitness of midwives to safely deliver babies. Percival Willoughby wrote his *Observations on Midwifery* in the 1660s for the express purpose of granting a much-needed education to midwives, a point he stressed repeatedly throughout the book.[59] *The English Midwife Enlarged* included a dialogue between a midwife and a doctor in which the midwife thanked the doctor for the directions he gave her concerning labor and delivery and requested further training from him: 'Sir I so well approve of your last Nights discourse, that I must humbly entreat you, that you would be pleased to afford me your Instructions in the safe performance of my Art.' The dialogue is telling in that it exemplified the ideal relationship (according to doctors) between midwives and medical men in which the learned practitioner imparted knowledge to the humble and grateful midwife.[60]

Physicians therefore justified their publication of books on the subject of midwifery by repeatedly stating that they were publishing in order to instruct, and thereby 'To discharge our consciences for the good of the Nation,' and to protect the country from 'unfortunate practisers.'[61] Physicians claimed to write their books on midwifery as a direct result of the 'many sad and incommodious things [that] are wont to happen to women with child' when they are brought 'into the world by ignorance and carelessnesse.' They maintained it was their Christian duty to do so.[62] Percival Willughby's previously mentioned *Observations on Midwifery* reads like a collection of horror stories about births gone wrong thanks to the mishaps of midwives. Included is one story of how Willughby was called to help a poor woman too late, after the child was dead. The woman 'complained very sadly to me, how one of the midwives (that was a young woman) had afflicted her through much pulling and stretching her body.' He cited another instance where a woman wanted a male attendant when the birth was not proceeding well, but the midwife refused to summon one. Willughby also noted one such case in 1640 in which he was standing by, ready and willing to help if his expertise was needed. The aristocratic mother was in great pain and called out for his help, 'but the midwife would have had me put by, and said that my Lady must stay God's time and pleasure.' Willughby described how he forced his way in and swiftly delivered the lady of her child, proving the hero to the mother, much to the chagrin of the midwife who was depicted as ignorant, obstinate, and controlling. Willughby even included a disparaging comment about midwives from one of his patients, Mrs. Molyneux, who after five deliveries by midwives lamented 'they were all ignorant creatures,' who in any difficult birth could only 'haul and pull the woman's body, and the child by the limbs.'[63] There was even a patriotic slant to their arguments, since safer outcomes during childbirth increased the numbers and health of the country. In *Health's Grand Preservative: or the Womens best Doctor* the author professed his treatise to be for the good of 'all that Love their Health,' but to be particularly necessary for women, 'on whose good or ill Constitutions the Health and Strength, or Sickness and weakness of all Posterity does in a more especial manner depend.'[64] Physicians' writing on the subject of midwifery served several purposes: the texts made the physician seem knowledgeable on the subject and charitable in his intention to share knowledge with those who required his tutelage, while simultaneously discrediting the expertise of the midwife.

In addition to questioning midwives' skill, physicians also addressed their moral fitness. Physicians once again assumed an air of superiority, this time in counseling them on proper behavior, implying that advice was needed. The moral character of the midwife had always been of prime importance, ostensibly due to the midwife's obligation to baptize infants in danger of dying before a priest could be summoned, and because midwives sometimes acted as witnesses of birth and inquisitors of laboring women.[65] Although the ideal midwife was morally sound, the popular imagination teemed with tales of wicked midwives that took on legendary proportions in the early modern period. Stories of morally bankrupt midwives lodging pregnant women for reprehensible purposes transcended national borders and excited the ire and imagination of the populace.[66] Midwives had a negative reputation for being drunkards, bawds, abortionists, and witches.[67] Such unsavory characteristics were already present in the popular imagination, making the job of belittling midwives much easier. Physicians could simply support the already-present fears.[68] Physicians were not concocting stories about murderous midwives in their medical tracts: they had no need to do so. They were able to subtly hint at the midwife's reputation and rely on popular perception to carry the point. For instance, publications by physicians directed at midwives often stressed the importance of good moral conduct and instructed women on proper behavior. Physicians assumed an air of superior morality, in much the same way that they touted their superior learning. They instructed midwives to

respect two things above all, your Consciences and Credits; and principally to the first; and to that end, for all the Treasure in the World, to give no Medicine to cause a Woman to miscarry of her Child; but

119

prudently send such kind of People to the Learned Physitian to deal with…Have a great care whom you lay in your Houses, for fear of encouraging naughty Woman.[69]

While not directly invoking the sensational cases of morally bankrupt midwives, such a warning assumed that midwives could benefit from a reminder of the proper moral behavior that their position required and served to further highlight the distinction between the learned male physician and the female midwife.

Evidence that the public was aware of the difference in the job of the physician as opposed to that of the female healer appears in the books written by lay healers themselves. In her research on books written for women, many of whom were not written by physicians, Suzanne Hull found that medical writing geared toward women persistently depicted women as inferior to men, who were their natural teachers.[70] The books did not intend to educate women to be physicians. Instead, they made a clear distinction between 'kitchen physick' and the 'art' of the physician. For example, in *The English Housewife*, first published in 1615 and intended for the wives of small farmers, physic was included in the skills a housewife should master, along with 'cookery, banqueting-stuff, distillation, perfumes, wool, hemp, flax, dairies, brewing, baking, and all other things belonging to a household.' Yet her 'virtue in physic' should be limited to 'knowing how to administer many wholesome receipts or medicines for the good of [her family].' Any additional knowledge would prove useless, as the authors admitted: 'We must confess that the depth and secrets of this most excellent art of physic is far beyond the capacity of the most skilful woman, as lodging only in the breast of the learned professors; yet … our housewife may from them receive some ordinary rules and medicines.'[71] While it might be helpful for a woman to possess basic medical knowledge for aiding her family, she should remember that her knowledge of physic was a far cry from that of the skillful physician.

This attitude can be found in the lay population of the seventeenth century as well, as evidenced by the literate and educated Ferrar sisters, who became proficient at treating surgical problems. Despite the women's proven success in surgery and treating the most unpleasant wounds, the family patriarch, their uncle Nicholas Ferrar, forbade the daughters from 'meddling' with physic. His reasoning was that physic 'required ye best art, long experience, deep judgement and maturity.'[72] Healing was a vocation that could be mastered, even by women, but physic required additional traits such as judgment more often associated with men than women. Nicholas Ferrar's opinion about the work of a physician demonstrates that there was a difference in the lay public's mind between the job of the physician and other healing tasks.

This is precisely the message that physicians were trying to convey in their printed works. In their quest to close ranks against competitors, physicians essentially defined themselves by contrast. Godly physicians were the polar opposite of unlearned healers, who possessed 'neither conscience, learning, art, nor Feare of God; nor never had good tutor to instruct them.'[73] Thus, the most important component in defining their unique offering was their university education, in which learning and morality were both essential elements. It was their education that formed them as moral authorities and that would consequently enable them to assume a position of public trust.[74]

Medical education was not just theoretical but had real significance to the patient, as the formally-educated physician incorporated learning and good judgment in terms of choosing the ideal course of treatment, both of which contributed to his ability to understand each patient's unique constitution.[75] His advice was tailored for each patient and covered the specifics of how to set up one's house, from construction to organization of the household, as well as how to behave in a manner pleasing to God.[76] Physicians gave counsel, not just medicine. They were interested in reforming the habits of their patients by stressing the connection of health and virtue, teaching and persuading those who consulted them about how they should regulate their lives. Only an upright and learned person could be trusted to give such advice about life. Consequently, physicians argued that a learned health advisor must be not only knowledgeable, but also must possess excellent judgment, and judgment in turn required that the character as well as the knowledge of the advisor be outstanding.[77] Because their education made them both virtuous and learned, physicians thought of themselves as members of a grave and dignified profession, distinct from all other healers in both their approach to health and in their theories on disease. They even attempted to convey their dignified nature to the public through their outward appearance, imitating the dress and demeanor of high church officials.[78]

In light of the esteem in which physicians held their profession and their lauding of its significance in God's plan, it must have seemed inconceivable to them that merely reading books on medicine in the vernacular or even in Latin could be sufficient to make men into knowledgeable physicians.[79] As Harold Cook has argued, this attitude of self-importance among physicians helps explain why such pretenders were criticized by physicians for their folly in thinking their study could rival a formal education. As one physician asserted, 'It is a great error on such men, that do dream that the art of physick may be easily attained unto: so that if they have gotten two or three chemical medicines, without any other grounds; they profess themselves to be great Doctors and cunning physicians.'[80] Dr. Jonathan Goddard pointed out the absurdity of imposters (in this case apothecaries) who 'make ostentations of being the masters of all the secrets and practice of all the Physicians of London…as if the Art of Physick, or one half of it, was the Knowledge of Recipes to cure diseases.'[81] Thus, physicians stridently criticized empirics who gave 'a pill for every ill' as lazy, greedy, and ignorant, as there was a great deal more to medicine than prescribing remedies.

The long years of education, and the moral authority that went along with it, were what enabled learned physicians to offer advice to their patients and were crucial, they argued, to a successful outcome. As the physician John Cotta noted, 'the dignitie and worth of Physicks skill consisteth not (as is imagined commonly) in the excellence and preeminence of remedies but in their wise and prudent use.'[82] Even good remedies, according to Cotta, could prove harmful if recommended by the unlearned.[83] A physician's education was of paramount importance in understanding disease: 'What though they can judge of the gout, the palsy and the dropsy? So can simple women do: but judge rightly of the causes and differences of these disasters…, that requireth Art, which is not in any Empiric.'[84]

Printing in the vernacular allowed physicians to stress the superiority of the art of physic as they practiced it, over the empiric's peddling of nostrums or the unlearned practitioner's potentially dangerous attempts at healing. The dissemination of medical knowledge taking place throughout the century was not a deathblow to the profession. Physicians did not sit passively by while empirics raised their pens--they joined in the writing of vernacular medical texts. By doing so, they transformed the publishing boom into an opportunity to distinguish themselves in contrast with their competition as the best choice for a favorable outcome. They warned readers about the threat to public health that all books by uneducated healers posed, even as they touted their own publications as an act of charity for those who could not find or afford a physician.

Rhetoric about empirical healing versus the role of an educated physician was an important element in physicians' struggle to distinguish themselves from their competition. Had they not chosen to utilize the possibilities introduced by the printing press, they could have conceivably become increasingly antiquated and unnecessary in the eyes of the public. Publications by physicians would become even more essential when trying to convince patients to rely on their services with an affliction that was as shameful as it was dreaded in seventeenth-century England: the pox.

Notes

1 John Archer, *Every Man His Own Doctor, Compleated with an Herbal Shewing, First, How Every One May Know His Own Constitution and Complexion by Certain Signs: Also, the Nature and Faculties of All Food...* (1673).

2 W. Eamon, *Science and the Secrets of Nature: Books of Secrets in Medieval and Early Modern Culture* (Princeton: Princeton University Press, 1994), 234. On increasing literacy, see M. Spufford, *Small Books and Pleasant Histories: Popular Fiction and Its Readership in Seventeenth-Century England* (London: Methuen and Company, 1981).

3 L. Beier, *Sufferers and Healers: The Experience of Illness in Seventeenth-Century England* (New York: Routledge, 1987), 33.

4 W. Eamon, *Science and the Secrets of Nature: Books of Secrets in Medieval and Early Modern Culture*, 260-1.

5 W. Eamon, *Science and the Secrets of Nature: Books of Secrets in Medieval and Early Modern Culture*, 261-2.

6 On changes in the commercialization of medicine, see J. Brewer, 'Commercialization and Politics,' in N. McKendrick, J. Brewer, and J.H. Plumb (eds), *The Birth of a Consumer Society: The Commercialization of Eighteenth-Century England* (Bloomington: Indiana University Press, 1982) and W. Birken, 'The Social Problem of the English Physician in the Early Seventeenth Century,' *Medical History* 31 (April 1987).

7 On the importance of the printing press to early modern culture, see E. Eisenstein, *The Printing Press as an Agent of Change*, vol. 2 (Cambridge: Cambridge University Press, 1979).

8 Laura Gowing has noted that the change began in the sixteenth and seventeenth centuries. The growing interest in dissection and anatomical study and the scientific innovations of the seventeenth century ushered in a market for a new genre of medical texts, from cheap palm-sized books to costly folio treatises. L. Gowing,

Common Bodies: Women, Touch, and Power in Seventeenth-Century England (New Haven: Yale University Press, 2003), 17. For a discussion of printed medical works and the movement to free medical knowledge during the civil war, see P. Crawford, 'Attitudes to Menstruation in Seventeenth-Century England,' *Past and Present* 91 (1981), 48. Paul Slack studied the effect on published medical works during the Tudor period and has identified 153 titles published between 1486 and 1605. He confirms Gowing and Crawford's contention that medical literature during the seventeenth century found a market and grew in numbers. P. Slack, 'Mirrors of Health and Treasures of Poor Men: The Uses of the Vernacular Medical Literature of Tudor England,' in C. Webster (ed.), *Health, Medicine, and Mortality in the Sixteenth Century* (New York: Cambridge University Press, 1979), 238-9.

9   R. Porter and D. Porter, *In Sickness and in Health: The British Experience 1650-1850* (London: Fourth Estate, 1988), 274.

10   H. Cook, 'Good Advice and Little Medicine: The Professional Authority of Early Modern English Physicians,' *The Journal of British Studies* 33, no. 1 (January 1994), 1.

11   J. Goeurot, *The Regiment of Life*, trans. T. Phayer (1544), Translator's Preface. Cited in L. Beier, *Sufferers and Healers: The Experience of Illness in Seventeenth-Century England*, 21.

12   For example Archer, *Every Man His Own Doctor, Compleated with an Herbal Shewing, First, How Every One May Know His Own Constitution and Complexion by Certain Signs : Also, the Nature and Faculties of All Food ...,* Christopher Wirtzung, *The General Practise of Physicke* (1605) and T. Tryon, *The Good House-Wife Made a Doctor* (1692).

13   T. Tryon, *A Pocket-Companion; Containing Things Necessary to Be Known, by All That Values Their Health and Happiness: Being a Plain Way of Nature's Own Prescribing, to Cure Most Diseases in Men, Women and Children, by Kitchen-Physick Only* (1694).

14   On easing the afflictions of the poor and needy see Anon., *The Treasurie of Commodious Conceits, and Hidden Secretes, Commonlie Called the Good Huswives Closet of Provision, for the Health of Her Houshold...* (1591), and Anon., *The Treasurie of Hidden Secrets* (1627). For examples of target audiences see William Salmon, *Iatrica, Seu, Praxis Medendi, the Practice of Curing Being a Medicinal History of above Three Thousand Famous Observations in the Cure of Diseases* (1681).

15   For an example of an overt attempt to bypass the physician see

W.M., *The Queens Closet Opened. Incomparable Secrets in Physick, Chirurgery, Preserving, Candying, and Cookery* (1655). Texts such as this one were quite popular, as attested to by the fact that there were many different versions of *The Queen's Closet* published throughout the seventeenth century. For an example of a more subtle approach see W. Salmon, *The Family-Dictionary, or, Household Companion* (1696), A2 and O. Wood, *An Alphabetical Book of Physicall Secrets* (1639).

16 W.M., *The Queens Closet Opened. Incomparable Secrets in Physick, Chirurgery, Preserving, Candying, and Cookery.*

17 T. Elyot, *The Castle of Helth* (1541), A3-4.

18 T. Elyot, *The Castle of Helth* (1541), A3-4.

19 L. Beier, *Sufferers and Healers: The Experience of Illness in Seventeenth-Century England*, 20.

20 For an example of physicians trying to shroud their activities in secrecy and the mystery of Latin, see E. Maynwaring, *Medicus Absolutus. The Compleat Physitian* (1668), 150.

21 L. Fioravanti, *A Short Discourse of the Excellent Doctor...* trans. John Hester (1580). Cited in L.Beier, *Sufferers and Healers: The Experience of Illness in Seventeenth-Century England*, 20.

22 C. Severn (ed.), *The Diary of the Reverend John Ward [1648-79]* (London: 1839), 242. For more on Sydenham's approach to medicine, see A. Cunningham, 'Thomas Sydenham: Epidemics, Experiment and the "Good Old Cause,"' in R. French and A. Wear (eds), *The Medical Revolution of the Seventeenth Century* (New York: Cambridge University Press, 1989).

23 J. Sharp, *The Midwives Book* (1671), Introduction. See also the midwife Margaret Stephens, *The Domestic Midwife* (1795), 105. Cited in J. Donnison, *Midwives and Medical Men: A History of Inter-Professional Rivalries and Women's Rights* (London: Heinemann, 1977), 34.

24 E. Cellier, *A Letter to Dr. ----* (1680). In their study of the 1582 *The Monument of Matrones*, a book of prayers for women, Colin Atkinson and William Stoneman assert that the section of prayers for midwives reflects a high degree of pride and professionalism, in which midwives are depicted as strong, capable women, proud of their profession. C. Atkinson and W. Stoneman, 'These Griping Greefes and Pinching Pangs: Attitudes to Childbirth in Thomas Bentley's the Monument of Matrones (1582),' T. Bentley, *The Monument of Matrones* (1582), 200-201. The anonymously published *The Mid-wives Just Petition* of 1643 provides

evidence that seventeenth-century midwives considered themselves
a distinct group of professionals central to women's fertility and
childbirth. In the document they are petitioning the government to put
an end to the war in order save their trade and ultimately the future
of the country, as men who are absent from their wives because they
are fighting in wars are not impregnating them. Anon., *The Mid-Wives
Just Petition: Or, a Complaint of Divers Good Gentlewomen of That Faculty.
Shewing the Whole Christian World Their Just Cause of Their Sufferings in
These Distracted Times, for Their Want of Trading. Which Said Complaint They
Tendered to the House on Monday Last, Being the 23. Of Jan. 1643* (1643).

25 J. Archer, *Every Man His Own Doctor, Compleated with an Herbal Shewing,
First, How Every One May Know His Own Constitution and Complexion by
Certain Signs: Also, the Nature and Faculties of All Food...* (1673). See also
Anon., *Every Woman Her Own Midwife* (1675), for a similar take on the
genre.

26 W. Eamon, *Science and the Secrets of Nature: Books of Secrets in Medieval and
Early Modern Culture*, 95. H. Cook, *The Decline of the Old Medical Regime in
Stuart London* (Ithaca: Cornell University Press, 1986), Chapter One.

27 J. Hart, *The Anatomie of Urines* (1625), A4.

28 N. Culpeper, *The English Physitian: Or an Astrologo-Physical Discourse of the
Vulgar Herbs of This Nation* (1652).

29 N. Culpeper, *The English Physitian: Or an Astrologo-Physical Discourse of the
Vulgar Herbs of This Nation* (1652), A-B.

30 N. Culpeper, *Compleat Method of Physick, Whereby a Man May Preserve
His Body in Health; or Cure Himself, Being Sick, for Three Pence Charge, with
Such Things Only as Grow in England, They Being Most Fit for English Bodies*
(1652), A.

31 N. Culpeper, *Compleat Method of Physick, Whereby a Man May Preserve His
Body in Health; or Cure Himself, Being Sick, for Three Pence Charge, with Such
Things Only as Grow in England, They Being Most Fit for English Bodies*, B2.

32 See N. Culpeper, *Pharmacopoeia* (1649) and J. Axtell, 'Education and
Status in Stuart England: The London Physicians,' *History of Education
Quarterly* 10, no. 2 (Summer 1970), 150. For more on this see T. Brown,
'Word Wars: The Debate over the Use of the Vernacular in Medical
Writings of the English Renaissance,' *Texas Studies in Literature and
Language* 37, no. 1 (Spring 1995).

33 T. Brown, 'Word Wars: The Debate over the Use of the Vernacular in
Medical Writings of the English Renaissance,' 100.

34 J.S., *Children's Diseases, Both Outward and Inward* (1664), A4.

35 C. Wirtzung, *The General Practise of Physicke* (1605), A2. See also R. Porter, *Health for Sale: Quackery in England 1660-1850* (Manchester: Manchester University Press, 1989). See chapter 7 'The Quarrel of the Quacks' for examples from the primary sources and discussion.

36 J. Young, *Medicaster Medicatus, or a Remedy for the Itch of Scribling* (1685), 189.

37 For more on this see C. Gillispie, 'Physick and Philosophy: A Study of the Influence of the College of Physicians of London Upon the Foundation of the Royal Society.' *The Journal of Modern History* 19, no. 3 (September 1947) and C. Webster (ed.), *Health, Medicine, and Mortality in the Sixteenth Century* (New York: Cambridge University Press, 1979), (especially Paul Slack's contribution, 'Mirrors of Health and Treasures of Poor Men: The Uses of the Vernacular Medical Literature of Tudor England').

38 W. Birkin, 'The Royal College of Physicians of London and Its Support of the Parliamentary Cause in the English Civil War,' *The Journal of British Studies* 23, no. 1 (1983), 57.

39 J. Young, *Medicaster Medicatus, or a Remedy for the Itch of Scribling* (1685), 4.

40 J. Young, *Medicaster Medicatus, or a Remedy for the Itch of Scribling*, 2.

41 J. Securis, *A Detection and Querimonie of the Daily Enormities Comitted in Physick* (1566), B3.

42 A.K. Lingo. 'Empirics and Charlatans in Early Modern France: The Genesis of the Classification of the "Other" in Medical Practice,' *Journal of Social History* Vol. 19, No. 4 (Summer 1986), 583. Lingo is arguing for the situation in France, but her idea of framing competition as "other" holds true for England, as well.

43 J. Dryander, *Artzenei Speigel* (Frankfurt am Main: 1547), preface. Cited in W. Eamon, *Science and the Secrets of Nature: Books of Secrets in Medieval and Early Modern Culture*, 103.

44 H. Cook, 'Good Advice and Little Medicine: The Professional Authority of Early Modern English Physicians,' 18.

45 E. Dunk, *The Copy of a Letter Written by E.D. Doctour of Physicke to a Gentleman, by Whom It Was Published* (1606), 20-1. Cited in H. Cook, 'Good Advice and Little Medicine: The Professional Authority of Early Modern English Physicians,' 19.

46 W. Eamon, *Science and the Secrets of Nature: Books of Secrets in Medieval and Early Modern Culture*, 260-1.

47 L. Joubert, *Popular Errours*, trans. Gregory David de Rocher (Tuscaloosa: University of Alabama Press, 1989), 66, 69, 123, 172-3. Cited in W. Eamon, *Science and the Secrets of Nature: Books of Secrets in Medieval and Early Modern Culture*, 261.

48 J. Primrose, *Popular Errours. Or the Errours of the People in Physick*, trans. Robert Wittie (1651), 18, 42-8. Cited in W. Eamon *Science and the Secrets of Nature: Books of Secrets in Medieval and Early Modern Culture*, 263.

49 G. Keynes (ed.), *The Works of Sir Thomas Browne*, 4 vols. (Chicago: University of Chicago Press, 1964), 2: 25-30, in W. Eamon, *Science and the Secrets of Nature: Books of Secrets in Medieval and Early Modern Culture*, 263-4.

50 L. Joubert, *Popular Errours,* 66. Cited in W. Eamon, *Science and the Secrets of Nature: Books of Secrets in Medieval and Early Modern Culture*, 261.

51 L. Joubert, *Popular Errours,* 69, 123, 172-3. Cited in W. Eamon, *Science and the Secrets of Nature: Books of Secrets in Medieval and Early Modern Culture*, 261.

52 S. Mercurio, *De Gli Errori [Popolari D'italia]* (Venice: 1603), 1. Cited in W. Eamon, *Science and the Secrets of Nature: Books of Secrets in Medieval and Early Modern Culture*, 261-2.

53 J. Cotta, *A Short Discouerie of Seuerall Sorts of Ignorant and Vnconsiderate Practisers of Physicke in England with Direction for the Safest Election of a Physition in Necessitie* (1619)*, 25, 32-3.

54 C. Bently persuasively argues this point in 'The Rational Physician: Richard Whitlock's Medical Satires,' *Journal of the History of Medicine and Allied Sciences* 29 (1974), 180-185, 190-1.

55 C. Bently, 'The Rational Physician: Richard Whitlock's Medical Satires,' *Journal of the History of Medicine and Allied Sciences* 29 (1974), 190-1.

56 {Bannister, 1622 #474}, no pagination.

57 For additional examples see F.S. Mauriceau, *The Accomplisht Midwife, Treating of the Diseases of Women with Child, and in Child-Bed* (1673), P. Willughby, *Observations in Midwifery* (London: 1660's exact year not known), W. Salmon, *Pharmacopoeia Londinensis, or, the New London Dispensatory in Vi Books : Translated into English for the Publick Good... As Also, the Praxis of Chymistry, as Its Now Exercised Fitted to the Meanest Capacity* (1682), and D. Sennertus, *Practical Physick, or, Five Distinct Treatises of the Most Predominant Diseases of These Times the First of the Scurvy, the Second of the Dropsie, the Third of Feavers and Agues of All Sort, the Fourth of the French Pox, and the Fifth of the Gout, Wherein the Nature,*

Causes, Symptomes, Various Methods of Cure, and Waies of Preventing Every of the Said Diseases, Are Severally Handled, and Plainly Discovered to the Meanest Capacity (1676).

58   In the same book he praised them as 'worthy matrons' who 'are of the Number of those whom my Soul loveth, and of whom I make dayly mention in my Prayers.' N. Culpeper, *A Directory for Midwives: Or a Guide for Women. In Their Conception, Bearing and Suckling Children* (1651), A4.

59   P. Willughby, *Observations in Midwifery*.

60   Anon., *The English Midwife Enlarged, Containing Directions to Midwives; Wherein Is Laid Down Whatever Is Most Requisite for the Safe Practising Her Art* (1682), 33.

61   T.C. et al., *The Compleat Midwifes Practice* (1656), A2. See also T. Tryon, *A Pocket-Companion; Containing Things Necessary to Be Known, by All That Values Their Health and Happiness: Being a Plain Way of Nature's Own Prescribing, to Cure Most Diseases in Men, Women and Children, by Kitchen-Physick Only;* Physitian in the countrey (probably Dr. John Pechey), J. Pechey, *Some Observations Made Upon the Maldiva Nut Shewing Its Admirable Virtue in Giving an Easie, Safe, and Speedy Delivery to Women in Child-Bed / Written by a Physitian in the Countrey to Dr. Hinton at London, 1663* (1694); and E. Grey, *A Choice Manual of Rare Secrets* (1653).

62   Anon., *Every Woman Her Own Midwife*.

63   P. Willughby, *Observations in Midwifery*. Cited in A. Wilson, 'Participant or Patient? Seventeenth Century Childbirth from the Mother's Point of View,' in R. Porter (ed.), *Patients and Practitioners: Lay Perceptions of Medicine in Pre-Industrial England* (Cambridge: Cambridge University Press, 1985), 142-3. Mrs. Molyneux's comment was included in Willughby's text as proof that midwives were inferior, and is arguably biased, yet it is similar to a comment recorded by Ralph Josselin in his diary that after the birth of her eighth child, his wife Jane criticized the midwife for not having done 'her part,' as her labour was unusually 'sharp' and the baby appeared dead at birth. Cited in Beier, *Sufferers and Healers: The Experience of Illness in Seventeenth-Century England*, 186.

64   T. Tryon, *Healths Grand Preservative: Or the Womens Best Doctor* (1682).

65   L. Beier, *Sufferers and Healers: The Experience of Illness in Seventeenth-Century England*, 15. This explains in part why ecclesiastical licensing of midwives, unlike that of physicians and surgeons, was more concerned with their moral character than with their skill level.

66   See Anon., *The Murderous Midwife* (1673) and Anon., *The Cruel Midwife*.

129

Being a True Account of a Most Sad and Lamentable Discovery That Has Been Lately Made in the Village of Poplar in the Parish of Stepney (1693). See also P. Griffiths, *Lost Londons: Change, Crime and Control in the Capital City, 1550-1660* (New York: Cambridge University Press, 2008), 57-9.

67 T. Heywood, *The Wise-Woman of Hogsden* (1638), I, i. Cited in L. Beier, *Sufferers and Healers: The Experience of Illness in Seventeenth-Century England*, 29 and J. Lane, *The Making of the English Patient* (Stroud: Sutton, 2000), 31. Thomas Forbes argues that the low status of the midwife during this period was due to their association with witchcraft. T.R. Forbes, *The Midwife and the Witch* (New Haven: Yale University Press, 1966). See also W. Kerwin, 'Where Have You Gone, Margaret Kennix? Seeking the Tradition of Healing Women in English Renaissance Drama.' in L. Furst (ed.), *Women Healers and Physicians: Climbing a Long Hill* (Lexington: University Press of Kentucky, 1997), 96; B. Ehrenreich and D English, *Witches, Midwives, and Nurses: A History of Women Healers* (New York: Feminist Press, 1973); D. Harley, 'English Archives, Local History, and the Study of Early Modern Midwifery' *Archives* [Great Britain] 21, no. 92 (1994); and D. Harley, 'Ignorant Midwives--a Persistent Stereotype,' *Bulletin of the Society for the Social History of Medicine* 28 (1981). J. H. Aveling notes Visitation articles of 1559 included the question, 'Whether you know of any that do use charms, sorcery, enchantment,…witchcrafts, soothsayings, or any like crafts or imaginations invented by the Devil and specially in time of women's travail.' J.H. Aveling, *English Midwives: Their History and Prospects* (London: 1872), 2.

68 At least one famous physician, Sir Thomas Browne, not only supported witch-hunts, but his testimony at a trial in 1664 resulted in two women being convicted and hanged. D. Nagy, *Popular Medicine in Seventeenth-Century England* (Bowling Green: Bowling Green State University Popular Press, 1988), 52. H. Cook, *Trials of an Ordinary Doctor: Joannes Groenevelt in Seventeenth-Century London* (Baltimore: Johns Hopkins Univeristy Press, 1994), 108. For witchcraft during the period, see A. MacFarlane, *Witchcraft in Tudor and Stuart England* (London: Routledge and Kegan Paul, 1970) and C. Larner, *Enemies of God: The Witch-Hunt in Scotland* (1981).

69 Anon., *The English Midwife Enlarged, Containing Directions to Midwives; Wherein Is Laid Down Whatever Is Most Requisite for the Safe Practising Her Art*, A4. See the same warning in T.C. et al., *The Compleat Midwifes*

Practice, 120.

70 S. Hull, *Chaste, Silent and Obedient: English Books for Women, 1475-1640* (San Marino: Huntington Library, 1982).

71 K. Knight, 'A Precious Medicine: Tradition and Magic in Some Seventeenth-Century Household Remedies,' *Folklore (London, England)* 113, no. 2 (October 2002), 239. For additional primary source examples, see T. Dawson, *The Good Housewife's Jewel* (1596) and Hannah Woolley, *The Gentlewomans Companion* (1675).

72 B. Blackstine, ed., *The Ferrar Papers* (London: Cambridge University Press, 1938), 32. Cited in D. Nagy, *Popular Medicine in Seventeenth-Century England*, 64.

73 D. Harley, 'Spiritual Physic, Providence and English Medicine, 1560-1640,' in O.P. Grell and A. Cunningham (eds), *Medicine and the Reformation* (London: Routledge, 1993), 111.

74 H. Sacks, 'Parliament, Liberty, and the Commonweal,' in J.H. Hexter (ed.), *Parliament and Liberty from Queen Elizabeth I to the Civil Wars* (Stanford: Stanford University Press, 1991), cited in H. Cook, 'Good Advice and Little Medicine: The Professional Authority of Early Modern English Physicians,' 10.

75 F. Dawbarn, 'Patronage and Power: The College of Physicians and the Jacobean Court,' *BJHS* 31 (1998), 8. Dawbarn stresses the distinction between services provided by traditionally educated Galenic physicians versus the universal remedy pulled from the chest of a traveling quack.

76 See T. Brugis, *The Marrow of Physicke. Or, a Learned Discourse of the Severall Parts of Mans Body* (1640), T. Elyot, *The Castle of Helth* (1541); T. Venner, *A Plaine Philosophicall Demonstration Of...The Preservation of Health* (1628); and L. Lessius, *Hygiasticon: Or, the Right Course of Preserving Life and Health Unto Extream Old Age* (Cambridge: 1634).

77 H. Cook, 'Good Advice and Little Medicine: The Professional Authority of Early Modern English Physicians,' 13-6.

78 M. Pelling, 'Compromised by Gender: The Role of the Male Medical Practitioner in Early Modern England' in H. Marland and M. Pelling (eds), *The Task of Healing: Medicine, Religion and Gender in England and the Netherlands 1450-1800* (Rotterdam: Erasmus Publishing, 1996).' 102. Pelling notes that physicians had been trying to define themselves institutionally since the fifteenth century. They attempted to improve their status by associating themselves with larger groups in society. Lawyers were not a good choice because although they had achieved

worldly advancement, they had done so at the cost of losing the moral ground in contemporary opinion, and they were not associated with the universities, as physicians were. The clergy proved the better choice.

79   H. Cook, 'Good Advice and Little Medicine: The Professional Authority of Early Modern English Physicians,' 17-18.

80   P.P. Valentinus, *Enchiridion Medicum: Containing an Epitome of the Whole Course of Physic* (1608), 3 in L. Beier, *Sufferers and Healers: The Experience of Illness in Seventeenth-Century England*, 36.

81   J. Goddard, *Discourse on the Unhappy Condition of the Practice of Physic in London. And Offering Some Means to Put It into a Better; for the Interest of Patients, No Less, or Rather More, Than of Physicians* (1670). For additional analysis of this physician's views on medical practice in seventeenth-century London, see W.S.C. Copeman, 'Dr. Johnathan Goddard, F.R.S. (1617-1675),' *Notes and Records of the Royal Society of London* 15 (July 1960).

82   J. Cotta, *A Short Discouerie of Seuerall Sorts of Ignorant and Vnconsiderate Practisers of Physicke in England with Direction for the Safest Election of a Physition in Necessitie*, 43-44.

83   J. Cotta, *A Short Discouerie of Seuerall Sorts of Ignorant and Vnconsiderate Practisers of Physicke in England with Direction for the Safest Election of a Physition in Necessitie*, 18.

84   In L. Beier, *Sufferers and Healers: The Experience of Illness in Seventeenth-Century England*, 38.

PART II

THE DISTEMPERS

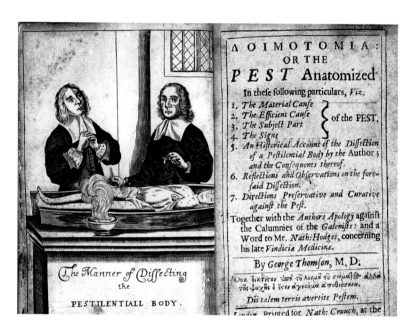

Figure 9: Two men dissecting a body with plague
Courtesy Wellcome Library, London

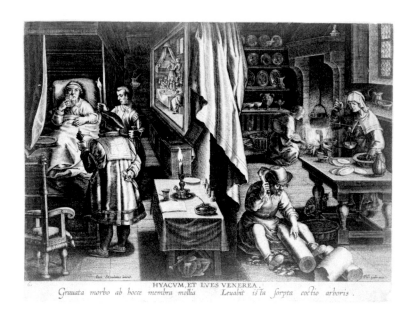

Figure 10: A man in bed suffering from syphilis, amidst a busy domestic scene
Courtesy Wellcome Library, London

5

'A Christian's Groans Under the Body of Sin'[1]:
The Pox and the Pious Physician

'Lues Venerea, a sickness very lothsome and odious, yea troublesome and dangerous, a notable testimonie of the just wrath of God against that sinne [lust]...which disease...raigneth ouer the face of the whole earth.'[2]

In early modern Europe, hospitals were charitable institutions, intended primarily to provide relief for the sick poor. Arguably, the most famous of them was the Hotel-Dieu in Paris. The hospital prided itself on its generosity towards and cure of all individuals with one notable exception: '[Hotel Dieu] receives, feeds, and tends all poor sufferers, wherever they come from and whatever ailment they may have, even plague victims—though not if they have the pox.'[3] As the hospital's exclusion of sufferers from the disease indicates, syphilis, or 'the pox,' as it was commonly called, was unlike any other illness.[4] The governors of the Westminster Infirmary in 1738 wrote in a similar vein that 'The Admission of Venereal Patients...[is] a Subversion of the Charity, or a Misapplication of the Money given in trust for the Poor... the Society [has] constantly rejected Venereal Patients for the very reason of Being Venereal'.[5] It was more than fear of contagion that differentiated syphilis. Plague was known to be contagious and was immensely feared, and yet plague patients were admitted.[6] Not all hospitals refused pox patients, yet for those pox patients treated in hospitals, cultural attitudes informed every aspect of their care.[7]

One facet of the pox that made it unique in seventeenth-century England was that most thought the disease was relatively new to Europe (introduced to England in the late fifteenth century). The newness of the disease meant that it was unstudied by the ancients. The challenge for seventeenth-century physicians lay in how to become knowledgeable about a disease that lacked a long-standing history. They would have to construct a history of the disease in order to incorporate it successfully into their realm of knowledge. Another challenge for physicians was the association of the pox with divine punishment for committing the sin of lust.[8] How were physicians supposed to justify treating a disease sent by God to punish a specific sin, particularly one that was self-inflicted through one's own sin and could have been avoided? They responded by drawing from and reinforcing their idea of themselves as moral arbiters in an attempt to assume a greater role in the regulation of public health.

Margaret Pelling has argued that venereal disease remains 'seriously underestimated' as a force in early modern England.[9] Certainly the pox had wide cultural and social repercussions that will be considered in this chapter; however, Pelling and other historians see the disease as a boon for unlicensed healers who could fill the gap between the need for medical care and the dearth of physicians who were available (or willing) to treat it.[10] While this assessment is accurate, her conclusion that because of these challenges the disease proved an unmitigated failure for physicians is not the only possibility. There is an argument to be made that the pox provided an opportunity for physicians--one that they capitalized on in order to advance their status and authority in the realm of public health.

Physicians certainly faced challenges in dealing with the pox. They had to compete with a bevy of irregular healers who were initially more receptive to the unique patient needs ushered in by the pox and whose use of empiric remedies seemed to threaten traditional Galenic medicine. However, many physicians proved flexible in accommodating their patients' needs, and they stressed their superior judgment and skill in managing difficult treatments that despite being empiric in origin could be better handled by a learned physician, or so the argument went. They also needed to explain a new disease, which necessitated constructing knowledge about it. Physicians enticed patients to trust them with the cure of the pox by developing medical theories to explain the disease's origin, history, and the manner in which it was contracted.[11] Garnering knowledge about a disease and demonstrating an ability to explain its qualities, cause, and spread had real value in terms of the establishment of authority for the profession. Knowledge about a disease is sometimes disregarded by modern historians who underestimate the cache that such an offering provided by making the bearer seem to be an expert about the disease.[12] Physicians took their cues on innovations such as patient privacy and the use of both mercury and guaiacum as remedies from empirics. Yet by choosing to focus on the illicit and sinful behavior of prostitution to explain the cause and spread of the disease, physicians were able to demonstrate actively their knowledge and expertise to the public regarding the French Disease.

The pox did not necessarily have a negative impact on the profession of medicine. There were contributions made by physicians in dealing with the disease that should contribute to an assessment of the disease's impact on the profession. Many physicians did treat pox patients, and some actively vied for their business. They developed medical theories about its history and etiology in order to bring the pox into their realm of knowledge, as the new disease did not readily fit into the framework of humoral medicine. Their theories meshed neatly with commonly held beliefs about the disease and its mode of transmission, so while they were hardly innovative, the lay community nonetheless readily accepted them.

The central beliefs about the pox, shared by medical and lay communities alike, were that it was a punishment sent from God, that it was a new disease, and that it resulted most frequently from illicit sexual intercourse. Each of these ideas is characterized by the following seventeenth-century physician's explanation of its origin and causes:

> The just punishment of God upon our sins hath for some hundred years since, produced a Disease unknown, as some think, to Antiquity, called the Venerian or French pox, which may be defined, An indisposition composed of all other Diseases and their Accidents, engendered by a contagious touch, but most commonly by impure Copulation, whence the Seed of several Men Fermenting, ariseth a Venenous either fixt, or volatile acid Salt, having usually its seat in gross and viscid Flegm, whence it proceeds to the Invasion of the other Humours.[13]

In deciding to treat the pox, physicians would have to deal with each of these challenges. They would have to justify treating a disease sent as a specific punishment for a specific sin, as well as incorporating a new disease into their traditional realm of knowledge. They would also have to manage the repercussions of a disease associated so closely with sexual sin, including the need to listen and respond to the unique demands for privacy from their fee-paying patients in response to the unprecedented degree of shame that an odious disease encompassed.

In the seventeenth century, many agreed that explorers returning from the New World brought the pox back to Europe. The Spanish physician Ruy Diaz de Isla in his 1539 *Treatise on the Serpentine Malady* was one of the first to have made this claim, as he had treated Columbus's pilot in 1493.[14] Ulrich von Hutten remarked in the sixteenth century that the only thing physicians could agree upon about the disease was its American origin.[15] The English physician Philip Barrough in 1596 also assumed an American origin: 'First the Spaniards borrowed it of the Indians, and brought it home in stead of their gold, and afterward Charles the fifth Emperour of Rome spread it around his Empire.'[16] From there it began spreading throughout Europe: 'French men caught it, when *Charles* the Eighth their King went against Naples. From whence the contagion spread it selfe throughout divers places of Europe.'[17] Contemporaries soon feared it was flourishing in England as well.

As a new disease, believed to be hitherto unknown to Europeans, the pox did not fit readily into physicians' traditional area of knowledge. Indeed, when the pox first appeared in Europe in the 1490s, physicians proved woefully lacking in their response to the disease. They were generally hesitant to treat it, in part because the pustules and ulcers associated with the disease would place it in the realm of the surgeon, trained to deal in outward appearances.[18] Additionally, the repugnant symptoms deterred some physicians from wanting to deal with it, as noted by the author of the tract *Prothylantinon*: 'the obscenity of it is the cause why Eminent Physicians meddle not with it, but have hitherto left the business wholly to Surgeons, Barbers, Tooth-drawers, and Mountebanks.' He added that while the pox is a 'nasty Disease,' it did not follow that physicians should think it beneath them to treat it.[19] The implication of the tract was that physicians *did* consider the disease too repulsive to 'meddle' with patients suffering from the pox.

By the seventeenth century lay and medical opinion alike held that the disease was rampant and spreading at an alarming pace. William Clowes, who spent ten years as a doctor at London's St. Bartholomew's Hospital, one of the two London hospitals that accepted pox patients, wrote at the close of the sixteenth century that one out of two patients admitted to the hospital suffered from the pox, and he claimed to have treated over a thousand patients in five years.[20] Since only a scant minority of the population ever set foot in a hospital, Clowes's experience was probably indicative of a much larger number of people who received care for the disease elsewhere.[21] The situation seemed to be getting worse, causing the surgeon Charles Peter in 1678 to dub the pox the 'domineering distemper of our age.'[22] In *Great Venus*

Unmasked (1672), Gideon Harvey wrote, 'this evil, instead of declining, assumeth a new growth even now in our days, infecting more in a day than were afflicted a century ago in a month.'[23] By the eighteenth century the author of *The Modern Syphilis* lamented that the disease was 'a Distemper so Notorious, as well as Universal, that it is now as great a Wonder to hear of many Persons, who never had it, or never used the Means to get it, as it was formerly to hear of any one labouring under it.'[24] These publications implied a fear shared by the public and medical community that the pox was entrenched in early modern English society.

Research supports these contentions and has suggested that the malady was even more widespread than anyone had suspected. For instance, Randolph Trumbach has concluded from his study of naval medical records that venereal disease was rampant among ships' populations.[25] Kevin Siena's research on the subject also points to extremely high rates of infection. Records of the royal hospitals reveal the pox was the single most common malady treated, accounting for twenty percent of admissions from 1600-1800. St. Bartholomew's and St. Thomas's records for the eighteenth century show that roughly one-fifth to one-quarter of all patients in hospitals were treated for the pox. Some years venereal patients accounted for as much as thirty percent of the hospital's patients.[26] The prevalence of the disease, or at the very least the perception that the disease was spreading at an alarming rate, posed a problem for physicians who were as a whole rather reticent to treat the disease until the seventeenth century.

Also problematic for physicians was the stigma attached to the disease. The frequency with which the pox struck seems not to have abated the repulsion people felt towards its sufferers or the shame that sufferers themselves felt. The abhorrent physical symptoms and the permanent disfigurement that tormented poxed patients led to both disgrace and disgust. Collapsed noses and balding heads were telltale signs of a disease sufferers would have preferred to keep hidden, but proved very difficult to conceal, particularly as the pox affected the most visible parts of the body. Margaret Pelling has noted that in the early modern period, medical practitioners and the lay population alike were very concerned with disfiguring conditions, especially those affecting the face.[27] Pelling has pointed to a court culture in London that stressed personal good looks and a society that still expected the individual to summarize his estate in his own person. It was a culture where a new flamboyance and even fastidiousness was required while at the same time it was still customary to seek the mind's construction in the face (and hands).[28] One of the reasons why the French disease was so abhorrent and therefore dreaded in seventeenth-century England was because its symptoms could be read quite literally upon a sufferer's face.

In the early modern period, people often thought physical deformity represented a defect of mind and moral nature. These ideas squared with contemporary notions surrounding the pox, which held that the deformity surrounding the disease represented vice as well as the pretensions and hypocrisies of urban life. There was a certain poetic justice regarding the fact that the pox did not spare the wealthy or famous but attacked the most prominent people in the most prominent way. This was noted in John Donne's wry explanation of why syphilis attacked the nose: 'It is reasonable that this disease should in particular men affect the most eminent and conspicuous part, which amongst men in generall doth affect to take hold of the most eminent and conspicuous men.'[29] It was ironic and unsettling that the disease transformed something so private into something so outwardly exposed. In a society conditioned to see God's hand in disease, the pox, with its disfiguring symptoms, must have seemed positively providential.

Adding to the feeling of exposure was the belief that God punished sexual sin with venereal disease. In fact, it is difficult to find any seventeenth-century English discussion of venereal disease that does not include this assertion in some form in both lay and medical texts.[30] The idea that God punished sin with disease was common thinking throughout the early modern period, and it was especially true for sexual sin, which 'God hath permitted…to raigne among them as a punishment for sinne' as well as a preventative measure to 'refraine the filthy lusts of men and women.'[31] Because the pox was believed to be brought upon the victims as the direct result of their actions, it was deemed to be a 'fit Sauce for that sweet sin of Letchery.'[32] It seemed divine justice to many that victims of the disease were suffering corporeal agony after indulging in illicit pleasures of the flesh. While any disease could be deemed God's wrath against a sinner, in the case of the pox, this potential was intensified both by the specificity of the disease for a particular sin and by the nature of contracting the disease. Obviously, there was a link between sexual activity and venereal disease, but more specifically, illicit sexual activity became associated with the disease. Consequently, in the seventeenth century prostitutes were most commonly associated with the spread of the pox.

The link between venereal disease and sexual intercourse was not clear when the disease first appeared in Europe; however, in the seventeenth century the link was firmly established. Contemporaries took notice of the fact that soldiers and prostitutes, traditionally associated with sexual license and moral disorder, were among its first victims. The link became even clearer as people observed that the disease's first sores often turned up on the genital organs. It was from there a short leap to associating the disease with the sin of lust. The loathsome symptoms were signs that the bodies of those struck with syphilis housed debauched and sinful souls. The godly surmised that the repulsive physical symptoms suffered by the syphilitic constituted an outward sign of greater moral corruption.[33] The divine Richard Baxter asserted that the French disease was a palpable manifestation of one's sinful state, leaving sufferers to 'go about stigmatized with a mark of Gods vengeance, the prognostick or warning of a heavier vengeance.'[34] The pox represented not just a physical disease but a spiritual one as well. It was as if God left His mark of displeasure on sufferers as a grotesque badge of sin.[35] It was impossible to conceal and impossibly shameful to exhibit.

Such stigmatization contributed to the disgust and disdain with which poxed patients were treated. Many assumed that the afflicted brought this suffering on themselves by enticing God's wrath. Claude Quetel has suggested that the seventeenth century brought 'a change in the moral landscape' with Englishmen coming to view the pox with increasing contempt.[36] This change was due in part to the association of the pox with prostitution. Once the venereal link was entrenched, ministers and medical men alike condemned patients with syphilis. John Calvin announced that with the introduction of the pox in Europe, 'God has raised up new diseases against debauchery,' and medical authorities concurred.[37] It was not just the connection with sexual intercourse that made it shameful to suffer from the disease, but the association with illicit sexual contact, which could harm a sufferer's reputation. Richard Baxter's *A Christian Directory* described the consequences of engaging in sinful sexual behavior on one's legacy:

> God hath added one concomitant plague not known before, called commonly, the *Lues Venerea,* the *Venereous Pox;* …[those suffering from the disease] leave an infamous name and memory, when they are dead, (if their sin was publickly known). Let them be never so great, and never so gallant, victorious, successful, liberal, and flattered or applauded while they lived, God ordereth it so, that Truth shall

141

ordinarily prevail, with the Historians that write of them when they are dead; and with all sober men, their names rot and stink, as well as their bodies.[38]

The shame to which Baxter referred could even tarnish the reputation of the surviving family members.[39] Raymond Anselement has noted that during a period in which the disease was allegedly commonplace, there was still a great deal of disapproval associated with syphilis, as evidenced by diary entries in which the authors unreservedly articulated their private disapproval.[40] Anselment has noted that moral condemnation was the reaction most common to those commenting on the suffering of others from the pox and that those connected to the afflicted individual responded with shame and guilt.[41] When Samuel Pepys was concerned that his brother had contracted the pox, he expressed his embarrassment at his brother's physical condition: 'If he lives, he will not be able to show his head—which will be a very great shame to me.' After his brother and the doctor both swore that he did not have the pox, Pepys confessed: 'All which did put me into great comfort as to that reproach which was spread against him.'[42] Fears of shame and reproach by family members of the sufferers illustrate the power of the pox's stigma in seventeenth-century society.

When Pepys's wife, Elizabeth, suffered from a vaginal infection in November 1663, she and her husband were both concerned that those around them might assume she had the French pox. Elizabeth at first refused to allow a nurse to attend her, being 'loath to give occasion of discourse concerning it.' Pepys convinced the physician they hired to prescribe a treatment that the nurse could administer under the guise that 'it be only for the piles.' The physician and Pepys together maneuvered to guard Elizabeth's medical privacy. What they were trying to protect Elizabeth from was a disease stigma more powerful than most others in seventeenth-century society. Although other contemporary diseases and disorders brought embarrassment, it is difficult to find a contemporary condition worthy of comparison, in which sufferers regularly noted shame as a common illness experience.[43]

The embarrassment was just as real for the physicians themselves. The medical professor Eustachio Rudio impressed on his students the need to be cautious in their sexual habits so as not to join the one thousand medical men that he estimated infected with the disease: 'This warning right now I would have liked to intend for the health of physicians. For if it is shameful that others are deceived, it will be most shameful if those who profess the art of medicine are made to shipwreck.'[44] Evidence of the shame associated with the disease lay in its near invisibility as a cause of death in the London Bills of Mortality. It was common knowledge that syphilis was widespread throughout the seventeenth century, yet as the early demographer John Graunt realized, no one wanted to suffer the social stigma of admitting that his or her relative had died of it. Therefore, they often bribed searchers to attribute the death to other diseases, leaving him to conclude that only the most unfortunate '*hated* persons, and such whose very Noses were eaten off, were reported by the Searchers to have died of this too frequent malady.'[45] John Wynell commented on the 'mystery of concealment' regarding what he considered to be the gross underreporting of venereal diseases in the Bills of Mortality. In fact, he claimed to have written his tract on the pox as a response to the 'stupendous growth and spreading' of the disease.[46] The inherent desire to mask the disease and the consequent underreporting of it point to a level of ignominy associated with the pox not commonly seen in seventeenth-century diseases.

In sum, suffering from the French disease was not confined solely to physical symptoms, which could be agonizing and protracted, but also encompassed culturally encoded notions of shame and moral stigmatization, all of which added to the pain of pox patients in early modern England, and all of which influenced the way those who suffered sought treatment.[47] Physicians would have to adapt to meet the needs of these patients or be left behind by empirics who tended to be more responsive to patient demands.

Physicians eager to gain the business of the wealthy suffering from the pox changed the way they practiced medicine to suit the unique needs of these patients. The author of *The Honestie of this Age* noted that for the average patient, 'wee use plaine dealing, and call it the *poxe*, but in great personages, a little to guild ouer the loathsomenesse, wee must call it the *Gowt* or the *Sciatica*.'[48] At least for wealthier venereal patients, some physicians were willing to misdiagnose the pox, so great were the consequences of admitting to suffering from the disease. The moral background of the patient could also factor into a physician's diagnosis. As one eighteenth-century medical tract explained, if a patient presented with symptoms reminiscent of the pox and was deemed to be of 'sober discreet' character, he was diagnosed with scurvy. However, if he was 'inclined to wantonness by reason of his Youth, or sly Countenance,' then he was diagnosed with the pox.[49] Making sure that a patient received the appropriate diagnosis, when such a stigma accompanied a diagnosis of the pox, was a serious consideration for physicians.

As Kevin Siena has convincingly demonstrated, the pox challenged medical practitioners to change the way they offered their services in order to accommodate the disgrace faced by their patients. Perhaps the disgrace engendered by the disease was evidenced most notably by the fact that it spurred venereal patients to seek medical help differently from all other patients. Venereal patients in the seventeenth century demanded confidentiality and patient privacy from their healers.[50] This had never before been a consideration of physicians or of other groups of medical practitioners. Contemporaries dubbed the pox 'the secret disease,' and indeed, there was a considerable amount of secrecy that accompanied sufferers' experience. There are accounts of patients using secret entrances to medical practitioners' offices, seeking consultations in the dark of night, wearing masks to cloak their identity, having medicines sent through utmost secrecy, including resorting to using assumed names.[51]

Medical practitioners recognized the unique needs of venereal patients and responded accordingly. Some began to advertise their ability to be discreet and offered the highest level of confidentiality to their patients. While the disease might have prompted secrecy, the array of advertisements all over London attested to its ubiquity. From handbills to street hawkers, booksellers in coffee shops and advertisements in the periodical press, remedies for the pox were everywhere.[52] Significantly, the advertisements of physicians, surgeons, and empirics were not markedly different from one another. Members from all three touted their therapeutic efficacy and used lay testimony.[53]

Kevin Siena has analyzed the bevy of medical advertisements of Stuart London in which healers of all kinds, including physicians, were vying for business from people with syphilis. These advertisements show that healers specializing in the treatment of venereal disease were among the first practitioners to promise patient confidentiality, while not a single nonvenereologist made a similar claim. These venereologists considered privacy so important that they situated the promise at the top of their bills, along with other crucial selling points, such as the effectiveness and rapidity of their treatments.[54] For instance, when advertising his antivenereal pill, the surgeon Charles Peter was typically discreet: 'I could quote vast numbers of People that have been cured by them, to my great pleasure and profit (but Silence in such cases is and always shall be my resolution.)'[55] It is important to note here that such restraint represented a departure from the manner in which physicians and healers advertised remedies for other types of diseases. It was customary for those who chose to advertise their healing services to state the names of individuals who could act as references. Yet for syphilis, their ability to protect the identity of past patients was a selling point.[56] The desire for secrecy by paying patients was so intense that it actually altered the way those who purported to cure the disease offered their services, both physicians and non-physicians alike.

The same patient base that required false diagnosis of the pox was also desirous of privacy in the treatment of syphilis. Their unique needs affected the types of cures that medical practitioners offered, as wealthy patients wanted to be treated for the disease without anyone knowing it. Physicians and non-physicians alike offered this option. The physician Nicholas Culpeper included a section in his book entitled, 'To Cure the Said French Disease a more private way, with great Secrecy.' The chapter contained a remedy to promote salivation without keeping patients from their daily business.[57] Many tracts on syphilis at least acknowledged that patients desired privacy, especially those whose reputations stood to be ruined by an admission of syphilis. As the surgeon Charles Peter explained, such a person

> cannot have the conveniency of all things requisite, without rendering him liable to a discovery, which Accident may appear as terrible to him, as the *Pox* it self, and whose Reputation may be utterly destroyed by this unhappy, and perhaps never before perpetrated Crime.[58]

His use of the word *crime* indicates the degree of ignominy toward the French disease that was prevalent among the medical and lay community alike. Because an admission of the pox could have damaging repercussions not only for the sick individual, but for the family reputation as well, there were powerful incentives to avoid any association with the disease.

The unique needs of venereal patients changed the way physicians practiced medicine and advertised their services. However, it is important to note that these changes were not exclusive to learned physicians. One man was so concerned about avoiding the black mark to his reputation that the pox would render that he paid a quack twenty-five guineas for his treatments, ten for its cure and fifteen for secrecy.[59] The impetus for altering the way physicians treated their patients and the institution of discretion and patient privacy actually came from other venereologists, many of whom had not received a formal medical education. Siena, in fact, does not distinguish between physicians and others types of practitioners who treated venereal disease when discussing new marketing techniques that evolved to provide for the unique needs of venereal patients. These changes, therefore, did not benefit physicians disproportionately more than other healers, particularly since non-physicians tended to be quicker to alter their treatments and methods in response to the medical marketplace.

However, by the seventeenth century many physicians did treat the pox.[60] There was money to be made in curing the disease, as evidenced by the objections of physicians to the unlicensed practitioners who 'in this Selfish Age' find the business of offering remedies for the pox 'very Gainful.'[61] The amount of advertising carried out by myriad healers, physicians and non-physicians alike, to lure those suffering from the pox also attested to this fact.

There were many treatment options available to those suffering from syphilis in seventeenth-century England. Remedies ranged from the fairly benign, if ineffective, treatments derived from the Galenic model including baths, chicken broth, bloodletting, and syrups, as well as the use of guaiac bark. Some healers, including physicians, utilized dangerous procedures, including mercury cures, cauterizing ulcers with white-hot irons, and trepanation (employed to relieve the headaches associated with the disease).[62] Physicians therefore faced a great deal of competition from surgeons, apothecaries, and innumerable irregular and unlicensed healers who offered a variety of remedies for curing the pox. These competitors had several advantages. They were not encumbered with the lengthy regimen and individualism that characterized the learned physician's approach to patient care. Furthermore, they could suggest a specific remedy directed at the disease rather than at the individual patient that was the same for everyone. An empirical remedy therefore tended to be less expensive and quicker than the treatments offered by physicians.[63]

Moreover, the most common treatments employed by all types of healers were derived from empirical remedies. For example, empirical practitioners initially promoted non-Galenic treatments derived from guaiac wood. Decoctions made from the bark of guaiacum, a wood imported from Hispaniola, was extolled as 'a soveraine remedy against the French-pox,' one that 'doth wonderfully cure.'[64] Guaiacum was an essential part of mixtures such as 'Moses Water.' Full courses of 'wood treatment,' administered by physicians and non-physicians alike, involved elaborate medical regimens including sweating, semi-fasting, and internal and external administration of guaiacum. However, enthusiasm for guaiacum had diminished since its introduction in the early sixteenth century although the sweating and purging promoted by guaiacum, along with sarsaparilla and china root, were still the preferred relief, especially in the early stages of the disease.[65] The treatment that soon gained the upper hand was mercury, either used as an external ointment or ingested, depending on the healer.[66] Mercury treatments were the standard of care for most cases of the pox by the latter half of the seventeenth century, for reasons described later in this chapter.

The fact that learned physicians could offer nothing decidedly different in the way of remedies placed them in a difficult position. For two centuries, physicians had attempted to consolidate their position at the top of the medical ladder, arguing that their medicine, being rational and learned, was the best. It was an extremely important part of their medical code *not* to use empirical remedies, which had no justification in reason or learning, the two principle characteristics of university medicine. Unlicensed healers used empirical remedies, and physicians associated them with a lack of education, lack of experience, and sometimes outright fraud. Roger French has emphasized the significance of the distinction in the minds of physicians between themselves as professionals and the remedies they offered, versus their unlearned competition and their empirical remedies: 'It was professionally important—it was ethical—not to associate with apothecaries or surgeons and not to practice their trades; the learned and rational physician had to be socially, intellectually and financially superior.'[67] Of course, having anything in common with unlearned healers who were not even part of the tripartite medical hierarchy was even more out of the question. Since all types of practitioners used remedies derived from the same basic ingredients, physicians faced the difficult task of distinguishing their treatment for the pox from surgeons, unlearned healers, and the opportunists who offered patients what they wanted: privacy and a quick cure. Physicians had to make the claim that they alone were qualified to devise the correct remedy for a specific patient, thereby undermining their competitors.[68]

Incorporating the pox into physicians' realm of knowledge, addressing the unique needs of patients suffering from the disease, accounting for their initial ambivalence about treating the pox, and stressing the superiority of their remedies derived from empirical treatments all posed serious problems for university-educated physicians. They would have to respond to the disease in a way that made them appear as experts in the treatment of the pox and as actively battling the disease. Physicians relied on their wisdom and good judgment to differentiate themselves from their competition in the cure of a disease where the physical was so clearly entwined with the spiritual and in which the treatment could be as dangerous and unpleasant as the disease itself.

Physicians touted their expertise in the cure of the pox, but their success in the battle to combat the disease was not impressive. Both Keith Thomas and Roy Porter have suggested that early modern medicine was 'losing the struggle against disease,' particularly severe epidemics like syphilis and plague.[69] In making such a statement, they are alluding to the lack of unique therapies developed by physicians and their inability to curb its spread. However, physicians offered more than just treatments for the pox: they managed to explain a disease that was mysterious and hitherto unknown in terms of traditional Galenic medicine, and they argued that they were the most qualified to treat it. Supplying information about the disease conformed to contemporary notions of how authority and expertise were established and helped physicians seem knowledgeable and competent.[70]

Physicians wrote copiously on the pox. In fact, the quantity of medical literature on the subject is second only to that written on the plague.[71] The sheer magnitude of their publications on the pox helped physicians assume an air of authority, just as garnering knowledge about the disease made them appear successful.[72] Patient expectations are culturally constructed and change over time. In the case of the pox, or any distemper, patients expected that the physician they employed was part of a learned profession that retained esoteric knowledge about diseases and their cures. Part of fulfilling patient expectations in seventeenth-century England involved providing knowledge about the disease, including supplying it with a name.

Without a proper name, the disease did not fit neatly into the traditional humoral medical system. Giving the disease a formal name allowed physicians to gain access to what Roger French and Jon Arrizabalaga have termed the 'technical stock in trade of the rational physician and his traditional learning.'[73] This learning was based on Galenic medical theory and proved the physician's greatest resource and was recognized by everyone who had been through a university arts course. There was power and authority in such a system of knowledge because it could explain medical particulars in terms of an entire world picture, one that French and Arrizabalaga maintain was complex enough to dazzle the layperson. Above all, physicians had to make the disease both a rational and learned business in order to bring it into their professional preserve and so maintain their claim that they alone had knowledge of it, comprised of both rational understanding and ancient writings.[74] This would take some effort since physicians had to incorporate the new disease into existing texts in order for Galenic theory to accommodate it. Physicians were, in fact, successful in developing medical theories about the origination and spread of the disease that meshed with their traditional Galenism.

While syphilis undoubtedly posed a challenge to Galenic medicine, it did not prove crippling to the system. Some historians have linked the decline of Galenism and the rise of modern medicine to scientific innovation, including disease theory. According to this line of argument, momentous breakthroughs such as advances in anatomy and the discovery of the circulation of blood by William Harvey in the early seventeenth century produced medical progress and resulted in a form of medicine based on experimental knowledge, observation, and experimentation that replaced a medicine of texts.[75] However, recent work on the history of science has tended to dispel the mystique of scientific progress as well as the timing of and rapidity implied in the term 'scientific revolution.'[76] The basic physiological concepts and associated therapeutic methods of Galenism—notably humoral theory and the practice of bloodletting to get rid of bad humours—had a continuous life extending from Greek antiquity into the nineteenth century.[77] As Mary Lindeman has explained, the system's ability to endure in part was based upon the fact that it was pliant:

> Far from being a rigid and immutable system, it proved especially adaptable; over the centuries it responded to challenges and even absorbed them. Thus the 'decline'of Galenism in academic medicine was a long, slow process that was just barely completed by 1800. There is some good evidence to suggest, moreover, that many of its canons, such as humoralism, persisted much longer.[78]

The flexibility of Galenism allowed its proponents to incorporate the pox into their traditional learning despite a lack of precedent.

Galenic physicians tended to view disease as a barometer of the body as a whole. When a patient suffered from scurvy, for example, the various individual symptoms that appeared, such as purple blotches on the skin, a fetid odor, the swelling of the gums and loosening of the teeth, lassitude, and fainting fits were surface manifestations of a disease in which physicians thought all symptoms were interlinked. Physicians disputed the ultimate cause, but many assumed that the root lay in a 'scorbutic constitution,' brought on through a complicated combination of poor life-style, bad air, bad morals, diet, and so on.[79] Physicians sought to understand how all the

149

symptoms worked together and to treat the body as a whole, rather than treating a single symptom with a single medicine. This was particularly important as medical theory held that distempers were mobile. Like an invading army, a malaise could surface in one location or organ and spread or retreat to another, thereby becoming more dangerous. For instance, if a cough moved from the throat to the lungs, it might become more worrisome. Therefore, all symptoms were significant and needed to be regarded in terms of their effect on the overall health of the individual. Parallel to this was the belief in the importance of forcing a disease out of the body, as poisons trapped within could prove damaging to an individual's health. Rather than allow disorders to remain latent, it was better to expel them with purges, phlebotomy, and sweats.[80]

Physicians utilized this traditional Galenic thinking in their explanation of the pox. Since contemporary medical writing held that symptoms of the disease were varied and mutable, Galenic explanation actually accommodated it quite well. The nebulous nature of the pox required a learned physician to sort out the symptoms. Medical texts loosely defined the disease as 'clap inveterate.' The symptoms of the early stages of the disease were often linked with or confused with gout.[81] A treatise on the cure of the 'French-Pockes' stressed that the disease was 'verie hard to be knowne from the Goute,' while the translation of *The whole worke of that famous chirurgion Maister Iohn Vigo* (1586) discussed gout under the section 'Of the French Pockes.'[82] English physicians acquainted with the long tradition of continental venereal disease studies understood that 'The Pox is an universal moveable Disease, caused by venomous infectious steems, and attended with the worst and mildest, most and fewest, changeable and uncertain symptoms of all kinds.'[83] Numerous medical works contained separate sections entitled 'Of Gonnorrhea,' 'For the running of the Raines,' and 'Of the French Pox,' often with no distinction maintained between the symptoms of the various categories.[84] William Salmon's chapter on gonorrhea characterized it as 'the beginning of the *French* Pox.'[85] Readers of Richard Bunworth's *A new Discovery of the French Disease and the Running of the Reins* (1662) were warned that if simple gonorrhea was left untreated 'either through negligence or bashfulness...it will certainly in a short time turn to the pox.'[86] Most medical authorities agreed that in its early stages, *lues venerea* was curable; however, once the disease was established, the majority admitted that the physician faced a difficult challenge, and a considerable number of them conceded that established cases were rarely cured.[87] Early intervention by a knowledgeable physician was imperative, or so the argument went.

Medical theory therefore delineated venereal diseases as exceedingly dangerous because of their metastatic nature, as these diseases spread throughout the body in some 'malignant,' 'corruptible,' or 'sequential' fashion, which explains why sufferers from venereal diseases sought help so quickly when compared with other medical complaints.[88] Physicians could claim that their expertise in discerning the complicated and changeable symptoms of syphilis was indispensable, as diagnosing the disease properly in its early stages proved essential to a successful outcome. The notion that simple complaints could evolve into the pox, and that the pox would only worsen if left untreated, was a powerful argument for physicians wishing to convince patients of their necessity. They were quick to warn readers of this danger: 'The Pox it self kils no man, but after a long Travail fixes at last upon one symptom, as a Pocky hectick, Ulcer of the Kidney or Bladder, Consumption of the Lungs, Meagrim, *Node*, *Tophe*, Dropsie, Night-pains, &c..'[89] Physicians thereby stressed the need to trust in their expertise, even after the initial stages of the disease had passed, since the danger could increase over time, as the pox 'yet continues, not in the open hostility it exercised before, but more treacherously and slily insinuates it self into the internal and fundamental parts of the Body.'[90] By all accounts, the pox was difficult to discern from other diseases. When making the case that they should be the ones entrusted with diagnosis of the disease, physicians were able to hearken back to their Galenic medical knowledge to present the pox as far more complicated than a disease whose sufferers could self diagnose with certainty. It was a disease that 'so many pretend to [cure], and so few do understand.'[91]

Expertise was particularly imperative given that the most common treatment for the pox in the seventeenth century was mercury, an extremely dangerous substance that could prove lethal if not dosed correctly. There were many forms of mercury available for use by all types of practitioners. A physician could administer mercury in a variety of ways, either internally by mouth or externally by frictions, fumigations, salivations, or applied as plasters.[92] Sufferers dubbed mercury the 'dreadfull remedy.' It was 'a desperate Cure for a desperate Disease.'[93] Some physicians, including Thomas Sydenham and Richard Wiseman, insisted that among available remedies, mercury alone could arrest the disease's progress. Medical theory held that the salivation its "right use" induced occurred when compounds of the metal rose to the brain and then fell like rain from the nose and mouth.[94] The side effects, however, could prove as dreadful as the disease itself.

Even the proponents of this 'most salubrious medicine' were wary of the awful side effects.[95] They had good reason to be, as a patient undergoing a mercury treatment might endure 'sweating' in which he or she was put in an enclosed room, swathed with a mercury ointment from head to foot, and left to sweat. This procedure was extremely uncomfortable for the patient and could prove lethal, as the patient might lose consciousness or suffer heart failure.[96] Even more common was mercurial salivation, in which physicians administered significant doses of mercury to patients with the intent of causing them to salivate profusely. Perhaps one of the reasons why this type of remedy was so popular was because promoting salivation was one of many ways by which early modern doctors tried to rid the body of infectious matter.

Physicians posited that salivation helped evacuate unwanted humours or 'poisons' from the body. Physicians monitored the amount of saliva or sweat their patients produced, often several pints per day. Thomas Sydenham, for example, insisted on about four pints every twenty-four hours. Mercurial treatments usually lasted four to six weeks and were notoriously uncomfortable for patients. The treatments produced appalling side effects including internal pain, intense nausea, and permanent damage to their mouths such as loss of teeth, gum damage, and the complete loss of the uvula, along with allegedly embarrassingly wretched breath.[97] Ulrich Von Hutten, who underwent the treatment, described the effect on patients:

> [their] Throats, their Lungs, with the Roofs of their Mouths, were full of Sores; their Jaws did swell, their Teeth loosen'd, and a stinking Matter continually was voided from these Places…which sort of Cure was indeed so terrible, that many chose rather to die than to be eased thus of their Sickness.[98]

In fact, there are accounts of patients who made this choice, such as the case of a woman whose symptoms returned after a course of salivation in 1710. When her medical practitioner suggested a second course, the thought 'so affrighted her, the last she underwent being so fresh in her Memory, that she resolved the contrary taking leave of him, and said she would rather chuse to dye.'[99] Another patient in 1721 declared he would 'sooner lose his Nose than take Physick.'[100] The terrible effects of the treatment were not lost on physicians, one of whom remarked that 'Under salivation [the patient] is ever dejected.' He described the misery involved, noting that the patient

152

can scarce ever close his eyes but the noisome slaver glides down into his stomach, makes him sick…[the patient] cannot be easy till he has disburthened his stomach of that load of saliva, that was swallowed during his sleep…Under a salivation palsies, numbness, deafness, contractions of the jaws, apoplexies, are often the unhappy consequences.[101]

The ill effects of mercurial salivation prompted the physician to admit, 'I am at a Loss to discover the true reason why the patient is so readily brought to submit to a salivation.'[102] In the seventeenth century the physician Gideon Harvey remarked, 'A Patient had better half hang himself than undergo this Cure, there being nothing comparable to the pain in their mouth, the anguish about their heart and sides, and the extream thirst.'[103] The fact that patients were, by and large, willing to undergo mercurial treatments attests to how frightened they were of leaving the disease untreated and to their eagerness to be rid of it.

The use of mercury for treating syphilis was also congruent with the public's expectations of the appropriate course of treatment for an excruciating and shameful disease. Dreadful diseases called for dreadful remedies, as echoed in *Hamlet*: 'Diseases desperate grown / By desperate appliance are relieved, / Or not at all.'[104] Contemporary medical thinking held that remedies were necessarily unpleasant, as the goal of physic was to eliminate unwholesome humours from the body. Both patient and doctor judged the efficacy of the cure by its ability to illicit a response from the body (usually through vomiting, purging, bleeding, or sweating). Moreover, enduring a horribly painful and expensive cure afforded some recompense for the sin with which God was punishing the sufferer. He or she was performing a sort of medical penance in enduring an unpleasant cure.[105] The fact that the typical course of mercury treatment lasted forty days invoked the feeling of a medical penance by imitating the length of the Lenten season. Bearing some degree of suffering in order to be cured seemed logical, as enduring the pain of healing was considered part of the scourge. This provided physicians with the opportunity to stress the importance of their unique expertise in the cure of such a terrible disease. For a disease whose cure could be as painful as the affliction itself, physicians argued that they were the only ones qualified to take on such a challenge.

Physicians were not the only healers using mercury cures for the pox. Many empirical healers used mercury for poxed patients as well. Physicians had much to gain by convincing patients that the efficacy of mercury cures depended upon the learning and experience of the healer administering the treatments. As dreadful as the disease was, 'so also is the cure abstruse, arduous, and difficult,' noted a physician in his tract on the pox.[106] Physicians stressed the necessity of trusting in the expertise of the learned medical professional: 'If it [mercury] is skillfully managed, it is by far the safest and most effectual Method of all.'[107] The correct choice of healer could keep them from 'perishing of the Pox, who might easily have been cur'd had they fallen into the hands of a skilful Physician.'[108] In his treatise on the pox, the physician L.S. included 'An *Advertisement*, wherein is discover'd the dangerous Practices of *Ignorant Pretenders* to the Cue of this *Disease*.' He advertised his own medicines just as he warned against the lack of skill and expertise of his competitors. He assured his readers that he had

> spent some years in studying to help you in this important Affair. And surely I may (without any breach of Modesty) pretend to some skill in this Business…For I have perus'd no less than three hundred sixty and eight Authors, who have learnedly treated this Disease …I have diligently compar'd what I read in Authors with what I daily observ'd in my own Patients.[109]

What he described were the ideal qualifications of a physician: one who combined real-world experience with copious study of the healing arts. He went on to tout his 'plentiful' experience in healing 'the worst of patients,' which he considered to be 'those who have been spoyl'd by Mountebankes and unskillful Surgeons.'[110] His writing was indicative of the belief held by many physicians that it took a wise and skilled medical professional to undo the mistakes made by the multitude of quacks plying their trade to a gullible public.

Although physicians considered a wise physician who combined book learning and practical experience the ideal choice, they were certainly not the only ones treating the public for the pox. Medical professionals voiced their concern that many empirics lacked the proper knowledge that treating such a complicated distemper required. Charles Peter lamented that of the 'great number of those that pretend to the Cure of this Distemper, I have found very few that could give a rational Account of it.'[111] Peter was amazed by the mischiefs many illiterate Persons have caus'd, by their ill-prepared Doses, many miserable Patients can witness...while we live in a Kingdom so well Furnished with Learned Physicians and Skilful Chyrurgeons, whose Knowledge in Anatomy, and daily Experience, make them the onely Persons capable of undertaking so dangerous a Malady.[112]

The physician John Archer professed to have written his book so that all could have proper medical knowledge, even those who had no access to 'a skillfull Doctor,' implying that self-dosing of mercury was preferable to going to an empiric, whom Archer delineated as an 'ignorant practitioner' who 'poysons the Body with Mercury.'[113]

People who used empirical remedies ran the risk of taking crude mixtures of mercury in the form of pills, a practice Gideon Harvey described as 'a most egregious veil for the shamefac'd Mounsieur.'[114] Empirics' uncontrolled mercury remedies were dangerous because the practitioner possessed no knowledge of medicine or the patient's individual constitution: 'Hence it is their Church-Yards are so well fill'd with dead Bodies, for they use it [salivation] … promiscuously without distinction, or consideration had of their peculiar and different cases.'[115] Other healers purposely set out to deceive patients, as lamented by one physician, who estimated that thousands of people every year lost their lives 'and ten thousands their noses' through the incompetence of healers who 'are full of words and promises, but without any Performance at all.'[116] Physicians' horror stories detailing quack calamities must have at the least given pause to pox patients considering their best recourse when faced with a shameful disease that often necessitated a frightening cure.

Physicians' writing stressed that it was imperative that sufferers not make the mistake of choosing the aid of the 'illiterate Rabble of Mountebanks, Toothdrawers, and Ignoramusses' who touted their skills in the treatment of the pox. Empirics, mountebanks, and other unlearned healers were lumped together in medical men's writing as 'pretenders' who offered cures that were more dangerous than the disease.[117] Gideon Harvey estimated that four out of five venereal cases were made worse by pretenders who attempted to take part in the lucrative treatments.[118] Albert Faber mourned the many patients of 'high and low degree' who 'commonly run the hazard of their lives' at the hands of 'Ignorants, Barber-Surgions and Mountebanks.'[119] The author of *The Tomb of Venus* described in vivid detail the unnecessary suffering that some of his patients endured in the name of treatments before they

155

came to him, giving the example of a married couple who both contracted the pox. They unwisely selected an unskilled healer who improperly managed their sweating cure. According to the author the husband and wife were 'kept in that Furnace of Affliction almost seven Weeks, but with what Success is dreadful to mention.' He detailed the outcome of their treatment and claimed to have been successful in curing them although he was not able to undo the damage already done by the previous healer.[120] Attempts to correct the mistakes resulting from empirics' improper handling of mercury was a common topic in physicians' tracts on the pox, such as John Archer's chapter on 'The Venereal Disease, not well Cured, or Mercury remaining in the Body.'[121] Physicians described the gruesome and painful nature of the disease as well as the unproductive suffering one could undergo at the hands of an unskilled healer to highlight the need for a skillful physician to alleviate the complicated and troublesome symptoms.

Physicians thereby used the danger inherent in mercury treatments to their advantage when attempting to justify themselves as the best choice of healers. They played on the sufferer's insecurity about submitting to a long, uncomfortable course of treatment by touting themselves as the most knowledgeable in administering mercury cures. Doing so not only helped them distinguish themselves from their competition but simultaneously gave them an opportunity to defend their methods against empirics who offered quick cures. Physicians cautioned the public that speedier treatments could prove even more dangerous than lengthier ones: '[The empiric] in three dayes may do you more hurt, than you shall ever [suffer] while you breath.'[122] The author of *The Tomb of Venus* bemoaned the treatment of the husband and wife whose ineptly handled mercury cure was previously described: 'And here I cannot but reflect a little upon the Management these People were under, the same thing being very common Abroad…most People striving who shall Cure quickest, not safest.'[123] In order to counteract such quick cures, physicians attacked not only the unskilled healer's use of mercury but also his or her ability to inflict more harm in a short amount of time than a proper physician would during a traditional forty-day treatment period. They thereby disparaged empirics, who otherwise excelled at developing and selling remedies for the pox.

The pox provided physicians with an opportunity to stress their higher level of expertise in dispensing the physic and in overseeing the sometimes long and drawn-out programs of treatments. Their knowledge also enabled them to explain why they chose to treat the disease in a particular person with a particular remedy, as well as knowing why God sent the disease and if He had left a cure close at hand.[124] Every patient was different and needed continuing advice as his case progressed—this was the type of care that physicians alone usually offered. By stressing the rational approach to the care of the pox as the optimal one, physicians transformed the empirical one-to-one relationship between disease and cure into a complex relationship between a diseased and idiosyncratic patient and a regimen of treatment, a relationship that they could claim only a learned physician could comprehend. [125] Whereas other venereologists offered a single cure-all for anyone suffering from the disease, physicians could tailor a program based on the individual needs of the patient. Other healers did not offer this.[126]

Although in their writing physicians were confident that their methods were the best, the pox was widespread and physicians proved inadequate in meeting the challenge of curbing it. While they were never able to meet this challenge successfully in the seventeenth century, they deflected some of the blame for not stemming its progress through their theories, which essentially held individual actions responsible for encouraging the spread of disease. By choosing to impugn behavior already deemed sinful by the public, physicians provided a logical explanation for the continuing increase in cases of the pox. Doing so gave an unfamiliar disease the familiar context of divine punishment for sinful behavior that meshed with the contemporary worldview. Paul Slack has pointed out that it was not enough to simply name and prescribe a remedy: 'Only if a disease was given a cause as well as a name and a cure could it be accounted for satisfactorily.'[127] Physicians' writing about the pox met this demand and made the illness less disturbing by setting it in the context of familiar assumptions.

In the seventeenth century, the pox was intimately linked to ideas about sin and illicit sexual behavior and was generally considered a justly deserved punishment from God for lascivious behavior: the disease 'GOD doth send… for a scourge to the people for whordness.'[128] The medical profession had the difficult task of responding to a disease that was repugnant, in both the physical and moral sense, and one that many feared to be infecting more and more people at an alarming rate. Physicians were not particularly successful at curbing the number of pox cases, and their treatments for the disease tended to be distressingly similar to those offered by lay healers.

Physicians proved able to adapt their therapeutics and to institute patient privacy as a result of the unique demands of sufferers of the pox, and doing so kept them competitive with empirics. Yet despite their limited offerings when compared to empirics, physicians wished the public to view them as experts in the care of the pox. The challenges that the disease posed to the medical profession has led some historians to conclude that syphilis was a failure for physicians and a bonanza for unlicensed healers of all kinds who could offer comparable care at a fraction of the price.[129] However, along with the challenges of the new disease, the pox offered physicians a unique opportunity to construct knowledge about its origination and spread. As the next chapter will demonstrate, they capitalized on this opportunity by choosing to explain the disease in medical terms that supported already–present misogynistic assumptions about the dangers of uncontrolled female sexuality. Physicians' picture of the pox made them successful in dealing with the disease, not because they developed any type of revolutionary treatment methods, but because their attempts to name and explain the pox mitigated fears and provided comfort through explanation. These familiar assumptions held that in the majority of cases, the disease was punishment from God, and therefore was preventable if the population refrained from engaging in sinful sexual behavior. Physicians' theories on and writing about the pox furthermore justified efforts to impose greater control over the lives of the lower classes forced to rely on public institutions to cure their syphilis.

Notes

1   C. Blackwood, *Some Pious Treatises Being 1. A Bridle for the Tongue: Or, a Treatise Directing a Christian How to Order His His [Sic] Words in a Holy Maner. 2. The Present Sweetness, and Future Bitterness of a Delicious Sin. 3. A Christians Groans under the Body of Sin. 4. Proving the Resurrection of the Same Body Committed to the Dust: Also, the Not Dying of the Soul within the Body. 5. Tractatus De Clavibus Ecclesiae* (1654), title page.

2   W. Clowes, *A Profitable and Necessarie Booke of Observations* (1596). See also W.Clowes, *A Short and Profitable Treatise Touching the Cure of the Disease Called (Morbus Gallicus) by Unctions* (1579).

3   P.L. Allen, *The Wages of Sin: Sex and Disease, Past and Present* (Chicago: University of Chicago Press, 2000), 42.

4   The pox generally referred to syphilis, but there is some speculation by

historians that in some cases the disease might have been gonorrhoea or other sexually transmitted diseases, or even assorted urinary tract infections. The term syphilis was not often used during the period. It was more commonly referred to as the *lues venerea*, the pox, the French pox, or the French disease. The Bills of Mortality list the disease that we generally think of as syphilis as the French Pox.

5   Anon., *Some Reasons of a Member of the Committee, Etc. Of the Trustees of the Infirmary in James Street Westminster, near St. James Park, for His Dividing against the Admission of Venereal Patients* (1738). Cited in K. Siena, *Venereal Disease, Hospitals and the Urban Poor: London's 'Foul Wards,' 1600-1800* (Rochester: University of Rochester Press, 2004), 1, 3. Siena notes that despite the prevailing morality against venereal patients, they were not always rejected by hospitals. He goes so far as to say that 'early London hospitals treated venereal patients as a rule, not an exception.' As this chapter will demonstrate, they did so not out of charity alone, but with the aim of reforming the behaviour that led to the disease.

6   For a background to syphilis, see K. Kiple, ed., *The Cambridge World History of Human Disease* (Cambridge: Cambridge University Press, 1993) and C. Clayton Dennie, M.D., *A History of Syphilis* (Springfield: Charles C. Thomas, 1962).

7   K. Siena, *Venereal Disease, Hospitals and the Urban Poor: London's 'Foul Wards,' 1600-1800* (Rochester: Rochester Studies in Medical History. University of Rochester Press, 2004), 12.

8   K. Siena, *Venereal Disease, Hospitals and the Urban Poor: London's 'Foul Wards,' 1600-1800*, 65.

9   M. Pelling, 'Medicine and the Environment in Shakespeare's England,' in M. Pelling (ed.), *The Common Lot: Sickness, Medical Occupations and the Urban Poor in Early Modern England* (London: Longman, 1998), 28.

10   See for example A. Wear, 'Medical Ethics in Early Modern England,' in A. Wear, J. Geyer-Kordesch, and R. French (eds), *Doctors and Ethics: The Earlier Historical Setting of Professional Ethics* (Amsterdam: Rodopi, 1993) and M. Pelling, 'Appearance and Reality: Barber-Surgeons, the Body and Disease,' in L. Beier and R. Finlay (eds), *London 1500-1700: The Making of the Metropolis* (New York: Longman, 1986).

11   There is a debate over whether syphilis was new to Europe in the late fifteenth century, but for the purposes of this chapter, the salient point is that most early modern English men and women believed that the disease was new. For a discussion of this, see B. Baker, and G.

Armelagos, 'The Origin and Antiquity of Syphilis: Paleo-Pathological Diagnosis and Interpretation,' *Current Anthropology* 29, no. 5 (1988); F. Livingstone, 'On the Origin of Syphilis: An Alternative Hypothesis,' *Current Anthropology* 32, no. 5 (1991); and J. Arrizabalaga, 'Syphilis,' in K. Kiple (ed.), *The Cambridge World History of Human Disease* (Cambridge: Cambridge University Press, 1993).

12 M. Pelling, 'Appearance and Reality: Barber-Surgeons, the Body and Disease,' 10, 96 and also C. Webster (ed.), *Health, Medicine, and Mortality in the Sixteenth Century* (New York: Cambridge University Press, 1979).

13 J. S., M.D. *A Short Compendium of Chirurgery Containing Its Grounds & Principles : More Particularly Treating of Imposthumes, Wounds, Ulcers, Fractures & Dislocations : Also a Discourse of the Generation and Birth of Man, Very Necessary to Be Understood by All Midwives and Child-Bearing Women: With the Several Methods of Curing the French Pox, the Cure of Baldness, Inflammation of the Eyes, and Toothach, and an Account of Blood-Letting, Cup-Setting, and Blooding with Leeches* (1678).

14 R. Diaz de Isla, *Treatise on the Serpentine Malady* (1539). Cited in R. Porter, *The Greatest Benefit to Mankind* (New York: W.W. Norton & Company, 1997), 174. See also I.F. Nicholson, *The Modern Syphilis: Or, the True Method of Curing Every Stage and Symptom of the Venereal Disease* (1718), 4-5.

15 U. Von Hutten, *De Morbo Gallico. A Treatise of the French Disease, Publish'd above 200 Years Past* (1730).

16 P. Barrough, 'The Sixth Booke Containing the Cure of the Disease Called Morbus Gallicus, in *The Methode of Physicke* (1596), 361-2.

17 T. Beard, *The theatre of Gods judgements wherein is represented the admirable justice of God against all notorious sinners* (1642), 252.

18 R. French and J. Arrizabalaga, 'Coping with the French Disease: University Practitioners' Strategies and Tactics in the Transition from the Fifteenth to the Sixteenth Century,' in R. French, J. Arrizabalaga, A. Cunningham and L. Garcia-Ballester (eds), *Medicine from the Black Death to the French Disease* (Aldershot: Ashgate, 1998), 252.

19 S. *Prothylantinon, or, Some Considerations of a Notable Expedient to Root out the French Pox from the English Nation with Excellent Defensive Remedies to Preserve Mankind from the Infection of Pocky Women : Also an Advertisement, Wherein Is Discover'd the Dangerous Practices of Ignorant Pretenders to the Cure of the Disease* (1673), A5.

20 W. Clowes, *A Briefe and Necessarie Treatise, Touching the Cure of the Disease*

Called Morbus Gallicus, or Lues Venerea, by Vnctions and Other Approoued
Waies of Curing: Nevvlie Corrected and Augmented by William Clowes of
London (1585). St. Thomas Hospital also received syphilis patients.

21 M. Pelling, 'Appearance and Reality: Barber-Surgeons, the Body and
    Disease,' 97-98. Pelling provides a detailed analysis of William's
    Clowes's treatment of syphilis in seventeenth-century England.

22 C. Peter, *A Description of the Venereal Disease: Declaring the Causes, Signs,
    and Effects, and Cure Thereof. With a Discourse of the Most Wonderful
    Antivenereal Pill* (1678), 9.

23 G. Harvey, *Great Venus Unmasked, or, a More Exact Discovery of the
    Venereal Evil, or French Disease Comprizing the Opinions of Most Antient and
    Modern Physicians with the Particular Sentiment of the Author Touching the Rise,
    Nature, Subject, Causes, Kinds, Progress, Changes, Signs, and Prognosticks of
    the Said Evil : Together with Luculent Problems, Pregnant Observations, and the
    Most Practical Cures of That Disease, and Virulent Gonorrhoea, or Running of
    the Reins* (1672), 97.

24 I.F. Nicholson, *The Modern Syphilis* (1718), 1.

25 R. Trumbach, *Sex and the Gender Revolution*, vol. 1, *Heterosexuality and the
    Third Gender in Enlightenment London* (Chicago: University of Chicago
    Press, 1998).

26 K. Siena, *Venereal Disease, Hospitals, and the Urban Poor: London's 'Foul
    Wards,' 1600-1800* (Rochester: University of Rochester Press, 2004), 4,
    42.

27 M. Pelling, 'Appearance and Reality: Barber-Surgeons, the Body and
    Disease,' 89. See also Roy Porter, *Bodies Politic: Disease, Death, and Doctors
    in Britain, 1650-1900* (London: Reaktion Books, 2001), 35-88 and
    S.M. Grieco, 'The Body, Appearance and Sexuality,' in *Renaissance and
    Enlightenment Paradoxes*, N.Z. Davis and A. Farge (eds), (Cambridge,
    MA: Belknap Press, 1993), 46-64. Pelling points out that these attitudes
    were not confined to any one class, whether rural or urban, but that
    urban life added new dimensions to attitudes about the body, as the city
    became the main arena for competition among social aspirants. As a
    note of interest, in the late medieval period, adulteresses across Europe
    were often marked by having their noses chopped off, a punishment
    which must have seemed like a similar penalty. Noses were linked to
    sexuality. Indeed, medieval scholars stressed the connection between a
    person's nose and his or her sexual activities. See V. Groebner, *Defaced:
    The Visual Culture of Violence in the Late Middle Ages* (New York: Zone

Books, 2004), 72-3.

28 M.Pelling, 'Appearance and Reality: Barber-Surgeons, the Body and Disease,' 89-92. Pelling notes this increased sensitivity to defect or deformity was similarly represented in Elizabethan and Jacobean clothing, which concealed much of the body from public view. It was also a factor in personal grooming, as during the Jacobean period, men's hair was allowed to grow longer and more of women's hair was in view, just when it seemed that the likelihood of hair loss by disease was at its greatest. Wigs rapidly evolved to fill the gap.

29 Quoted in R. Anselment, *The Realms of Apollo: Literature and Healing in Seventeenth-Century England* (Newark: University of Delaware Press, 1995), 137.

30 Peter Lewis Allen provides a concise overview of the relationship between syphilis and sin in the minds of early modern people in the chapter, 'The Just Rewards of Unbridled Lust: Syphilis in Early Modern Europe,' found in P.L. Allen, *The Wages of Sin: Sex and Disease, Past and Present* (Chicago: University of Chicago Press, 2000).

31 P. Lowe, *An Easie, Certaine, and Perfect Method, to Cure and Preuent the Spanish Sicknes Wherby the Learned and Skilfull Chirurgian May Heale a Great Many Other Diseases* (1596).

32 Paracelsus, *An Excellent Treatise Teaching Howe to Cure the French-Pockes with All Other Diseases Arising and Growing Thereof, and in a Manner All Other Sicknesses. Drawne out of the Bookes of That Learned Doctor and Prince of Phisitians, Theophrastus Paracelsus. Compiled by the Learned Phillippus Hermanus, Phisition and Chirurgion,* trans. John Hester (1590). For this idea explored in the secondary literature, see R. Davenport-Hines, *Sex, Death and Punishment: Attitudes toward Sex and Sexuality in Britain since the Renaissance* (London: Collins, 1990).

33 P.L. Allen, *The Wages of Sin: Sex and Disease, Past and Present*, 42-3.

34 R. Baxter, *A Christian Directory, or, a Summ of Practical Theologie and Cases of Conscience Directing Christians How to Use Their Knowledge and Faith, How to Improve All Helps and Means, and to Perform All Duties, How to Overcome Temptations, and to Escape or Mortifie Every Sin: In Four Parts* (1673), 397.

35 P.L. Allen, *The Wages of Sin: Sex and Disease, Past and Present*, 42.

36 C. Quetel, *History of Syphilis*, trans. Judith Braddock and Brian Pike (Baltimore: Johns Hopkins University Press, 1990), 73-5.

37 P.L. Allen, *The Wages of Sin: Sex and Disease, Past and Present*, 42-3. J. Arrizabalaga, J. Henderson, and R. French, *The Great Pox: The French*

Disease in Renaissance Europe (New Haven: Yale University Press, 1997). For contemporary examples see Anon., *A Treatise Concerning the Plague and Pox* (1652) and Edwards, *A Treatise Concerning the Plague and the Pox Discovering as Well the Meanes How to Preserve from the Danger of These Infectious Contagions, as Also How to Cure Those Which Are Infected with Either of Them.* (1652).

38   R. Baxter, *A Christian Directory, or, a Summ of Practical Theologie and Cases of Conscience Directing Christians How to Use Their Knowledge and Faith, How to Improve All Helps and Means, and to Perform All Duties, How to Overcome Temptations, and to Escape or Mortifie Every Sin: In Four Parts* (1673), 397.

39   Kevin Siena likens syphilis to an ancient disease similarly associated with shame: 'Venereal patients were society's new lepers to be laughed at, their ulcers and collapsed noses unmistakable badges of shame.' K. Siena, 'Pollution, Promiscuity, and the Pox: English Venereology and the Early Modern Medical Discourse on Social and Sexual Danger,' *Journal of the History of Sexuality* 8, no. 4 (1998), 572. For a discussion on how the negative associations of leprosy may have been passed down to syphilitics, see S.N. Brody, *The Disease of the Soul: Leprosy in Medieval Literature* (London: Cornell University Press, 1974).

40   For instance, Edward Lake's diary discusses the suffering endured by the Countess of Danby because her elder son and his family were poxed. He offered little sympathy to the countess, remarking that her suffering was 'just recompense for her ill usage of her nearest relations.' G.P. Elliot (ed.), *Diary of Dr. Edward Lake* (London: Camden Society, no. 39, 1846), 16 in R. Anselment, 'Seventeenth-Century Pox: The Medical and Literary Realities of Venereal Disease,' *Seventeenth Century* [Great Britain] 4, no. 2 (1989), 143.

41   R. Anselment, *The Realms of Apollo: Literature and Healing in Seventeenth-Century England,* 143.

42   R. Latham, ed., *The Shorter Pepys* (Berkeley: University of California Press, 1985), 364-365. Excerpts are from March 14, 15-16, 1664.

43   Cited in Siena, *Venereal Disease, Hospitals and the Urban Poor: London's 'Foul Wards,' 1600-1800,* 38, 34-5.

44   E. Rudio, *De Morbus Occultis Et Venenatis* (Venice: 1604), 168-9. Cited in W. Schleiner, 'Moral Attitudes toward Syphilis and Its Prevention in the Renaissance,' *Bulletin of the History of Medicine* 68, no. 3 (1994), 403-404.

45   J. Graunt, *Natural and Political Observations Made Upon the Bills of Mortality,* Walter Willcox (ed.), (Baltimore: Johns Hopkins University

Press, 1939), 37. Graunt claimed that only 392 out of 229,250 people who died were recorded as having perished from syphilis. That represents only 0.0017 percent. Richard Baxter concurred that the legacy of those who died of syphilis was a grim one, as they 'leave an infamous name and memory, when they are dead, (if their sin was publickly known).' R. Baxter, *A Christian Directory, or, a Summ of Practical Theologie and Cases of Conscience Directing Christians How to Use Their Knowledge and Faith, How to Improve All Helps and Means, and to Perform All Duties, How to Overcome Temptations, and to Escape or Mortifie Every Sin: In Four Parts* (1673), 397.

46 J. Wynell, *Lues Venera, or a perfect cure for the French pox* (1660).

47 In the past, it has been argued that the social stigma associated with venereal disease was not present until the eighteenth century. For a refutation of this, see R. Anselment, 'Seventeenth-Century Pox: The Medical and Literary Realities of Venereal Disease.' Anselment uses literature to document that not only did seventeenth-century people fear the physical effects of syphilis, but that they also reacted to syphilis with shame and guilt.

48 Anon, *The Honestie of This Age* (1615).

49 *Medicina Flagellata or The Doctor Scarify'd* 1721, 18. Cited in P. Wilson, *Surgery, Skin, and Syphilis: Daniel Turner's London (1667-1741)* (Amsterdam: Rodopi, 1999), 70. It is worth noting that a similar situation occurred with lunacy. According to the bills of mortality; only paupers died by lunacy; everyone else received other diagnoses. See J. Boulton and J. Black, '"Those, that die by reason of their madness": Dying insane in London, 1629-1830,' *History of Psychiatry* 23.1 (March, 2012): 27-39.

50 K. Siena, 'The "Foul Disease" And Privacy: The Effects of Venereal Disease and Patient Demand on the Medical Marketplace in Early Modern London.' *Bulletin of the History of Medicine* 75: 2 (2001), 200-1.

51 P. Wilson, *Surgery, Skin, and Syphilis: Daniel Turner's London (1667-1741)*, 68.

52 P. Wilson, *Surgery, Skin, and Syphilis: Daniel Turner's London (1667-1741)*, 71.

53 J. Barry, 'Publicity and the Public Good: Presenting Medicine in Eighteenth-Century Bristol' in W. Bynum and R. Porter (eds), *Medical Fringe and Medical Orthodoxy, 1750-1850* (London: Croom Helm, 1987), 29, 32.

54 K. Siena, 'The "Foul Disease" And Privacy: The Effects of Venereal Disease and Patient Demand on the Medical Marketplace in Early Modern London,' 200.

55 C. Peter, *A Description of the Venereal Disease: Declaring the Causes. Signs, and Effects, and Cure Thereof. With a Discourse of the Most Wonderful Antivenereal Pill* (1678), 12.

56 K. Siena, 'The "Foul Disease" And Privacy: The Effects of Venereal Disease and Patient Demand on the Medical Marketplace in Early Modern London,' 200-1.

57 N. Culpeper, *Physical Receipts; or, the New English Physician* (1690), 46.

58 C. Peter, *Observations on the Venereal Disease, with the True Way of Curing the Same* (1686), 74.

59 Cited in P. Wilson, 'Exposing the Secret Disease: Recognizing and Treating Syphilis in Daniel Turner's London,' in Linda Merians (ed.), *The Secret Malady: Venereal Disease in Eighteenth-Century Britain and France* (Lexington: University Press of Kentucky, 1996), 68.

60 K. Siena examined the British Library's 512 medical advertisements from a variety of practitioners and found that more than half of them advertised treatment for the disease, more than 300 titles printed in London between 1650 and 1800, prompting him to pose the question, how many London physicians could afford *not* to treat the pox? The evidence from the handbills he researched shows that a significant portion of London physicians treated syphilis, and that they vied aggressively to attract pox patients. K. Siena, 'The "Foul Disease" And Privacy: The Effects of Venereal Disease and Patient Demand on the Medical Marketplace in Early Modern London,' 4. For the later period, see W. Bynum, 'Treating the Wages of Sin: Venereal Disease and Specialism in Eighteenth-Century Britain,' in W. Bynum and R. Porter (eds), *Medical Fringe and Medical Orthodoxy, 1750-1850* (London: Croom Helm, 1987).

61 F. J., *The Modern Syphilis* (1718). See also J. Wynell, MD, *Lues Venera Wherein the Names, Nature, Subject, Causes, Signes, and Cure, Are Handled, Mistakes in These Discovered, Rectified, Doubts and Questions Succinctly Resolved* (1660) and R. Bunworth, *A New Discovery of the French Disease and Running of the Reins Their Causes, Signs, with Plain and Easie Direction of Perfect Curing the Same* (1662), A6-7.

62 For a concise discussion of treatments of venereal diseases, see P.L. Allen, *The Wages of Sin: Sex and Disease, Past and Present* (Chicago:

University of Chicago Press, 2000), 51-54. For a contemporary account, see T. Sydenham, *A New Method of Curing the French-Pox Written by an Eminent French Author; Together with the Practice and Method of Monsieur Blanchard; as Also Dr. Sydenham's Judgment on the Same; to Which Is Added Annotations and Observations by William Salmon* (1690).

63   R. French and J. Arrizabalaga, 'Coping with the French Disease: University Practitioners' Strategies and Tactics in the Transition from the Fifteenth to the Sixteenth Century,' 255-6.

64   L. Coelson, *The Poor-Mans Physician and Chyrurgion* (1656), 392; G. Bruele, *Praxis Medicinae; or, the Physicians Practice* (1639), 392; and T. Brugis, *Vade Mecum; or, a Companion for a Chyrurgion* (1652), 124. Cited in J. Arrizabalaga, J. Henderson, and R. French, *The Great Pox: The French Disease in Renaissance Europe,* 141. On guaiacum as a cure for syphilis see R. Munger, 'Guaiacum, the Holy Wood from the New World,' *Journal of the History of Medicine,* 4 (1949).

65   M. Lindeman, *Medicine and Society in Early Modern Europe*, W. Beik and T.C.W. Blanning (eds), *New Approaches to European History* (Cambridge: Cambridge University Press, 1999), 57. Oswei Temkin has claimed that in the sixteenth century physicians individualized guaiac treatments to their patients, thus bringing them into the realm of traditional medical practice. O. Temkin, 'Therapeutic Trends and the Treatment of Syphilis Before 1900' in *The Double Face of Janus and Other Essays In the History of Medicine,* Owsei Temkin (ed.), (Baltimore: Johns Hopkins University Press, 1977), 472-484.

66   R. French and J. Arrizabalaga, 'Coping with the French Disease: University Practitioners' Strategies and Tactics in the Transition from the Fifteenth to the Sixteenth Century,' 255. Cures for syphilis derived from guaiac wood arrived in Europe in 1517 and were hailed as a new treatment for syphilis. Ulrich Von Hutten (who suffered with mercury cures) praised it as the mercy of God, although in actuality it had no effect against syphilis; it just induced sweating. See P.L. Allen, *The Wages of Sin: Sex and Disease, Past and Present,* 55. For a contemporary account of the merits of this treatment, see U. Von Hutten, *De Morbo Gallico. A Treatise of the French Disease, Publish'd above 200 Years Past* (1730); G. Harvey, *Great Venus: A New Method of Curing the French-Pox* (Amsterdam: 1690); and R. Bunworth, *A New Discovery of the French Disease and Running of the Reins Their Causes, Signs, with Plain and Easie Direction of Perfect Curing the Same* (1662). For secondary accounts of

guaiac bark see R. Munger, 'Guaiacum, the Holy Wood from the New World,' *Journal of the History of Medicine,* 4 (1949).

67 R. French and J. Arrizabalaga, 'Coping with the French Disease: University Practitioners' Strategies and Tactics in the Transition from the Fifteenth to the Sixteenth Century,' 251-2. For ethics behind this, see R. French, 'The Medical Ethics of Gabriele De Zerbi' in *Doctors and Ethics: The Earlier Historical Setting of Professional Ethics* A. Wear, J. Geyer-Kordesch, and R. French (eds), (Amsterdam: Rodopi, 1993), 74.

68 J. Barry, 'Publicity and the Public Good: Presenting Medicine in Eighteenth-Century Bristol,' 32.

69 R. Porter, *Disease, Medicine, and Society in England, 1550-1860* (Basingstoke: Macmillan, 1987), 16. A similar sentiment is expressed in K. Thomas, *Religion and the Decline of Magic* (New York: Scribner, 1971), 8-10.

70 J. Arrizabalaga, J. Henderson, and R. French, *The Great Pox: The French Disease in Renaissance Europe,* 9, 104, 121.

71 J. Arrizabalaga, J. Henderson, and R. French, *The Great Pox: The French Disease in Renaissance Europe,* 8. Lewis Jillings contends that by 1600 some 285 works on the disease had appeared. L. Jillings, 'The Aggression of the Cured Syphilitic: Ulrich Von Hutten's Projection of His Disease as Metaphor.' *The German Quarterly* 68, no. 1 (1995), 5.

72 J. Arrizabalaga, J. Henderson, and R. French, *The Great Pox: The French Disease in Renaissance Europe,* 17.

73 R. French and J. Arrizabalaga, 'Coping with the French Disease: University Practitioners' Strategies and Tactics in the Transition from the Fifteenth to the Sixteenth Century,' 252-4.

74 R. French and J. Arrizabalaga, 'Coping with the French Disease: University Practitioners' Strategies and Tactics in the Transition from the Fifteenth to the Sixteenth Century,' 252, 254.

75 M. Lindeman, *Medicine and Society in Early Modern Europe,* 66.

76 S. Lawrence, *Charitable Knowledge: Hospital Pupils and Practitioners in Eighteenth-Century London* (Cambridge: Cambridge University Press, 1996), 20.

77 N. Sirasi, *Medieval and Early Renaissance Medicine: An Introduction to Knowledge and Practice* (Chicago: University of Chicago Press, 1990), 97, 70-1.

78 M. Lindeman, *Medicine and Society in Early Modern Europe,* 67-8.

79 R. Porter and D. Porter, *In Sickness and in Health: The British Experience*

1650-1850 (London: Fourth Estate, 1988), 142-3.

80 R. Porter and D. Porter, *In Sickness and in Health: The British Experience 1650-1850*, 142-3.

81 P. Levens, *A Right Profitable Boole for All Diseases Called, the Path-Way to Health* (1632), 50 and C. Peter, *Observations on the Venereal Disease, with the True Way of Curing the Same*, 56.

82 P. Hermanni, *An Excellent Treatise Teaching Howe to Cure the French-Pockes*, trans. Iohn Hester (1590), 4 and J. de Vigo, *The Whole Worke of That Famous Chirurgion Maister Iohn Vigo*, trans. Bartholomew Traheron (1586), 262-69.

83 G. Harvey, *Little Venus Unmask'd; or, a Perfect Discovery of the French Pox* (1670), 25. Cited in R. Anselment, *The Realms of Apollo: Literature and Healing in Seventeenth-Century England* (Newark: University of Delaware Press, 1995), 136-7.

84 M. Nedham, *Medela Medicinae* (1665), 83-4 and R. Williams, *Physical Rarities* (1652), 84.

85 W. Salmon, *Select Physical and Chyrurgical Observations* (1687), 227.

86 R. Bunworth, *A New Discovery of the French Disease and Running of the Reins Their Causes, Signs, with Plain and Easie Direction of Perfect Curing the Same*, 60.

87 R. Anselment, *The Realms of Apollo: Literature and Healing in Seventeenth-Century England*, 141. See for example N. Culpeper, *Culpeper's School of Physick* (1659), 358; N. de Blegny, *New and Curious Observations Concerning the Art of Curing the Venereal Disease, and the Accidents It Produces* (1676), 45; L.S., *Profulacticon: Or Some Considerations of a Notable Expedient to Root out the French Pox from the English Nation. With Excellent Defensive Remedies to Preserve Mankind from the Infection of Pocky Women* (1673), A4; and J. Pechy, *The Store-House of Physical Practice* (1695), 506.

88 P. Wilson, *Surgery, Skin, and Syphilis: Daniel Turner's London (1667-1741)*, 70-71 see also M. Nicolson, 'The Metastatic Theory of Pathogenesis and the Professional Interests of the Eighteenth-Century Physician,' *Medical History* 32 (1988), 281.

89 G. Harvey, *Little Venus Unmask'd; or, a Perfect Discovery of the French Pox*, 72.

90 M. Nedham, *Medela Medicinae*, 36.

91 Anon., *An advertisement at the blew ball in Great Knight-Rider-Street, by Doctors Commons Back-gate liveth a physician which hath a pill far beyond any medicament yet ever known, or at least published; which cureth those diseases so*

many pretend to, and so few do understand, called, the French Pox and gonorrhea... (1675)

92 P. Wilson, *Surgery, Skin, and Syphilis: Daniel Turner's London (1667-1741)*, 74-5.

93 R. Anselment, *The Realms of Apollo: Literature and Healing in Seventeenth-Century England*.

94 See for example J. Wynell, MD, *Lues Venera Wherein the Names, Nature, Subject, Causes, Signes, and Cure, Are Handled, Mistakes in These Discovered, Rectified, Doubts and Questions Succinctly Resolved* (1660), 73, 71.

95 T. Sydenham, *The Entire Works of Dr. Thomas Sydenham*, trans. John Swan (London: R. Cave, 1763), 352 and R. Wiseman, *Severall Chirurgicall Treatises* (1676), 278. Harvey recognizes its 'salubrious nature' in G. Harvey, *Little Venus Unmask'd; or, a Perfect Discovery of the French Pox*, 118. See also T. Brugis, *Vade Mecum; or, a Companion for a Chyrurgion*, 278 and J. Pechy, *The Store-House of Physical Practice*, 508-9.

96 R. French and J. Arrizabalaga, 'Coping with the French Disease: University Practitioners' Strategies and Tactics in the Transition from the Fifteenth to the Sixteenth Century,' 272.

97 See P. Wilson, *Surgery, Skin, and Syphilis: Daniel Turner's London (1667-1741)*, 161-6; O. Temkin, 'Therapeutic Trends and the Treatment of Syphilis before 1900,' 521-2; R. French and J. Arrizabalaga, 'Coping with the French Disease: University Practitioners' Strategies and Tactics in the Transition from the Fifteenth to the Sixteenth Century,' 272; and P.L. Allen, *The Wages of Sin: Sex and Disease, Past and Present*. For a primary source example see Jean Astruc's notes on the care of specific patients. J. Astruc, *A Treatise of Venereal Diseases, in Nine Books*, trans. William Barrowby (1754), 183-92.

98 U. Von Hutten, *De Morbo Gallico. A Treatise of the French Disease, Publish'd above 200 Years Past*. 9.

99 Anon., *The Tomb of Venus* (1710), 66-70.

100 Cited in K. Siena, *Venereal Disease, Hospitals and the Urban Poor: London's 'Foul Wards,' 1600-1800*, 24.

101 N. Robinson, *A Treatise of the Venereal Disease* (1736), 302-3.

102 N. Robinson, *A Treatise of the Venereal Disease* (1736), 259. Cited in K. Siena, *Venereal Disease, Hospitals and the Urban Poor: London's 'Foul Wards,' 1600-1800*, 24.

103 G. Harvey, *Little Venus Unmask'd; or, a Perfect Discovery of the French Pox*, 93. See also W. Salmon, *Select Physical and Chyrurgical Observations*, 262.

104 W. Shakespeare, "Hamlet," in *The Complete Pelican Shakespeare* Alfred Harbage (ed.) (New York: Viking Penguin, 1969), IV.iii. 9-11.

105 In addition to these beliefs, patient expectations sometimes held that just completing the course of the cure amounted to a successful cure, regardless of the eradication of the disease. For more on this, see L. Merians (ed.), *The Secret Malady: Venereal Disease in Eighteenth-Century Britain and France* (Lexington: University Press of Kentucky, 1996).

106 J. Astruc, *A Treatise of Venereal Diseases, in Nine Books,* I. 235.

107 J. Astruc, *A Treatise of Venereal Diseases, in Nine Books,* I. 235.

108 L.S., *Profulacticon: Or Some Considerations of a Notable Expedient to Root out the French Pox from the English Nation. With Excellent Defensive Remedies to Preserve Mankind from the Infection of Pocky Women,* A4-A5.

109 L.S., *Profulacticon: Or Some Considerations of a Notable Expedient to Root out the French Pox from the English Nation. With Excellent Defensive Remedies to Preserve Mankind from the Infection of Pocky Women,* A2.

110 L.S., *Profulacticon: Or Some Considerations of a Notable Expedient to Root out the French Pox from the English Nation. With Excellent Defensive Remedies to Preserve Mankind from the Infection of Pocky Women,* A2.

111 C. Peter, *A Description of the Venereal Disease: Declaring the Causes, Signs, and Effects, and Cure Thereof. With a Discourse of the Most Wonderful Antivenereal Pill,* 10.

112 C. Peter, *A Description of the Venereal Disease: Declaring the Causes, Signs, and Effects, and Cure Thereof. With a Discourse of the Most Wonderful Antivenereal Pill* (1678), 4.

113 J. Archer, *Secrets Disclosed; or, a Treatise of Consumptions; Their Various Causes and Cure* (1693), A4.

114 G. Harvey, *Little Venus Unmask'd; or, a Perfect Discovery of the French Pox,* 102.

115 Anon., *The Tomb of Venus,* 8-9.

116 L.S., *Prothylantinon, or, Some Considerations of a Notable Expedient to Root out the French Pox from the English Nation with Excellent Defensive Remedies to Preserve Mankind from the Infection of Pocky Women: Also an Advertisement, Wherein Is Discover'd the Dangerous Practices of Ignorant Pretenders to the Cure of the Disease,* A4-A5.

117 U. Von Hutten, *De Morbo Gallico. A Treatise of the French Disease, Publish'd above 200 Years Past,* 31 and L.S., *Prothylantinon, or, Some Considerations of a Notable Expedient to Root out the French Pox from the English Nation with Excellent Defensive Remedies to Preserve Mankind from the Infection of Pocky*

Women: Also an Advertisement, Wherein Is Discover'd the Dangerous Practices of Ignorant Pretenders to the Cure of the Disease. The quack was typically held to be dangerous because he cared more about memorizing the Latin names of disease than understanding their proper cures, so that he has 'more Hard words than a Juggler, and uses them to the same Purpose, to amuse and beguile the Ignorant or unwary, first of their Wit, and next of their Mony.' Anon., *The Character of a Quack Doctor, or, the Abusive Practices of Impudent Illiterate Pretenders to Physick Exposed* (1676).

118 G. Harvey, *The Conclave of Physicians in Two Parts, Detecting Their Intrigues, Frauds, and Plots, against Their Patients, and Their Destroying the Faculty of Physick: Also a Peculiar Discourse of the Jesuits Bark, the History Thereof, with Its True Use and Abuse* (1686), 39.

119 A.O. Faber, *Alberti Ottonis Fabri Medici Regii Exer. Suec. Paradoxon De Morbo Gallico Libr. Ii, or, a Paradox Concerning the Shameful Disease for a Warning to All against Deceitful Cures*, trans. Johan Kauffman (1662), C2.

120 Anon., *The Tomb of Venus,* 61-2.

121 J. Archer, *Secrets Disclosed, or, a Treatise of Consumptions; Their Various Causes and Cure* (1693), 1.

122 L.S., *Prothylantinon, or, Some Considerations of a Notable Expedient to Root out the French Pox from the English Nation with Excellent Defensive Remedies to Preserve Mankind from the Infection of Pocky Women,* A4-A5. For the empiric's point of view, see R. *Health for Sale: Quackery in England 1660-1850* (Manchester: Manchester University Press, 1989), chapter 5. See also W. Bynum, 'Treating the Wages of Sin: Venereal Disease and Specialism in Eighteenth-Century Britain.'

123 Anon., *The Tomb of Venus,* 62. See also A.O. Faber, *Alberti Ottonis Fabri Medici Regii Exer. Suec. Paradoxon De Morbo Gallico Libr. Ii, or, a Paradox Concerning the Shameful Disease for a Warning to All against Deceitful Cures / Translated out of the High-Dutch by Johan Kauffman* (1662).

124 J. Arrizabalaga, J. Henderson, and R. French, *The Great Pox: The French Disease in Renaissance Europe,* 114, 282, 17, 19.

125 R.French and J. Arrizabalaga, 'Coping with the French Disease: University Practitioners' Strategies and Tactics in the Transition from the Fifteenth to the Sixteenth Century,' 256-7.

126 It was not just quacks that physicians cautioned against as dangerous due to their lack of knowledge, but the general public, as well. See for example R. Wittie, *Popular Errours. Or the Errours of the People in Physick*

(1651).

127 P. Slack, 'Mirrors of Health and Treasures of Poor Men: The Uses of the Vernacular Medical Literature of Tudor England,' in C. Webster (ed.), *Health, Medicine, and Mortality in the Sixteenth Century* (New York: Cambridge University Press, 1979), 268.

128 P. Lowe, *An Easie, Certaine, and Perfect Method, to Cure and Preuent the Spanish Sicknes Wherby the Learned and Skilfull Chirurgian May Heale a Great Many Other Diseases,* Sig. B2v.

129 M. Pelling, 'Appearance and Reality: Barber-Surgeons, the Body and Disease,' 96. Margaret Pelling asserts that barber-surgeons rapidly assumed the dominant role in the treatment of the disease, 10. See also C. Webster (ed.), *Health, Medicine, and Mortality in the Sixteenth Century* (New York: Cambridge University Press, 1979).

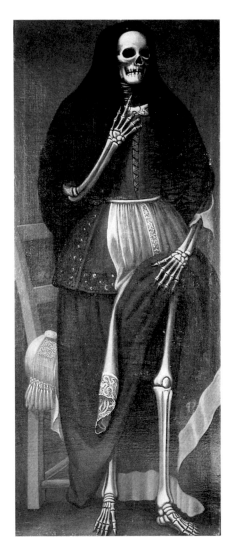

Figure 11: A skeleton as a woman warning of the dangers of fornification
Courtesy Wellcome Library, London

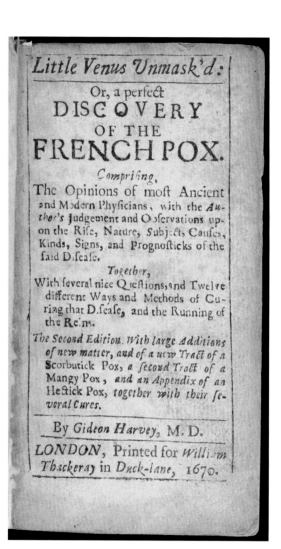

Little Venus Unmask'd:

Or, a perfect
DISCOVERY
OF THE
FRENCH POX.

Comprising,
The Opinions of most Ancient
and Modern Physicians, with the *Author's* Judgement and Observations upon the Rise, Nature, Subject, Causes,
Kinds, Signs, and Prognosticks of the
said Disease.

Together,
With several nice Questions, and Twelve
different Ways and Methods of Curing that Disease, and the Running of
the Reins.

*The Second Edition. With large Additions
of new matter, and of a new Tract of a
Scorbutick Pox, a second Tract of a
Mangy Pox, and an Appendix of an
Hectick Pox, together with their se-
veral Cures.*

By *Gideon Harvey,* M. D.

LONDON, Printed for *William
Thackeray* in *Duck-lane,* 1670.

Figure 12: Titlepage: Little Venus unmask'd
Courtesy Wellcome Library, London

6

'The Baneful Source of all our Woe'[1]:
Women and the Pox

'The very name Pox, sounds terrible to English Ears, and makes an Impression of Horrour upon us. For this aggregative Evil is like Pandora's Box, out of which all other Diseases and Mischiefs issue.'[2]

The French pox was a dreaded disease[3] In seventeenth-century England, it was associated with illicit sexual behavior and was considered shameful. The pox also stigmatized its victims with distressing physical symptoms. Sufferers were compelled to seek medical assistance for the disease, although many did not enlist the aid of a university-educated physician, opting instead for a lay or empiric healer. As the previous chapter demonstrated, physicians utilized remedies that were largely empiric in origin, but they argued that their education and the wisdom it afforded enabled them to offer their patients the safest and most efficacious course of treatment. They made few claims about successfully curbing the spread of the disease, but they theorized about the disease and brought it into their realm of knowledge.

Constructing knowledge about the disease proved helpful to their professional status in that they chose to use the threat of the pox to support proscriptive attitudes towards certain segments of the population that were deemed threatening to the social order. Specifically, physicians chose to stress promiscuous women in general, and prostitutes in particular, as the vector of infection, theorizing that their bodies were designed to spread the disease to men who were unable to resist them.[4] Physicians' theories about prostitution and the pox contributed to the attitudes toward and treatment of those infected, particularly indigent sufferers reliant on charitable care. Physicians' willingness to write in English, coupled with their decision to withhold information from the public that could lead to immoral decisions while simultaneously elevating themselves as moral authorities, provided physicians with another avenue to become experts in a disease in which the public mind so clearly linked sin and divine retribution.

English physicians' writing on the subject of the French pox stressed the disease's association with divine retribution for the sin of lust and its link with prostitution. These treatises, which are primarily health guides written for lay readers, demonstrate that physicians were fashioning a new, more inclusive role for themselves as moral guides. Because they focused on prostitution to explain the spread of the pox, physicians' tracts on the disease were brimming with moral platitudes about avoiding the terrors of the pox by avoiding the sin of fornication, and they were equally adamant that lifestyle choices contributed both to the infection and to its severity once contracted.[5] Moralizing about venereal disease by the medical community was not a forgone conclusion, as evidenced by the reaction of other countries' medical professions.[6] In his comparative study of syphilis in European countries, Winfried Schleiner reached the conclusion that 'Continental perceptions of morality [were] less pronounced and narrow than those in England.' He noted a lesser degree of moral conviction evident in Italian syphilographers who willingly shared prophylactic measures in comparison with English surgeons and physicians writing on the subject, who were 'imbued with values that make them view almost every aspect of the disease through a moral lens.'[7] Why did English physicians focus on this particular aspect of the disease, to the point where they chose not to include common preventative measures readily available in European medical works?

The decisions by medical men to concentrate on the sinful activities that led to venereal disease were part of the drive to control the behavior of the public, particularly the lower orders. Not surprisingly, the pox became an important factor in moral reform initiatives ranging from the eradication of prostitution to anti-wet nursing campaigns.[8] Medical opinions on ways in which the pox was spread and the means by which it could be prevented became part of the campaigns and exerted an influence on targeting and curbing society's vices.

Physicians overwhelmingly stressed sexual transmission and identified prostitutes as the most common vector of infection when explaining the French disease. In fact, the one major advancement in the study of the pox in the seventeenth century was the discovery of the venereal link. As the physician Jean Astruc explained, 'When the Venereal Disease made its first appearance in Europe, it was not known that the infection was propagated by Coition.'[9] By the seventeenth century, physicians had made the connection and were focusing on the venereal transmission of the disease. Most medical treatises cited lying with an infected woman as the most common means of contracting the pox. The treatises relegated other means of contraction to secondary importance.[10] In Girolamo Fracastoro's poem, *Syphilis sive Morbus Gallicus*, originally published in 1530, he did not stress the sexual transmission of syphilis. Instead, he blamed the disease on dangerous miasma. However, when Nahum Tate published the first English translation of the poem in 1686, he included a letter on syphilis in which the writer stated 'the baneful Source of all our Woe' was to be blamed upon 'That wheedling, charming Sex.'[11] English physicians concentrated on lust as the main cause for the spread of the pox, and blamed women, especially prostitutes, for inciting lust in men.[12]

The medical profession in England theorized that an inherently sinful activity usually propagated the French pox: sexual intercourse with prostitutes, and thereby gendered the disease. Anna Foa has argued that unlike many other diseases in the medieval and early modern periods, in the case of syphilis, European society did not seek out opportune scapegoats.[13] While this seems to have been true at first for syphilis, by the seventeenth century things had changed, in part because of the efforts of physicians to theorize on the ability of women, especially prostitutes, to spread the disease and even to engender it through their own sinfulness. In the seventeenth century, at least for England, the medical community made prostitutes the scapegoats for the spread of the pox.[14]

Medical theory delineated the link to prostitution through the putrefaction of seed theory posited by Nicholas de Blegny in the mid-seventeenth century that held prostitutes to blame for the disease. According to the theory, the pox was a 'contagious distemper…proceeding from the mixture and corruption of the seeds of divers persons received and contained in the womb of publick women.'[15] This theory was not just on the medical fringe; the medical community embraced it for over a century. The original translator of the treatise was Richard Boulton, a member of the Royal College of Physicians. Forty years after the translation, Boulton wrote of the ability of the female womb to produce venereal disease: 'When by the lasciviousness of a woman she admits too frequent congress with different persons, the course of nature is quite perverted and the semen…is vitiously depraved and too much exhalted by the extraordinary heat of the uterus.'[16] This theory was in agreement with what was already popularly believed to be the relationship between sinful actions and sexual intercourse: that prostitutes, the women guiltiest of sexual sin, in essence created the pox by the very act of their prostitution.

Influences of this theory can be found in medical treatises geared toward general readership, such as *A Short Compendium of Chirurgery,* which contained tips on curing various wounds, ulcers, and fractures, as well as the French pox. The chapter on venereal disease began by stating that the disease was just punishment from God for sin, and that it was most commonly transmitted 'by impure Copulation, whence the Seed of several Men Fermenting' produced an impure substance that infected the other humours.[17] Thomas Sydenham's *A New Method of Curing the French-Pox* related a similar medical theory:

'tis known, that if a Virgin, that is perfectly sound (if the Matter be so ordered as to free her from all suspicion of the Venereal Distemper) shall keep Company with half a dozen young Fellows, as sound as herself, and be debauched with them severally, time after time, some one or other of them shall quickly have the Pox, and all of them, by a repetition of Venereal Acts, shall at last be infected.[18]

Sydenham implied that promiscuity in women could actually produce the pox:

I suppose that [if] a common Woman has the Pox, and though she were not infected, if she has a particular Conversation [intercourse] with many Men, the mixture of so many Seeds does occasion such a Corruption in the Passage of the Matrix, that it degenerates into a proper virulent Ferment…[19]

According to such tracts, a woman's body became the locus of corruption and the vehicle of infection of others.[20] Her disease-spreading potential was not limited to sexual intercourse. Thomas Nedham warned that even when no penetration occurred, a woman could infect a man, as 'the Pocky Steams of the diseased woman do often evidently imprint their malignity on the genitals of the healthy play-fellow.'[21] Such theories invested a great deal of destructive power in unchaste women as disease-producing agents.

Some women were more dangerous than others. The physician Tobias

179

Whitaker explained in his treatise on venereal disease that certain women (he did not specify *which* women) had a 'venene temper contingent in them, as in Scorpions and Aspes and such other venomous creatures.' The 'pollution' within them was 'natural nourishment to themselves and poison to others.'[22] Thus, such women, though not infected themselves, 'do abbreviate the lives of all men that have any congregation with them.'[23] Even more disconcerting, certain types of behavior, when taken to the extreme, could increase the probability of infection with the disease. For example, chaste kissing was not dangerous, but lascivious kissing could spread the pox. Moderate copulation was safe, but overindulgence could result in one or both partners coming down with the pox.[24] This made sense in a system of Galenic medicine wherein moderation in all things was essential to the maintenance of good health. Such reasoning was consistent with a worldview that connected moral with physical health.

Physicians' theories also held that diseased female sexuality had greater ramifications for the public health in general. A lewd woman could negatively affect the physical environment by being both morally and physically diseased. This was due to the belief that if the population was not clean and continent, disease could result.[25] In the case of the pox, the link between spiritual and physical corruption was clear. Contemporary medical theory maintained that the pox was spread by 'seedlets of contagion' that were infective agents, not in the sense of germ theory, but as entities that corrupted the air. The contemporary concept of 'contagion' was that it was a synonym for staining, both in the literal sense of the air and in the metaphorical sense of moral pollution.[26] Therefore, even if prostitutes were not directly responsible for spreading the pox, they still polluted the moral atmosphere.

Given the above examples, it is not surprising that medical theories blaming prostitutes for the pox were considered by the medical community and the lay public alike as plausible and credible. Such theories (specifically Blegny's putrefaction of seed theory) were not met with shock but rather widespread agreement, or at least acknowledgment of the soundness of their principles. The theories seemed reasonable since early modern society had long feared the destructive capabilities of uncontrolled female sexuality. These anxieties now focused on a particular disease and were perpetuated in medical discourse.[27]

For instance, medical theories that held women to blame for the pox mirrored misogynistic biblical views of women. Ruth Mazo Karras has argued that misogyny constituted a significant part of the church's teaching about women. Particularly in late medieval England, those negative views primarily concerned women's sexuality.[28] Women were lustful and therefore dangerous to men. Karras has asserted that women's lust became a focal point in order to displace onto them the responsibility for the sins of men who could not control their own temptations. The placing of blame also indicated a real fear of women--that they would disrupt the established order of society by leading men astray, by causing bastards to inherit, or by destroying clerical celibacy. Prostitutes were only the most extreme examples of a general female tendency to lustfulness.[29] Such messages appear in the tracts of theologians and were copiously transmitted to the laity through sermons, both printed and oral, didactic treaties, and devotional texts written in the vernacular in fourteenth and fifteenth centuries and copied for use by the laity. Karras has noted that the many printed editions of some attest to their popularity and that the effects of the availability of these model sermons, compendia, and other pastoral works indicate the development of a common pool of moral teaching, 'a truly mass literature in which one form or other reached absolutely everybody.'[30] In short, there existed by the seventeenth century a tradition of placing the blame of sexual sin on women as temptresses long before physicians' theories blamed them as well.

Representations of filthy harlots infecting generations of Englishmen were common literary currency that had repercussions on the way all members of society, medical and non-medical alike, viewed the disease.[31] Thomas Nashe's *Pierce Peniless, His Supplication to the Devil* included the following rant against pox-harboring prostitutes: 'Our uncleane sisters [prostitutes]... speedily carry them to hell, there to keepe open house for all yonge devils that come, and not let our ayre bee contaminated with theyre six penny damnation any longer.' Shakespeare linked prostitutes with venereal disease in several of his plays. In *Troilus and Cressida*, Thersites catalogued a list of diseases associated with prostitution, most notably the French pox. In *Pericles*, when Marina was imprisoned in a brothel, she remarked that in such places, 'Diseases have been sold dearer than physic.'[32] Whether attending a play or reading a medical tract, the public was exposed to the belief that prostitution spread dangerous diseases that threatened the health of the realm.

Contributing to the potential dangers of prostitution was the difficulty of discerning whether or not lewd women harbored disease, particularly if they appeared healthy. Shakespeare's *Timon of Athens* highlighted the destructive power of prostitutes who only appeared sound: 'This fell whore of thine / Hath in her mor destruction than thy sword, / For all her cherubin look.'[33]

181

Contemporary misogynistic tracts also warned young men of the perils of fair-looking prostitutes:

> *Angels* they may seem in Dress, and meen,
> But could you view the frightful *Fiend* within,
> Who whets their lewd desires, and *eggs* them on,
> To act those Mischiefs they too oft have done;
> Not *Midnight Spectres,* nor sad *Scenes* of *War,*
> Would half so dreadful to your Sense appear…
> Breath breath a while, my over-heated *Muse,*
> Before you enter their accursed *Stews;*
> *Where* Aches, Buboes, Shankers, Nodes *and* Poxes,
> Are hid in Females Dam'd *Pandora*'s Boxes.[34]

Physicians' medical treatises echoed the danger fair-looking women might conceal. Titles such as *Great Venus Unmasked* implied that the masked Venus was responsible for destruction , while *The Tomb of Venus* suggested a similar fate for those who were unknowingly drawn in.[35] Other tracts warned unsuspecting males to beware the hidden danger: 'In Women the Disease resteth in their secret Places, wherein are little pretty Sores, full of venomous Poison, being very dangerous for such as unknowingly meddle with them.'[36] Some physicians cautioned that prostitutes' ability to inflict harm was proportional to their own degree of infection: '[The pox], when contracted from these infected Women, is so much the more grievous, by how much they are more inwardly corrupted and polluted therewith.'[37] In short, the more diseased the prostitute, the more dangerous the disease for the man she contaminated.

Most dangerous of all were prostitutes who purposely concealed their disease in order to continue practicing their trade. Tracts described such women as 'cunning,' 'lustful,' and 'beguiling.'[38] They were predators who were damnable most of all for luring respectable young men to debauchery.[39] In *The Crafty Whore,* the 'Crafty devices,' responsible for the 'Ruine of many rich and ancient families' were revealed for the 'benefit of all, but especially the younger sort.'[40] *Strange & True Newes* described a prostitute who turned madam after she was too poxed to lure men. Her house of ill repute alone was responsible for undoing more youngsters than 'half the houses in the city of London.' According to the tract, she grew more devious every day, as she profited from men's misery.[41] Women like this were 'vultures,' responsible for the downfall of many families. Their deceit and lack of remorse regarding the lives they destroyed made them unworthy of sympathy and deserving only of disgust and outrage from the reader. Medical tracts also focused on the suffering of male victims of the pox while virtually ignoring the suffering that infected prostitutes endured.

The suffering of men who contracted the disease through dalliances with prostitutes received the attention of medical writers, who generally assumed a male audience.[42] The physician and author of *Prothylantinon* blamed 'pocky women' for the miseries humanity endured from venereal disease.[43] The Spanish physician Gaspar Torrella wrote that men endured more physical pain than women who had the pox because men had a hotter complexion. He advised men to avoid infected women. The reverse was not necessary because the uterus was cold, dry, and dense; therefore, it was not easily damaged. Consequently, it would take repeated sexual contact with infected males for a woman to contract the disease.[44] Ideas such as this one offer a glimpse into the manner in which medical theory mirrored popular beliefs about the spread of diseases and the suffering endured by people with the disease.

Significantly, the suffering that these diseased prostitutes endured was not a common theme in popular representations of the pox, either.[45] Instead, the focus was on the misery prostitutes caused men, as illustrated in Thomas Dekker's *The Honest Whore*.[46] Count Hippolito asserted 'there has been known / As many by one harlot, maimed and dismembered, / As would ha' stuffed an hospital.'[47] A similar notion was echoed in the tract *The Female Fire-Ships*, which categorized prostitutes as 'True *Canibals,* who can with ease devour, / A dozen Men while Time shapes out an Hour.'[48] In Thomas Dekker's *Newes from Graves-ende* prostitutes were depicted as possessing no fear of the pox, but rather a type of moral immunity to it: 'Knowing their deaths come o're from *France*: / Tis not their season now to die, / Two gnawing poisons cannot lie, / In one corrupted flesh together.'[49] Again, there was no mention of the prostitutes' battle with the pox. They were the agents of infection rather than sufferers of the same disease as their male counterparts.

As Kevin Siena has demonstrated, the growing tendency on the part of physicians to associate women with syphilis validated in medical theory what the lay culture already believed.[50] By portraying sexually active women as responsible for the pox in corporeal, scientific terms, physicians were seizing upon the existing cultural beliefs that women and their sexuality were inherently dirty and that uncontrolled sexually active women were dangerous to society. Their motivation, according to Siena, was professional self-promotion. In restating these ideas in university discourse, physicians were attempt-

183

ing to present themselves as reputable and secure a position in a competitive field by transcribing into theory beliefs that the populace already held.[51] Contemporary culture clearly played a role in the development of physicians' theories about the spread of the pox, as medical theories are social constructs. They are not immune to popular ideas; rather, they simultaneously inform and are influenced by popular notions. Reflecting already existent and commonly held popular beliefs was part of the process of physicians building their reputation as learned, rational, and trustworthy.

In her work on the construction of knowledge, Barbara Shapiro found that the scientific revolution ushered in changes in beliefs not only about the nature of the physical world but also, and more fundamentally, in beliefs about what methods were best for finding truth.[52] By the seventeenth century, truth had a distinct moral element to it in determining whom to believe. Steven Shapin has further developed this concept. He argues that truth during this period was dependent upon 'morally textured' relationships between people and upon notions of authority and trust. In the seventeenth century, as in society today, people learned about the world not necessarily through personal observation but by accepting the testimony of others whom they trusted as authorities.[53] In the scientific culture of Restoration England, virtue and morality encumbered trust. As Thomas Hobbes in *Leviathan* astutely observed, 'In Beleefe are two opinions; one of the saying of the man; the other of his virtue.'[54] Virtue was an essential determinant of trust. It was also much easier to attain if one had gentlemanly status, as Shapin has argued.[55] Such status could be conferred either by gentlemanly birth or by virtue and learning, and so the circular logic of what constituted authority and the right to be believed was based upon a mixture of interdependent factors revolving around virtue, morality, and gentlemanly status.[56]

The seventeenth-century physician found himself in a nebulous position in terms of establishing authority in such a society. His university training certainly augmented his credibility, but there was a decent chance that he was not considered a gentleman by those around him. As previous chapters have demonstrated, physicians as a group were nervous about status for themselves as individuals and for their profession, and they were interested in establishing themselves as guardians of medicine informed by morality. Given Shapiro and Shapin's work on the factors behind conceptions of truth and credibility, along with the challenges that 'new diseases' presented to the medical profession, it is logical that physicians were self-aware of the necessity of developing new medical theories to make them seem knowledgeable about the disease. In this way, they could protect their claim to expertise in the field of etiology and continue to improve their status and authority in society in general.

The combination of research by historians studying truth and those studying venereal disease during the period have made it unfeasible to view medical theories on the pox as works of impartial science. The theories were informed by popular perceptions about the disease and its transmission that physicians then put into scientific terms. This manner of theory making is, at its core, decidedly conservative. It reinforced traditional views and beliefs, and as this chapter will demonstrate, quite consciously served the needs of authority at the expense of the urban poor. Physicians' response to the challenge of the pox was multi-faceted but purposeful in that it helped them as a profession appear to be actively battling the pox according to contemporary expectations. They named and explained the disease, they emphasized its complicated nature and the possible dangers of the treatments, and they focused on its spread through prostitution. The culmination of their efforts was advice to the public on physical as well as moral steps that could be taken to avoid the pox, advice that further solidified the position of the physician as a medical and moral authority.

In their publications on the subject of venereal disease, particularly those geared toward general readership, physicians envisioned themselves as responsible for more than just the health of their patients. Physicians regarded their job as exceedingly important to both the physical and moral aspects of their patients and the community as well. Such a perception is evident in the grappling over how much knowledge about preventing the pox physicians should make available to the public, as they considered it imperative to bear in mind any moral implications that their advice might have on the actions of the lay population.

In fact, a major part of their rhetorical battle against the pox involved *not* providing information to the public about how to avoid the disease. This may seem counter-intuitive, given the perceived epidemic of the pox, yet withholding information complemented physicians' interest in the moral aspects of caring for their patients' health by advising them to eschew sinful behavior that could lead to illness. Physicians assumed the role of moral arbiters in determining what information should be kept from the public--a role all the more important given the influx of vernacular works discussed in chapter four that made medical knowledge accessible to the reading public. The translator of Nicholas de Belgny's work felt compelled to apologize

185

for 'Englishing' the text and carefully edited parts of the work that he did not consider appropriate for an English audience.[57] Marchamont Nedham reverted to Latin on occasion in his treatise on the pox, 'partly for modesties sake, and partly because such Cautions may prove an encouragement to wickedness.'[58] Sharing preventative measures with the lay population essentially meant that medical practitioners had chosen to 'prostitute their Conscience.'[59] They thereby couched their refusal to share preventative measures in terms of their moral obligation to their patients.

In their writing on the pox, medical men often felt compelled to consider carefully what type of information they should offer for public consumption. In particular, they excluded any information that might encourage lustful behavior, by 'acquainting the World with the Effects of it [syphilis], and the way to get out of the Labyrinth which it generally leaves Men in.'[60] When it came to the pox, they were more cautious about sharing preventatives with the general public than they were with other diseases because they feared encouraging lust. Dr. James Cooke cautioned that the diverse ways in which earlier continental authorities offered to prevent the possibility of infection 'should not be taught, lest [they] should invite [men] To Lust, and so procure sinning with the more wretched freedom.'[61] The physicians Gideon Harvey and John Marten desisted from publishing any information about the disease that might 'lessen the deterrent force of fear.'[62] In *Two Treatises. The First of Venereal Pox*, the authors asserted that it was possible to teach men how they might 'enter the most infected whores' without contracting the pox, but they could 'say nothing of such medicines in good conscience.' In the tract, the authors of some treatises encouraged other physicians and surgeons not to make known such medicine to 'lustful people' and not to make themselves 'fosterers of lust.'[63] It is for this reason that physicians claimed to withhold some knowledge about the disease, such as the ability to tell 'whether Artifice were not used, to patch up a Mistress for the Battle.' It was more productive to encourage the reader to avoid the sinful behavior altogether.[64] The message put forth in some medical texts intended for the general public was that although physicians were capable of supplying the reader with a considerable amount of knowledge about the French pox, it was their moral imperative not to do so.

Rather than offering preventative measures, their tracts more often encouraged readers to 'abstain from whores, and to remember that Whoremongers and Adulterers the Lord will judg, who yet is wont also to punish them in this Life, with that most filthy disease.'[65] Physicians could then advise men to avoid infection by avoiding such women, as did the physician Philip Barrough, whose tract warned men that 'There be devilish women desirous to be handled and dealt withal, who will beautifie themselves, to inflame mens hearts to lust towards them; abandon these your company, and thrust them out of doors and house.'[66] The English translation of Daniel Sennert's *A Method of Curing the French Pox* included a discussion of whether or not preventative measures against the French pox even existed. The author concluded that 'All such Preservatives, to speak properly, are nothing else but Impostures.' The reason for this is that God would not allow such things:

> Seeing that it [the pox] is commonly the reward of the Sin of Fornication, which God has always had in Abomination, and that that Distemper may be avoided by Continence, which is true Preservative, it seems that it was no ways necessary that God should create a specific Preservative against that.[67]

Preventative measures, as far as the publications of English physicians were concerned, meant eschewing sinful behavior that could lead to disease. William Clowes stressed virtuous conduct as the most effective form of disease prevention:

> Forasmuch as the best avoiding and curing of everie disease, consisteth in shunning and removing the cause thereof, I wish all men generally, especially those which be infected, to loathe, detest, hate, and abhorre that striking sinne that is the original cause of this infection, and to praie earnestly to God the heavenly Physition and Chirurgeon, for his gratious assistance to the perfect amendment of life, the most safest and surest waie to remove it.'[68]

Since disease was deemed to be a manifestation of sin, the avoidance of sin would prove the most powerful means of preserving one's health. John Archer made this point in his 'Epistle to the Reader' with a succinct statement about the medical effects of immoral behavior: 'Away then with that necessity of dying at such a time, when a man is cut off for his wickedness, or by his foolish intemperance; for the wise man said, Be not wicked or foolish over-much, why wilt thou die before thy time?'[69] Archer's message was that choosing moral behavior had a definite effect on one's earthly life, as well as afterlife.

Although prevention of syphilis through virtuous behavior may have been the ideal, it was never fully realized, resulting in infected individuals seeking advice on treatment options. Physicians then had to determine what information about treating the disease should be provided to the public, so that physicians could ease patients' suffering, while simultaneously being careful not to encourage 'rogues and idle persons…to wallow in the muck' and continue to engage in the same type of sinful behavior that first made them sick.[70] These writers made a distinction, therefore, between providing information on prophylactic measures that might encourage lustful behavior and carefully measured information regarding descriptions of and treatment options for the pox. The physician Joseph Cam was disinclined to reveal ways to avoid the disease or how to spot it in others, as this could encourage vice. However, he found it permissible to 'give a Description how a Patient may know his Degree of Infection, and how reasonable it may be for him to make a serious Application in Season.'[71] John Archer similarly acknowledged that he meant for his tract to educate the afflicted on their medical condition, not to share remedies, as the latter could prove dangerous information in the hands of the public:

> Though I shew not the materials for Cure, I mean Physick, yet the sick have sufficient benefit, if they understand how to be cured safely, which is to be understood by those Physicians which by long and daily practice know how…it is safest to keep Knives out of Childrens hands lest they endanger their Lives; but the knowledge of the Disease, and how to judge of your condition, I think absolute necessary for every Patient and Physician.[72]

The author also felt compelled to justify curing the disease by pointing out that although the pox was chiefly contracted through copulation with an infected lover, there were 'many other ways that honest and innocent persons of both Sexes are and may be infected,' among them passing the disease between an infant and wet nurse or sharing a cup with an infected person.[73] Physicians' writings portrayed these methods of contraction as exceptions, rather than the rule.[74] The exceptions, nonetheless, allowed physicians to divide sufferers into two groups: those who had contracted the pox through the 'filthy, rotten burning of harlots' (or the 'harlots' themselves) and those who had contracted it through no fault of their own.[75] Physicians could justify treating the disease in order to aid the latter. The former, particularly prostitutes, should be cured only for the greater good: preventing the spread of the pox to the innocent.

In sum, physicians were reticent about sharing prophylactic measures with the public and hesitant about disclosing remedies for fear of encouraging lust. They were, however, far more comfortable concentrating their efforts on the necessity of curbing prostitution in order to control the spread of the pox. Focusing on the disease-spreading potential of women, particularly unchaste women, offered several advantages. Primarily, it gave physicians a subject upon which they had a great opportunity to expound. It was easy for physicians to moralize about the sinfulness of the disease if they blamed prostitutes as the vector of infection and as temptresses who were adept at luring otherwise chaste men to sin, particularly as prostitutes were generally not fee-paying patients of physicians.

Additionally, the magnitude of the problem of prostitution in seventeenth-century England actually worked to the advantage of physicians. Physicians generally agreed that the pox was rampant, but if prostitution was the root cause, blame for its spread should be placed on the women practicing it and the magistrates who failed to put a stop to it. Letters and diaries recorded lay impressions of widespread prostitution and the ruin that it caused. The author of a poetical letter of warning to a young man coming to the 'wicked town' of London depicted the city as being overrun by prostitutes eager to trade money for venereal disease. The tract yielded social commentary on prostitution as so popular and so unchecked by civic authority that it even went on in churches. However, the places most likely to see such women 'sell[ing] their Rotten Ware' were gathering places like alehouses where whoring was so common it had become a 'fashionable vice.'[76] It was not just in London where such things occurred, but wherever there was the deadly mixture of alehouses and prostitutes, as lamented by a widow who was incensed by the sins being committed in her neighborhood: 'I am ashamed to think that in *Taunton* there should be so many Alehouse-haunters and Tiplers... and unclean and wanton Wretches...Many of them proclaim their sin like *Sodom,* and carry their deadly Leprosie in their foreheads.'[77] There was a feeling among the lay population that prostitution had grown out of control and that civic authorities were incapable of controlling its spread. Most writers did not attempt to estimate the exact number of prostitutes plying their trade but instead referred to the 'incredible numbers' of them roaming the streets or lamented that their town was 'overstocked with harlots.'[78]

Although London authorities officially closed the stews in 1546, pros-

189

titution still flourished, leading to the enactment of a drastic law under Oliver Cromwell in an attempt to curb prostitution. Under the 1650 Commonwealth Act 'for the suppressing of the abhominable and crying sins of incest, adultery and fornication wherewith this land is much defiled and Almighty God highly displeased,' adultery and incest were punished with the death penalty. Those convicted of fornication were jailed for three months, and brothel keepers were to be whipped, set in the pillory, and marked with a hot iron on the forehead with a 'B,' for a first offense and put to death for a second offense.[79] The law was only in effect for a decade, but Keith Thomas has pointed out that the act's failure was due to logistics and that the act represented popular support for safeguarding the family against the disruptive effects of sexual license.[80]

Linking prostitution to syphilis, and claiming that the disease could not be curbed unless prostitution was eradicated, helped physicians become more involved in governing the public health of England by supporting anti-prostitution campaigns. These campaigns, which included anti-prostitution measures but sought to curb other types of immoral behavior as well, were often organized through the Societies for the Reformation of Manners. The campaigns were already underway throughout much of the seventeenth century, gaining ground by the closing decades for reasons of economic upheaval and social disorder discussed in the upcoming chapter.

The first of the Societies for the Reformation of Manners formed in 1691. The largest efforts centered in London although there were similar societies in towns throughout England. While laws had long been in place to regulate moral offences, including prostitution, enforcement tended to be lax. The Societies were attempts by private individuals to ensure that moral legislation was rigorously enforced.[81] Groups of citizens, including many dissenters, formed Societies for the express purpose of rooting out public sinners, securing warrants against them from magistrates, and assisting constables in arrests.[82] Any citizen could swear out a warrant and have a local constable serve it. The Societies printed and distributed packets of blank warrants in order to streamline the process. They also hired messengers to deliver the warrants to magistrates.[83]

Although the Societies for the Reformation of Manners attacked vice in general, at the center of the movement was a desire to suppress immorality, particularly prostitution.[84] The majority of the prosecutions aided by the Societies were for 'lewd and disorderly practices,' the common law offence under which prostitution was punished.[85] The courts prosecuted an average of 1,330 people per year for this offence in the years for which the reports survive between 1708 and 1724. In fact, in every year records exist, this was the most numerous offence, some years outnumbering all others. The vast majority of those accused of lewd behavior and disorderly practice were women. The list of offenders in the 1693 London judicial records reveals that most were accused of 'nightwalking' and picking up men. The literature of the Societies depicts women as actively seeking to spread immorality. It is telling that the reformers focused their efforts against prostitution on prostitutes and not their clients or the proprietors of brothels.[86] Like physicians whose writings blamed prostitutes for luring men to debauchery, social reformers largely blamed the problem of prostitution on the women who practiced it rather than the individuals who ran the brothels or the men who frequented them.

The Societies focused on street prostitutes because the major motivation behind the reform movements was to attack problems of poverty, crime, and disorder in London—problems that appeared to be spiraling out of control at the end of the seventeenth century and into the eighteenth century. Prostitution was both a symptom and cause of the problems.[87] Prostitution was especially heinous because it spread venereal disease, thereby destroying the health of soldiers and sailors and killing innocent wives. It is significant that the reformers were actively pursuing enforcement of the laws against the social immorality of lewdness rather than the private vice of fornication. Prostitution upset the social order: the husbands who visited brothels broke marriage vows and created discord in their families. Servants who stole from their masters to pay for prostitutes similarly upset the social order. Additionally, moral reformers pointed to the economic disruptions caused by prostitution.[88] Brothels were depicted in the sermons and pamphlets produced by the Societies for the Reformation of Manners as nurseries of crime: 'Here 'tis that Bodies are Poxt and Pockets are pickt of considerable Sums..all leading to the great Disturbance and Disquietment of Their Majesties peaceable Subjects.'[89] In short, 'lost women', as they were often referred to in anti-prostitution tracts, made attractive targets for the reformers because they were so easily viewed as enemies of public order.[90]

This perhaps accounts for the wide appeal that the Societies held. Their efforts to tighten the law against sexual offences in the 1690s were part of a broad popular movement for moral reform. Prior to the somewhat organized efforts by the Societies, there had been spontaneous efforts by various parishes across the country to prosecute those accused of immoral behavior.[91] These efforts increased with the accession of William and Mary, as the godly worried that while the Restoration signaled a sign from God that England was favored, Restoration society was not godly. John Milton noted that there was a 'general complaint' of increased vice in England, and he mentions 'Whoredom' among the most common and concerning.[92] He was not alone in fretting about the moral health of English society. In 1690, William III wrote to the bishop of London about his concern for the notorious 'overflowing of vice' and the need for 'a general reformation of the lives and manners of all our subjects.'[93] William's letter satisfied the Societies for the Reformation of Manners' imperatives to press for the issuing of Royal Proclamations against vice and immorality. Queen Mary also obliged by issuing one in 1691. In it she urged Justices of the Peace to enforce laws against immorality. She also issued letters asking Justices of the Peace to crack down on vice and urging all citizens to report information against offenders to the proper authorities. The queen's proclamation is significant in that it represented a strong endorsement of the strategy of the Societies for the Reformation of Manners. Queen Anne regularly issued similar proclamations during her reign, testifying to the support that the Societies enjoyed at high levels. They also managed to procure the signatures of twenty-nine Lords Temporal and nine Lords Spiritual on a declaration endorsing the Societies' strategies.[94] The Societies were successful in garnering support because they were articulating an overarching fear that morality was in serious decline in Restoration England.

The Societies certainly were not without critics. They were controversial, yet their overall aim of enforcing public morality and thereby enforcing public order fit contemporary sensibilities. Although little is known about the membership of the Societies, historians have established that there was a small stratum of urban gentlemen and a wider base of urban petty bourgeoisie who were members. They have also demonstrated that the intensely moralistic middle classes largely supported the Societies in their endeavors.[95] The powerful support that the Societies enjoyed translated to considerable success against public debauchery. In the years that the Societies functioned, from 1690-1738, they were responsible for over 100,000 prosecutions for moral offences, mainly in and around London.[96]

It is interesting that these campaigns were taking place at the end of the century. They serve as a reminder that looking only at the scientific revolution for clues about the role of the physician in society can result in an overly secular picture of late seventeenth-century English society. The Societies included both Anglicans and Dissenters among their supporters. Personal piety was extremely important to both groups.[97] This is the backdrop against which physicians were writing about the pox.

Religion and morality play a strong role throughout the century, albeit with differing motivations and in differing forms. The Societies for the Reformation of Manners certainly were different from the Puritan experiments in social control earlier in the century. The motivation of the former was more secular than the latter. Although the Societies couched their aims in moralistic terms, a key component was the maintenance of public order through policing immoral activity. As Alan Hunt has asserted, moral regulations such as anti-prostitution campaigns reveal deep social anxieties, in this case about women's uncontrolled sexuality. Their efforts were not isolated but projects of moral regulation aimed at governing others.[98] The Societies for the Reformation of Manners linked the providential rationale seamlessly to a more immediate and direct benefit: public order.[99]

Moral reform efforts manifested as both a religious imperative and a medical project to achieve a common goal: protection of men, and in turn innocent families, from the scourge of syphilis.[100] If disease was God's vengeance, then it should be met with a combination of appropriate religious actions and practical social actions, as long as God approved the latter.[101] Kevin Siena has stressed the complicity of the medical profession in such efforts and demonstrated how 'medical authorities employed the frightening image of venereal disease to help create and enforce danger beliefs aimed at policing behavior.'[102] In the case of the pox, the targeted behavior was prostitution. Medical literature helped establish and support proscriptive attitudes toward female promiscuity, which could threaten the male hierarchy and the social order. By stressing the disease-polluting potential of women posited in medical theory, physicians linked a social danger to sexual danger.[103] Physicians did not limit their input to theorizing, but they went a step further in suggesting practical solutions for dealing with prostitution.

Outrage over the threat that sexual misconduct posed to society spurred medical men to suggest various ways of dealing with the problem. One idea proposed by a medical practitioner was to transport 'those pernicious Animals, Common *Pockie* and *Incurable Prostitutes*' to the West Indies. He reasoned that this was the charitable thing to do, as the climate there was more conducive to curing the disease.[104] William Clowes stressed the importance of curbing prostitution to control the pox and encouraged magistrates to seek the 'correction and punishment of this filthie vice.'[105] In 1660 a group of noteworthy physicians, including Nicholas Culpeper, Daniel Sennert, and Abdiah Cole, complained that citizens still tolerated the stews. They reasoned that if authorities used as much diligence to restrain 'rambling whoring' as they did to expel those infected with plague, they might be able to eradicate the disease.[106] They lamented that authorities did not use proper diligence, resulting in moral scandal:

> Prostitutes swarm in the streets of this metropolis to such degree, and bawdy-houses are kept in such an open and public manner, to the great scandal of our civil polity, that a stranger would think that such practices, instead of being prohibited, had the sanction of the legislature, and that the whole town was one general stew.[107]

Thomas Nash echoed this idea, commenting on the shady reputation of the city's suburbs by musing: 'London, what are thy suburbs but licensed stews?'[108] Blaming the pox on prostitution allowed physicians to complain that civic authorities were not doing enough to curb prostitution and therefore helped physicians defend themselves against criticism that they were the ones responsible for failing to curtail the disease.[109]

Physicians' efforts to prevent the spread of the pox became one of keeping Adam from succumbing to Eve. They were engaged in fighting the ultimate losing battle, as they themselves recognized. Physicians pointed out that they could do little to restrain the inevitability of men failing to resist prostitutes: 'For many do indulge in this brutish Passion, that as soon as they are out of the Physician's Hands, they run presently into the Arms and Embraces of infected Courtizans.'[110] Physicians used this argument repeatedly to prevent condemnation for not proving more effective in quelling the spread of disease:

> Who can but wonder, but that miserable man should be…so absorpt in Sensuality, as for one moment of vanishing pleasure, to involve himself in such an Abyss of lasting Miseries? But when I consider the Imperious and charming Power of a Good Face, and bewitching Artifaces of Women, and Man's natural Propension to Venus…it draws me from Admiration to Commiseration. For we are all…subject to the same Propensions and Inclinations of Nature.[111]

The likelihood that men would yield to the temptation of women served an additional purpose in that it allowed physicians to morally condemn prostitution yet sympathize with their male patients who had become victims of their 'natural Propension to Venus.' By portraying the situation as one of inevitability that men would lust and women would take advantage of them, particularly men of 'greenness of years' and 'vehemency of temptation,' physicians were able to claim that there was little they could do to halt the spread.[112] They depicted their efforts as Herculean and of biblical importance; any gains made were admirable, but physicians could not reasonably expect a total victory. Physicians were working to protect families and the social order by denouncing prostitution and attempting to persuade men to eschew lustful behavior, even though they were making little actual progress.

The pox added urgency to the traditional moral arguments against prostitution.[113] Physicians' texts that held prostitutes responsible for engendering and spreading the disease bolstered anti-prostitution campaigns' purpose by linking control over the spread of the pox with greater social control that sought to discourage illicit sex and the disorder that was associated with it. However, social control, as physicians, moralists, and civic authorities envisioned it, was clearly meant for the poor. They were the ones traditionally associated with disorder and vice. Nowhere is this expectation more evident than in the vastly different experiences of wealthy versus indigent patients suffering from the pox in seventeenth-century England. Research has shown that all patients desired confidentiality in their diagnosis and treatment. Shame was an integral part of the experience of syphilis--not one that was socially or economically determined. What *was* determined by these factors was whether privacy was an option in their treatment.[114] For the poor, it usually was not.

Those who could not afford to pay for medical services were forced to fall back on the medical resources available to them by their parish under the Elizabethan Act of 1601.[115] This typically meant admittance to the parish workhouse, where they were given rudimentary care for their disease. If their symptoms did not abate, they might be sent to one of the two London hospitals that treated venereal patients, St. Thomas or St. Bartholomew. At this level of care, privacy was not a luxury provided for patients. The indigent sick lined up at the gates of the hospital and had to disclose the nature of their illness in order to be admitted. If it was later discovered that they had misrepresented their ailment, they were forced to leave the hospital. The temptation to lie about the venereal nature of their disease proved a compelling one, since 'foul' patients, as they were referred to, were treated differently

195

from 'clean' ones. Hospitals who accepted patients suffering from the pox segregated them from all other patients, even those known to be contagious. At St. Bartholomew they were lodged offsite at old leper houses converted to venereal wards and threatened with expulsion should they break quarantine.[116] At St. Thomas 'cured' venereal patients were publicly whipped before leaving the hospital. At neither institution were they allowed back if they became re-infected, as the pox was considered a curable disease, so to experience symptoms again meant that the patient had returned to his or her sinful ways. At both institutions, mercury treatment was the norm, even when salivation was becoming less common for private patients, who pressured their medical practitioners to dispense gentler guaiacum treatments. This fact has led Oswei Temkin to surmise that the rougher mercury cures were a kind of social discipline, meted out as moral punishment to the indigent sick, as mercury was used almost exclusively at public institutions by the end of the seventeenth century.[117]

The treatment regime for poor men and women was the same because the central aims of the hospitals were to segregate venereal patients from the rest of society, to compel patients to express repentance for the sinful actions that made them sick, and to offer thanks for their benefactors who enabled them to be cured.[118] In the eighteenth century charities set up exclusively for the shelter and reclamation of prostitutes would appear. The first of its kind was the Magdalen Hospital, established mid-century.[119] Such institutions continued to stress repentance, piety, and continence for their inmates.[120] Socio-economic status, therefore, superseded even gender in determining how sufferers reliant on public health care were treated.

Understanding the intended outcome of treating venereal patients helps to explain why they were admitted in the first place. After looking at the ledgers of St. Bartholomew and St. Thomas hospitals, Kevin Siena has concluded that the answer lies in the sheer magnitude of the infected. The records indicate that 'poverty and the pox represented a major social problem in early Stuart London.'[121] In reaching such a conclusion, he has countered arguments by Randolph Trumbach and Edward Shorter that it was a disease largely confined to the upper echelons of society prior to the eighteenth century. Siena maintains that it was absolutely rife among the London poor long before 1690, as evidenced by hospital records that indicate throngs of poor Londoners applied week after week for a bed in the 'foul wards.'[122] It was simply too big a problem to be ignored, and one that people preferred not to have staring them in the face quite literally when they walked the streets.

Reactions to the disease at the parish level, therefore, were in large part motivated by the desire to rid the streets of repugnant victims of the pox as much
as by the desire to procure medical assistance for them.[123]

Hospitals in essence incarcerated the poxed poor.[124] By segregating the
'foul' from the public, hospitals symbolically and literally kept the contagion
of immorality away from the general public. The forced repentance with
which patients had to comply, along with the whippings for St. Thomas patients, were purposely public because they served another symbolic purpose:
as a deterrent from sexual sin. Kevin Siena has argued that the punishments
enforced by the hospitals were not just intended to make patients see the error of their ways but served the same social function as other public punishments and shaming rituals central to social policing efforts in the period. The
fact that contemporaries saw prostitution, immorality, and vice in general as
spiraling out of control by the end of the century encouraged the drive to
clear the diseased poor from the streets and use them as examples to deter
others, particularly the baser sort who were considered more vulnerable to
temptation.[125]

Such attempts at social discipline were not intended for the upper classes, as they would not have been dependent on hospital care. The forced
repentance and public whippings to which pox patients in hospitals were
subjected were clearly intended for the lower orders whose disease placed
an economic strain on the parish's resources. Anyone, rich or poor, could be
guilty of the sin of lasciviousness that led to the pox, and physicians' moralizing about the sins leading to venereal disease were ostensibly addressed to
all, but the lower class sufferers of the disease were the ones who were forced
to forgo privacy and face the derision of their benefactors. The moralizing
about and treatment of the pox, therefore, were at least somewhat determined by socio-economic factors.

However, gender should not be taken out of the equation, even for
the poorest segment of the population receiving hospital care for the pox.
For example, the charitable eighteenth-century Lock Hospital in London re-
leased men after treatment, yet women were compelled to go to the Lock's
sister institution, the Lock Asylum for the Reception of Penitent Women,
where they received additional spiritual cleansing. The proffered reason for
the lengthened healing process was that women needed the means to support themselves in order to prevent their return to prostitution.[126] The Lock
Asylum was therefore meant to ensure that they could be financially cared
for after their release, ideally married off, and would be spiritually recovered

197

enough to ensure that they did not return to their old ways. Linda Merians has suggested that the tendency to blame women for the spread of venereal disease was 'ever present and increasing' even into the eighteenth century. [127] Women, and especially prostitutes, posed a danger to society due to their potential to spread disease and therefore needed to be handled carefully. The literature generated by the Lock Asylum clearly made such a connection: 'A Common prostitute is an evil to the community not dissimilar to a person infected with the plague; who, miserable himself, is daily communicating the contagion to others, that will propagate still wider the fatal malady.'[128] In the seventeenth century, such thinking helped physicians walk the fine line between moralizing about the disease and alienating potential patients. By blaming prostitutes, both for engendering the disease and tempting men, physicians helped displace culpability from their wealthy patients to that segment of society who could not afford their services.[129] In doing so, they helped enforce the moral link with the pox that made social control of the lower orders more justifiable, a program that actually placed them in sympathy with a large segment of the population who shared their concerns about morality and public order.

The French pox differed from other diseases due to the temptation to moralize about those infected with the disease to an extent rarely seen with other ailments. Medical practitioners have by no means been immune to assigning guilt and blame to their venereal patients. From the early seventeenth-century surgeon William Clowes who referred to his pox patients as those 'wicked and sinful people,'[130] to the nineteenth century Dr. Samuel Solly, president of the Royal Medical and Chirurgical Society, who reported to a government committee that syphilis was self-inflicted, avoidable by refraining from sexual activity, intended as a punishment for sins, and therefore not to be interfered with, physicians have long been judgmental in their reaction to patients suffering from venereal disease.[131] However, while seventeenth-century physicians offered advice on avoiding disease by living a life of continence and piety, they insinuated that women were responsible for the spread of the pox. In his treatise on venereal disease, the physician John Wynell included in his 'To the reader' section a sympathetic view of the unfortunate fate that befell so many blameless men:

For (in this wanton, painting, patching, perfuming, issuing age) a man knows not whom or what he takes, to himself or his son, in marriage, a blessing, or a curse. Whereby not onely are our own bodies are endangered, damnified; but posterity, primarily, fundamentally, corrupted, extirpated.[132]

He made sure to allude to the culpability of the wives by lamenting that the husband and wife must then live 'an uncomfortable life together…(like two dogs in a chain, ever snarling)…and all because abusefull deceit in the marriage.'[133]

While Wynell wrote about women in general, he awarded prostitutes the lion's share of guilt in spreading venereal disease. In their writings about prostitution, physicians broadened the scope of their responsibilities beyond individual patient-doctor relationships. They thereby further differentiated their services and their position in society from the competition by defining their role in terms of larger issues of public health: targeting those who spread the disease and developing information about the disease. Doing so lent physicians an air of authority, as well as afforded them an opportunity to balance their duty to help those who were suffering while not encroaching on God's duty to punish people for sinful behavior. This sort of medical morality was pragmatic, as medical professionals attempted to convince the public that they could be trusted guardians of public morality. Combining medicine and morality corresponded to the worldview of seventeenth-century England, that health equaled morality and morality equaled health. The medical profession did not create a new set of moral values but largely accepted the traditional view that the health of one's body and one's soul were intimately connected. Their striving to have a voice in the morality of the nation as it pertained to the health of the nation helped them extend their realm of influence into the public's most intimate behavior, carving a greater niche for themselves in the public health of the nation as a whole. It is to this concept of public health as it pertains to epidemics of bubonic plague that the next chapter will be dedicated.

Notes

1   G. Fracastoro, *Syphilis Sive Morbus Gallicus*, trans. Nahum Tate (1686), 336.

2   L.S., *Prothylantinon, or, Some Considerations of a Notable Expedient to Root out the French Pox from the English Nation with Excellent Defensive Remedies to Preserve Mankind from the Infection of Pocky Women : Also an Advertisement, Wherein Is Discover'd the Dangerous Practices of Ignorant Pretenders to the Cure of the Disease* (1673), 13.

3   The pox generally referred to syphilis, but there is some speculation by historians that in some cases the disease might have been gonorrhoea or other sexually transmitted disease, or even assorted urinary tract infections. The term syphilis was not often used during the period. It was more commonly referred to as the *lues venerea*, the pox, the French pox, or the French disease. The Bills of Mortality list the disease that we generally think of as syphilis as the French Pox.

4   K. Siena, 'Pandora's Pox: The Medical Presentation of Women in Early Modern Venereological Tracts.' Thesis (M.A.)–University Of Rochester, 1993.

5   See L. Jillings, 'The Aggression of the Cured Syphilitic: Ulrich Von Hutten's Projection of His Disease as Metaphor,' *The German Quarterly* 68, no. 1 (1995) and C. Whitbeck, 'Causation in Medicine: The Disease Entity Model,' *Philosophy of Science* 44, no. 4 (December 1977).

6   See S. Watts, *Disease, Power, and Imperialism* (New Haven: Yale University Press, 1997).

7   For example, Paul Ricius, Professor of Medicine at Padua, ridiculed priests for espousing moral views of syphilis. Winfried Schleiner, 'Moral Attitudes toward Syphilis and Its Prevention in the Renaissance,' *Bulletin of the History of Medicine* 68, no. 3 (1994), 397, 409. For more on syphilis and morality, see J.D. Oriel, *The Scars of Venus: A History of Venereology* (London: Springer-Verlag, 1994).

8   See the work of R. Davidson and L. Hall (eds.), *Sex, Sin, and Suffering: Venereal Disease and Eurorpean Society since 1870* (London: Routledge, 2001) and P. Baldwin, *Contagion and the State in Europe, 1830-1930* (Cambridge: Cambridge University Press, 1999).

9   J. Astruc, *A Treatise of Venereal Diseases, in Nine Books,* trans. William Barrowby (1754), I. 117.

10   N. Culpeper, D. Sennert, and A. Cole, *Two Treatises. The First of the Venereal Pocks. The Second Treatise of the Gout* (1660); J. Marten, *A Treatise of All the Degrees and Symptoms of the Venereal Diseases, in Both Sexes* (London: 1708); G. Harvey, *Great Venus Unmasked* (1672); E. Maynwaringe *The History and Mystery of the Venereal Lues* (1673); and C. Peter, *A Description of the Venereal Disease* (1678).

11   G. Fracastoro, *Syphilis Sive Morbus Gallicus*, trans. Nahum Tate (1686), 336.

12   See for instance G.Harvey, *Great Venus Unmasked, or, a More Exact Discovery of the Venereal Evil, or French Disease Comprizing the Opinions of Most Antient and Modern Physicians with the Particular Sentiment of the Author Touching the Rise, Nature, Subject, Causes, Kinds, Progress, Changes, Signs, and Prognosticks of the Said Evil : Together with Luculent Problems, Pregnant Observations, and the Most Practical Cures of That Disease, and Virulent Gonorrhoea, or Running of the Reins* (1672).

13   A. Foa, 'The New and the Old: The Spread of Syphilis (1494-1530),' in E. Muir and G. Ruggiero (eds), *Sex and Gender in Historical Perspective: Selections from Quaderni Storici* (Baltimore: Johns Hopkins Press University Press, 1990), 27.

14   O. Temkin's research suggests that more moralizing on the disease occurred after this connection was made. O. Temkin, 'On the History of "Morality and Syphilis,"' in *The Double Face of Janus and Other Essays in the History of Medicine* (Baltimore: Johns Hopkins University Press, 1977) and O. Temkin, 'Medicine and the Problem of Moral Responsibility,' in *The Double Face of Janus and Other Essays in the History of Medicine* (Baltimore: Johns Hopkins University Press, 1977). Lewis Jillings discusses victim blaming in regard to syphilis, along with medical metaphors and the invocation of the 'plague mentality,' through which decadent and corrupt people get their comeuppance through the scourge of God, all of which are ideas that have influenced this chapter. L. Jillings, 'The Aggression of the Cured Syphilitic: Ulrich Von Hutten's Projection of His Disease as Metaphor,' *The German Quarterly* 68, no. 1 (1995). See also S. Sontag, *Illness as Metaphor* (New York: Vintage, 1979) and R. Porter, *Disease, Medicine, and Society in England, 1550-1860* (Basingstoke: Macmillan, 1987).

15   N. de Blegny, *New and Curious Observations Concerning the Art of Curing the Venereal Disease, and the Accidents It Produces* (1676), 3. There was also

a theory, first attributed to Paracelsus, which held that the pox came about from fornication between a prostitute and a leper. Paracelsus, *An Excellent Treatise Teaching Howe to Cure the French-Pockes with All Other Diseases Arising and Growing Thereof*, trans. John Hester (1590). This theory is mentioned in Peter Lowe, *An Easie, Certaine, and Perfect Method, to Cure and Preuent the Spanish Sickness* (1596).

16   R. Boulton, *Physico-Chirurgigal Treatise of the Gout, the King's Evil, and the Lues Venerea* (1714), 252.

17   J. S. *A Short Compendium of Chirurgery Containing Its Grounds & Principles* (1678), 114.

18   T. Sydenham, *A New Method of Curing the French-Pox* (1690), 3.

19   T. Sydenham, *A New Method of Curing the French-Pox* (1690), 20.

20   W. Schleiner, 'Moral Attitudes toward Syphilis and Its Prevention in the Renaissance,' *Bulletin of the History of Medicine* 68, no. 3 (1994), 185-6. See P. Desault, *A Treatise on the Venereal Distempers, Containing a Method of Curing It without Salivation, Danger, or Great Expense*, trans. Andree John (1738).

21   T. Needham, *A Treatise of a Venereal Consumption and the Venereal Disease* (1700), 6.

22   T. Whitaker, *An Elenchus of Opinions Concerning the Cure of the Small Pox Together with Problematicall Questions Concerning the Cure of the French Pest* (1661), 97.

23   T. Whitaker, *An Elenchus of Opinions Concerning the Cure of the Small Pox Together with Problematicall Questions Concerning the Cure of the French Pest*, 111-112.

24   W. Bynum, 'Treating the Wages of Sin: Venereal Disease and Specialism in Eighteenth-Century Britain,' in W. Bynum and R. Porter (eds), *Medical Fringe and Medical Orthodoxy, 1750-1850* (London: Croom Helm, 1987), 13.

25   In times of plague as well as pox, it was thought that moral pollution had a tangible, physical effect on the health of the population. For more on this see J. Arrizabalaga, J. Henderson, and R. French, *The Great Pox: The French Disease in Renaissance Europe* (New Haven: Yale University Press, 1997), 269.

26   J. Arrizabalaga, J. Henderson, and R. French, *The Great Pox: The French Disease in Renaissance Europe*, 35, 166-167.

27   K. Siena, 'Pandora's Pox: The Medical Presentation of Women in Early

Modern Venereological Tracts,' 98.

28 R.M. Karras, *Common Women: Prostitution and Sexuality in Medieval England* (New York: Oxford University Press, 1996), 102-3.

29 R.M. Karras, *Common Women: Prostitution and Sexuality in Medieval England*, 107-8, 111-112. Women often acted as the upholders of this patriarchal moral code. See J.M. Bennett, 'Feminism and History,' *Gender and History [Great Britain]* 1 (1989), 259-263; L. Gowing, *Domestic Dangers: Women, Words, and Sex in Early Modern London* (Oxford: Clarendon Press, 1996), 3; and A. Fletcher, *Gender, Sex and Subordination in England, 1550-1800* (New Haven: Yale University Press, 1995), xvi.

30 Some of the more popular ones include A. Carpenter, *Destructorium Vitiorum, or Destroyer of Vice* (1429) and 'The Prick of Conscience,' a poem that survives in 114 manuscripts. R. Lewis and A. McIntosh, *A Descriptive Guide to the Manuscripts of the Prick of Conscience* (Oxford: Society for the Study of Medieval Languages an Literatures, 1982), 1-2. For more examples see J. Coleman, *Medieval Readers and Writers, 1350-1400* (New York: Columbia University Press, 1981), 23. Cited in R.M. Karras, *Common Women: Prostitution and Sexuality in Medieval England,* 104-105.

31 Disease metaphors were popular literary devices during this period, and the pox lent itself to such uses because it was so richly metaphoric. Early modern writers commonly depicted disease as the enemy to be overcome, a foreign agent or 'other' who debilitates, causing suffering, pain, and sometimes death for its victims. In the case of syphilis, the imagery was slightly different. Pox metaphors portrayed the perception of danger cloaked within the female body in a very literal sense. For a more complete discussion of syphilis as a metaphoric disease, see S. Gilman, *Disease and Representation: Images of Illness from Madness to Aids* (New York: Ithaca, 1988); Susan Sontag, *Aids and Its Metaphors* (New York : Farrar, Straus, Giroux, 1988); and S. Sontag, *Illness as Metaphor* (New York: Farrar, Straus, 1977).

32 Each of the above examples quoted in J.C. Adams, *Shakespeare's Physic, Lore and Love* (Upton-upon-severn: SPA Limited, 1989), 52, 57, 59. For links between the writing of Shakespeare and syphilis, see J. Fabricius, *Syphilis in Shakespeare's England* (London: Jessica Kingsley Publishers, 1994); W. Clemen, *The Development of Shakespeare's Imagery* (London: Methuen, 1987); E. Partridge, *Shakespeare's Bawdy* (London: Routledge,

1956); and C. Spurgeon, *Shakespeare's Imagery and What It Tells Us* (Cambridge: Cambridge University Press, 1935).

33   W. Shakespeare, 'The Life of Timon of Athens' in *The Complete Pelican Shakespeare*, ed. Alfred Harbage (New York: Viking Penguin, 1969), IV.iii. 61.

34   R. Ames, *The Female Fire-Ships. A Satyr Against Whoring* (1691).

35   G. Harvey, *Great Venus Unmasked* (1672) and Anon., *The Tomb of Venus* (1710).

36   U. Von Hutten, *De Morbo Gallico. A Treatise of the French Disease, Publish'd above 200 Years Past* (1730), 7.

37   U. Von Hutten, *De Morbo Gallico,* 7.

38   P. Aretine, *Strange &Amp; True Nevves from Jack-a-Newberries Six Windmills* (1660), A2.

39   Anon., *Antimoixeia: Or, the Honest and Joynt Design of the Tower Hamlets for the General Suppression of Bawdy Houses, as Encouraged by the Publick Magistrates* (1691). The line reads, 'Impudent Harlots [who] by their Antick Dresses, Painted Faces, and Whorish Insinuations, allure and tempt our Sons and Servants to Debauchery.'

40   Anon., *The Crafty Whore: Or, the Mistery and Iniquity of Bawdy Houses Laid Open,* (1658).

41   P. Aretine, *Strange &Amp; True Nevves from Jack-a-Newberries Six Windmills, or, the Crafty, Impudent, Common-Whore (Turned Bawd) Anatomised and Discovered in the Unparralleld Practises of Mris Fotheringham ... With Five and Twenty Orders Agreeed Upon by Consent of Mris Creswell, Betty Lawrence ... With Divers Others for Establishing Thereof* / Published by Way of Admonition to All Persons to Beware of That House of Darkness (1660), A2.

42   C. Peter, *A Description of the Venereal Disease*, 8. Peter commented on the fury of the disease: 'Oh, how intolerable are the pains that many poor wretches endure by this Distemper, especially in the night, at which time it most boldly walks its Rounds to afflict poor Mortals!' Another physician compared the pox to Pandora's box, 'out of which all other Diseases and Mischiefs issue,' in order to stress the varied and agonizing suffering that its victims endured. The author asserts, 'When a man is attaqu'd with the Pox, he has not one single Disease alone, but a Legion of Maladies presently after seize his miserable Body,' and proceeds to list an entire page of them, from headaches to stoppage of urine. L.S., *Profulacticon: Or Some Considerations of a Notable Expedient*

to Root out the French Pox from the English Nation. With Excellent Defensive Remedies to Preserve Mankind from the Infection of Pocky Women (1673), 13-14.

43 L.S., *Prothylantinon, or, Some Considerations of a Notable Expedient to Root out the French Pox from the English Nation with Excellent Defensive Remedies to Preserve Mankind from the Infection of Pocky Women : Also an Advertisement, Wherein Is Discover'd the Dangerous Practices of Ignorant Pretenders to the Cure of the Disease.*

44 Quoted in J. Arrizabalaga, J. Henderson, and R. French, *The Great Pox: The French Disease in Renaissance Europe,* 123.

45 There are, of course, some empathetic portrayals of prostitutes, and these also tend to be formulaic. They generally follow the pattern of the repentant woman, yearning for forgiveness. See for example Anon., *The Poor Whore's Lamentation, or, the Fleet-Street Crack's Complaint for Want of Trading to the Tune of the Guinea Wins Her* (1685).

46 For further discussions of *The Honest Whore* and prostitution, submission, and social control, see A. Conway, 'Defoe's Protestant Whore,' *Eighteenth-Century Studies* 35, no. 2 (2002); K. Jackson, 'Bethlem and Bridewell in the "Honest Whore" Plays,' *Studies in English Literature 1500-1900* 43, no. 2 (2003); and B. Kreps, 'The Paradox of Women: The Legal Position of Early Modern Wives and Thomas Dekker's "the Honest Whore,"' *English Literary History* 69, no. 1 (2002).

47 T. Dekker, 'The Honest Whore.--Part the First,' in Ernest Rhys (eds), *The Best Plays of the Old Dramatists: Thomas Dekker* (New York: Charles Scribner's Sons, 1900), II.i. Bellafront alludes to the hidden danger of disease inherent in the prostitute when she attempts to persuade the men around her to forsake harlots: 'Worse than the deadliest poisons, they are worse: / For o'er their souls hangs an eternal curse' T. Dekker, 'The Honest Whore.--Part the First,' III.iii.

48 R. Ames, *The Female Fire-Ships. A Satyr Against Whoring* (1691).

49 T. Dekker, *Newes from Graves-Ende* (1604), sig. F2v.

50 K. Siena, 'Pandora's Pox: The Medical Presentation of Women in Early Modern Venereological Tracts,' v-vi. For a discussion of syphilis as portrayed in seventeenth-century literature, with particular emphasis on the works of William Shakespeare and Thomas Dekker, see M. Healy, *Fictions of Disease in Early Modern England* (New York: Palgrave, 2001), particularly chapter 4 'The Pocky Body: Part I' and chapter 5 'The Pocky Body: Part II.' See also J.D. Rolleston, 'Venereal Disease in

Literature,' *British Journal of Venereal Diseases* 10 (1934). and B.F. Leavy, *To Blight with Plague: Studies in a Literary Theme* (New York: New York University Press, 1992).

51 K. Siena, 'Pandora's Pox: The Medical Presentation of Women in Early Modern Venereological Tracts,' v-vi.

52 B. Shapiro, 'Law and Science in Seventeenth-Century England,' *Stanford Law Review* 21, no. 4 (April 1969) and B. Shapiro, *Probability and Certainty in Seventeenth-Century England: A Study of the Relations between Natural Science, Religion, History, Law, and Literature* (Princeton: Princeton University Press, 1983), in which her focus is on the profession of law, although it is possible to draw parallels with medicine.

53 S. Shapin, *A Social History of Truth: Civility and Science in Seventeenth-Century England* (Chicago: Chicago University Press, 1994), 27.

54 S. Shapin and S. Schaffer, *Leviathan and the Air-Pump: Hobbes, Boyle, and the Experimental Life* (Princeton, 1985), 250.

55 Shapiro differs from Shapin in that she does not consider social rank to have been as essential a component of trustworthiness, but rather that expertise, experience, and opportunity were at least of equal importance. B. Shapiro, *A Culture of Fact: England, 1550-1720* (Ithaca: Cornell University Press, 2000), 139.

56 S. Shapin, *A Social History of Truth: Civility and Science in Seventeenth-Century England.* These factors would later be replaced by the specialist's expertise. See also S. Shapin and S. Schaffer, *Leviathan and the Air-Pump: Hobbes, Boyle, and the Experimental Life,* in which they first attempt to show how the production of scientific knowledge was dependent upon (or tied up with) social order. On construction of knowledge in the Italian context, see B. Dooley, *The Social History of Skepticism: Experience and Doubt in Early Modern Culture,* vol. 2, *The Johns Hopkins University Studies in Historical and Political Science* (Baltimore: Johns Hopkins University Press, 1999).

57 Cited in R. Anselment, *The Realms of Apollo: Literature and Healing in Seventeenth-Century England* (Newark: University of Delaware Press, 1995), 140.

58 M. Nedham, *Medela Medicinae,* 72. Cited in R. Anselment, *The Realms of Apollo: Literature and Healing in Seventeenth-Century England,* 140.

59 Anon., *A Method of Curing the French Pox* (1690), 117.

60 C. Peter, *A Description of the Venereal Disease,* 12.

61 Cited in R. Anselment, *The Realms of Apollo: Literature and Healing in*

Seventeenth-Century England, 140.

62 Cited in R. Anselment, *The Realms of Apollo: Literature and Healing in Seventeenth-Century England,* 140. It was not unheard of for tracts to be published that offered to share preventatives, but these tended to be anonymous and comparatively scarce.

63 N. Culpeper, D. Sennert, and A. Cole, *Two Treatises. The First of the Venereal Pocks. The Second Treatise of the Gout,* 27-28.

64 J. Cam, *A Rational and Useful Account of the Venereal Disease: With Observations on the Nature, Symptoms, and Cure, and the Bad Consequences That Attend by Ill Management.* (1740), 5.

65 N. Culpeper, D. Sennert, and A. Cole, *Two Treatises. The First of the Venereal Pocks. The Second Treatise of the Gout,* 27-28.

66 P. Barrough, *The Method of Physic* (1652).

67 D. Sennert, *A Method of Curing the French Pox* (1690), 118, 120.

68 W. Clowes, *A Briefe and Necessarie Treatise, Touching the Cure of the Disease Called Morbus Gallicus, or Lues Venerea* (1585), Aiii-Aiiiv.

69 J. Archer, *Secrets Disclosed, or, a Treatise of Consumptions; Their Various Causes and Cure* (1693).

70 W. Clowes, *A Briefe and Necessarie Treatise, Touching the Cure of the Disease Called Morbus Gallicus, or Lues Venerea,* (1585), Aiiiv.

71 J. Cam, *A Rational and Useful Account of the Venereal Disease* (1740), C2.

72 J. Archer, *Secrets Disclosed, or, a Treatise of Consumptions; Their Various Causes and Cure,* 27.

73 J. Archer, *Secrets Disclosed, or, a Treatise of Consumptions; Their Various Causes and Cure,* 31-32. For a discussion of the connection between wet nursing and syphilis, see V. Fildes, *Wet Nursing* (Oxford: Basil Blackwell, 1988).

74 N. Robinson, *A Treatise of the Venereal Disease* (1763), J. Astruc, *A Treatise of Venereal Diseases, in Nine Books* (1754), C. Peter, *A Description of the Venereal Disease: Declaring the Causes, Signs, and Effects, and Cure Thereof. With a Discourse of the Most Wonderful Antivenereal Pill* (1678).

75 W. Bullein, *Bullein's Bulwarke of Defense against All Sicknesse, Soarenesse, and Woundes That Doe Dayly Assaulte Mankinde* (1579).

76 R. Ames, *The Female Fire-Ships. A Satyr Against Whoring.*

77 T. Alleine, *The Life & Death of Mr. Joseph Alleine, Late Teacher of the Church at Taunton* (1672).

78 Cited in T. Henderson, *Disorderly Women in Eighteenth-Century London* (New York: Longman, 1999), 177-8. Henderson also includes the

metaphorical description of the 'vast body of courtesans as plenty
as mackerel after thunder.' While uncovering seventeenth-century
contemporary estimates of the number of prostitutes in England
has proven to be difficult, Henderson notes that eighteenth-century
estimates in London ranged from 20,000 to 50,000.

79 Cited in J. Fabricius, *Syphilis in Shakespeare's England* (London: Jessica
Kingsley Publishers, 1994), 271.

80 K. Thomas, 'The Puritans and Adultery: The Act of 1650
Reconsidered,' in K. Thomas and D. Pennington (eds), *Puritans and
Revolutionaries: Essays Presented to Christopher Hill* (Oxford: Clarendon
Press, 1978), 259.

81 A. Hunt, *Governing Morals: A Social History of Moral Regulation*
(Cambridge: Cambridge University Press, 1999), 28.

82 E. Duffy, 'Primitive Christianity Revived; Religious Renewal in
Augustan England,' D. Baker (ed.), *Renaissance and Renewal in Christian
History* (Oxford: 1977), 293.

83 S. Burtt, 'The Societies for the Reformation of Manners: Between John
Locke and the Devil in Augustan England' in *The Margins of Orthodoxy:
Heterodox Writing and Cultural Response, 1660-1750* (New York, 1995),
152.

84 R. Shoemaker, 'Reforming the City: The Reformation of Manners
Campaign in London, 1690-1738,' in L. Davison, T. Hitchcock, T.
Keirn, R. Shoemaker (eds), *Stilling the Grumbling Hive: The Response
to Social and Economic Problems in England, 1689-1750* (New York: St.
Martin's Press, 1992), 100-101.

85 See for example Anon., *An Account of the Societies for the Reformation of
Manners in England and Ireland* (1701). Cited in T. Henderson, *Disorderly
Women in Eighteenth-Century London,* 87.

86 A. Hunt, *Governing Morals,* 35 and T. Henderson, *Disorderly Women in
Eighteenth-Century London,* 104-106.

87 T. Henderson, *Disorderly Women in Eighteenth-Century London,* 106-8 and
R. Shoemaker, 'Reforming the City: The Reformation of Manners
Campaign in London, 1690-1738,' 106. For prostitution and public
order, see M.E. Perry, '"Lost Women" In Early Modern Seville: The
Politics of Prostitution,' *Feminist Studies* 4, no. 195-214 (Feb. 1978).
Perry found that more emphatic control of prostitution was a result of
concern with increasing public disorder.

88 A. Hunt, *Governing Morals,* 29.

89   Anon., *Antimoixeria: or, the Honest and Joynt-Design of the Tower Hamlets for the General Suppression of Bawdy-Houses, as Encouraged by the Publick Magistrates,* (18 June 1691)

90   P. Griffiths, 'The Structure of Prostitution in Elizabethan London,' *Continuity and Change* 8, no. 1 (1993): 40, 48, 57. For contemporary examples see R. Greene, *A Disputation between a He-Cony--Catcher and a She-Cony--Catcher* (1592), 210, 213 and J. Taylor, 'A Bawd, a Vertuous Bawd, a Modest Bawd: As Shee Deserves, Reprove or Else Applaud,' (1630), 99, 103.

91   F. Dabhoiwala, 'Sex and Societies for Moral Reform, 1688-1800' in *The Journal of British Studies* 46:2 (April 2007), 297.

92   Cited in E. Duffy, 'Primitive Christianity Revived; Religious Renewal in Augustan England,' 288.

93   *His Majesty's Letter to the Lord Bishop of London* (1690), 15-16. Cited in J. Spurr, 'The Church, the Societies and the Moral Revolution of 1688' in *The Church of England, c. 1689-c.1833: From Toleration to Tractarianism* (New York 1993), 128.

94   A. Hunt, *Governing Morals,* 32-33.

95   A. Hunt, *Governing Morals,* 34 and S. Burtt 'The Societies for the Reformation of Manners: Between John Locke and the Devil in Augustan England,' in *The Margins of Orthodoxy: Heterodox Writing and Cultural Response, 1660-1750* (New York, Cambridge University Press, 1995), 154.

96   F. Dabhoiwala, 'Sex and Societies for Moral Reform, 1688-1800,' 318. Throughout these decades sexual immorality remained the most prominent target of metropolitan campaigners. In 1703, streetwalkers accounted for almost two-thirds of all committal to suburban houses of correction. F. Dabhoiwala, 302-303.

97   J. Spurr, 'The Church, the Societies and the Moral Revolution of 1688,' in *The Church of England, c. 1689-c.1833: From Toleration to Tractarianism* (New York: 1993), 138, 140.

98   A. Hunt, *Governing Morals,* 17, 9, 11.

99   S. Burtt, 'The Societies for the Reformation of Manners: Between John Locke and the Devil in Augustan England,' 153.

100 K. Siena, 'Pollution, Promiscuity, and the Pox: English Venereology and the Early Modern Medical Discourse on Social and Sexual Danger,' *Journal of the History of Sexuality* 8, no. 4 (1998), 571-2. See also A. Hunt, *Governing Morals.*

101 J. Arrizabalaga, J. Henderson, and R. French, *The Great Pox: The French Disease in Renaissance Europe,* 281.

102 K. Siena, 'Pollution, Promiscuity, and the Pox: English Venereology and the Early Modern Medical Discourse on Social and Sexual Danger,' 571-2.

103 T. Needham, *A Treatise of a Venereal Consumption and the Venereal Disease,* 553-555.

104 L.S., *Prothylantinon, or, Some Considerations of a Notable Expedient to Root out the French Pox from the English Nation with Excellent Defensive Remedies to Preserve Mankind from the Infection of Pocky Women.*

105 W. Clowes, *A Briefe and Necessarie Treatise* (1596), 1v.

106 N. Culpeper, D. Sennert, and A. Cole, *Two Treatises. The First of the Venereal Pocks. The Second Treatise of the Gout,* 13-14.

107 R. Dingley, *Proposals for Establishing a Public Place of Reception for Penitent Prostitutes* (1758), 1.

108 Cited in P. Griffiths, 'The Structure of Prostitution in Elizabethan London,' 54.

109 R. French and J. Arrizabalaga, 'Coping with the French Disease: University Practitioners' Strategies and Tactics in the Transition from the Fifteenth to the Sixteenth Century,' in R. French, J. Arrizabalaga, A. Cunningham and L. Garcia-Ballester (eds), *Medicine from the Black Death to the French Disease* (Aldershot: Ashgate, 1998), 252 and M. Pelling, 'Appearance and Reality: Barber-Surgeons, the Body and Disease,' in A.L. Beier and R. Finlay (eds), *London 1500-1700: The Making of the Metropolis* (New York: Longman, 1986), 101.

110 L.S., *Profulacticon: Or Some Considerations of a Notable Expedient to Root out the French Pox from the English Nation,* 15-16.

111 L.S., *Profulacticon: Or Some Considerations of a Notable Expedient to Root out the French Pox from the English Nation,* 14-15.

112 T. Needham, *A Treatise of a Venereal Consumption and the Venereal Disease.*

113 M.E. Perry, '"Lost Women" In Early Modern Seville: The Politics of Prostitution,' 137.

114 Economics come into play even with male visitors of prostitutes, as wealthier men could afford costly condoms (made from sheep's bladder) to help protect themselves from venereal disease. T. Henderson, *Disorderly Women in Eighteenth-Centiry London.* 38. Henderson notes that due to their cost (along with the widely held belief that prostitutes were barren) prostitutes typically did not purchase condoms

or require their patrons to do so in the seventeenth century. Siena has offered convincing evidence that 'class was no barrier to the impact of the pox on one's reputation.' K. Siena, 'The Clean and the Foul: Paupers and the Pox in London Hospitals, C. 1550-C.1700,' in *Sins of the Flesh: Responding to Sexual Disease in Early Modern Europe ed. Kevin Siena* (Toronto: Centre for Reformation and Renaissance Studies, Victoria University in the University of Toronto, 2005), 268.

115 K. Siena, *Venereal Disease, Hospitals, and the Urban Poor: London's 'Foul Wards,' 1600-1800* (Rochester: University of Rochester Press, 2004), 256-7.

116 K. Siena, 'The Clean and the Foul: Paupers and the Pox in London Hospitals, C. 1550-C.1700,' 264.

117 K. Siena, *Venereal Disease, Hospitals and the Urban Poor: London's 'Foul Wards,' 1600-1800,* 39, 94. O. Temkin, 'On the History of "Morality and Syphilis,"' 524. Siena qualifies Temkin's findings. His research showed that royal hospitals spared their patients mercury treatments, opting instead for the gentler guaiacum cures, but when finances became tight, they quickly switched back to mercury. Siena, 'The Clean and the Foul: Paupers and the Pox in London Hospitals, C. 1550-C.1700,' 274.

118 This is not to suggest that there were not differences in the experience of men versus women suffering from venereal disease, either in the seventeenth century or later. Feminist scholars have demonstrated how public health measures to control sexually transmitted diseases often aimed to regulate working class women's sexuality. See J. Walkowitz, *Prostitution and Victorian Society: Women, Class, and the State* (Cambridge: Cambridge University Press, 1980); L. Mayhood, *The Magdalens: Prostitution in the Nineteenth Century* (London: Routledge, 1990); and M. Spongburg, *Feminizing Venereal Disease: The Body of the Prostitute in the Nineteenth Century* (London: MacMillan, 1997).

119 S. Lloyd, '"Pleasure's Golden Bait": Prostitution, Poverty and the Magdalen Hospital in Eighteenth-Century London,' *History Workshop Journal,* no. 41 (1996), 54.

120 Donna Andrew has convincingly argued that the most thriving charities of the period combined elements of moral reform, public safety, and economic benefit (like the Magdalen Hospital). D. Andrew, *Philanthropy and Police* (Princeton, NJ: Princeton University Press, 1989), 8.

121 K. Siena, 'The Clean and the Foul: Paupers and the Pox in London

Hospitals, C. 1550-C.1700,' 266.

122 K. Siena, *Venereal Disease, Hospitals, and the Urban Poor: London's 'Foul Wards,' 1600-1800*, 10. In an effort to accommodate the large number of venereal patients, new institutions like Guy's hospital emerged in the eighteenth century and built venereal wards. Moreover, parish infirmaries cropped up all over London after 1720, but despite the increase in beds, there remained a pressing need for the Lock Hospital in 1747, as evidenced by the records of that hospital's lengthy waiting periods. R. Trumbach, *Sex and the Gender Revolution*, vol. 1, *Heterosexuality and the Third Gender in Enlightenment London* (Chicago: University of Chicago Press, 1998) 196-9. Edward Shorter also states that venereal disease remained on the margins of society prior to 1850. E. Shorter, *Women's Bodies: A Social History of Women's Encounter with Health, Ill-Health, and Medicine* (New Brunswick, NJ: Transactions Publications, 1991), 263-7.

123 R. French and J. Arrizabalaga, 'Coping with the French Disease: University Practitioners' Strategies and Tactics in the Transition from the Fifteenth to the Sixteenth Century,' 248.

124 K. Siena, 'The Clean and the Foul: Paupers and the Pox in London Hospitals, C. 1550-C.1700,' 264. The case was similar for the Magdalen Hospital. Stanley Nash found 'the most striking observation…is that to a large degree the Magdalen resembled the prison penitentiary.' S. Nash, 'Prostitution and Charity: The Magdalen Hospital, a Case Study,' *Journal of Social History* 17, no. 4 (Summer 1984), 623-4.

125 All in K. Siena, 'The Clean and the Foul: Paupers and the Pox in London Hospitals, C. 1550-C.1700,' 277. See also J. Arrizabalaga, J. Henderson, and R. French, *The Great Pox*.

126 K. Siena, *Venereal Disease, Hospitals and the Urban Poor: London's 'Foul Wards,' 1600-1800*, 214.

127 L. Merians, 'The London Lock Hospital and the Lock Asylum for Women,' in L. Merians (ed.), *The Secret Malady: Venereal Disease in Eighteenth-century Britain and France* (Lexington: University of Kentucky Press, 1996), 130.

128 Anon., 'An Account of the Institution of the Lock Asylum; for the reception of Penitent Female patients, when discharged from the Lock Hospital' (1793).

129 Surgeons were treating the indigent in hospitals. Physicians would not enter hospitals in significant number until the next century. See

S. Lloyd,"'Pleasure's Golden Bait": Prostitution, Poverty and the Magdalen Hospital in Eighteenth-Century London' and Siena, *Venereal Disease, Hospitals, and the Urban Poor: London's 'Foul Wards,' 1600-1800.*

130 W. Clowes, *A Briefe and Necessarie Treatise,* 150.

131 M.W. Adler, 'The Terrible Peril: A Historical Perspective on the Venereal Diseases,' in *British Medical Journal* (19 July 1980), 206-211. Dr. Solly's remarks were recorded in 1868. Adler also describes a twentieth-century physician writing to a patient, 'You have had the disease one year, and I hope it may plague you many more to punish you for your sins and I would not think of treating you,' 206.

132 J. Wynell, *Lues Venera, or a perfect cure for the French pox* (1660).

133 J. Wynell, *Lues Venera, or a perfect cure for the French pox.*

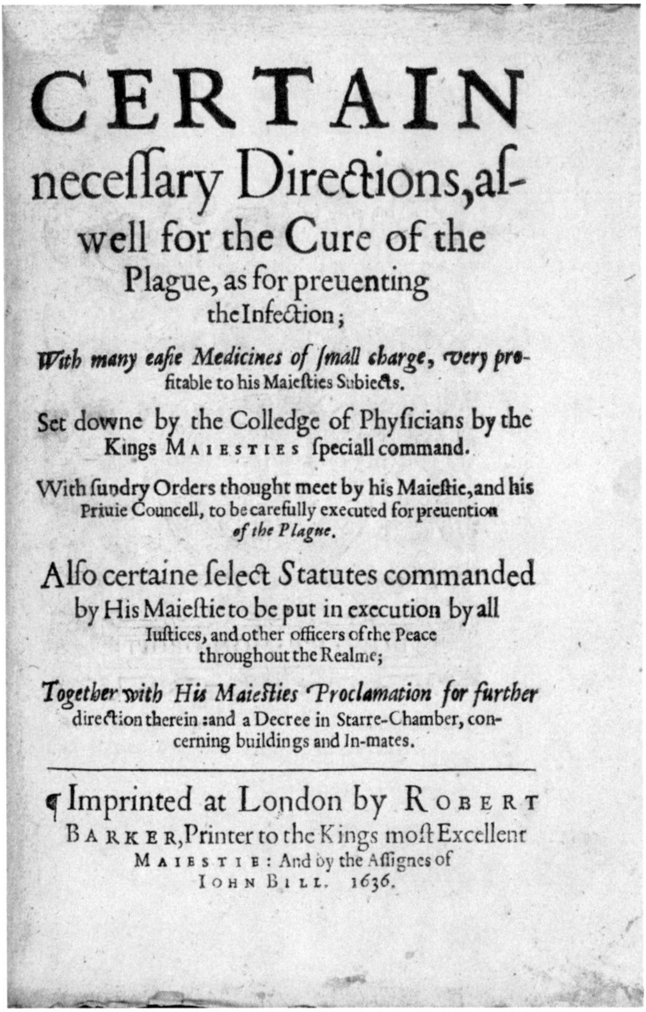

CERTAIN

neceſſary Directions, aſ-
well for the Cure of the
Plague, as for preuenting
the Infection;

With many eaſie Medicines of ſmall charge, very pro-
fitable to his Maieſties Subiects.

Set downe by the Colledge of Phyſicians by the
Kings MAIESTIES ſpeciall command.

With ſundry Orders thought meet by his Maieſtie, and his
Priuie Councell, to be carefully executed for preuention
of the Plague.

Alſo certaine ſelect Statutes commanded
by His Maieſtie to be put in execution by all
Iuſtices, and other officers of the Peace
throughout the Realme;

Together with His Maieſties Proclamation for further
direction therein : and a Decree in Starre-Chamber, concerning buildings and In-mates.

¶ Imprinted at London by ROBERT
BARKER, Printer to the Kings moſt Excellent
MAIESTIE : And by the Aſſignes of
IOHN BILL. 1636.

Figure 13: Titlepage: Certain necessary directions, as well for
the cure of the plague, as for preventing the infection with
many easie medicines of small charge, very profitable to His
Majesties subjects
Courtesy Wellcome Library, London

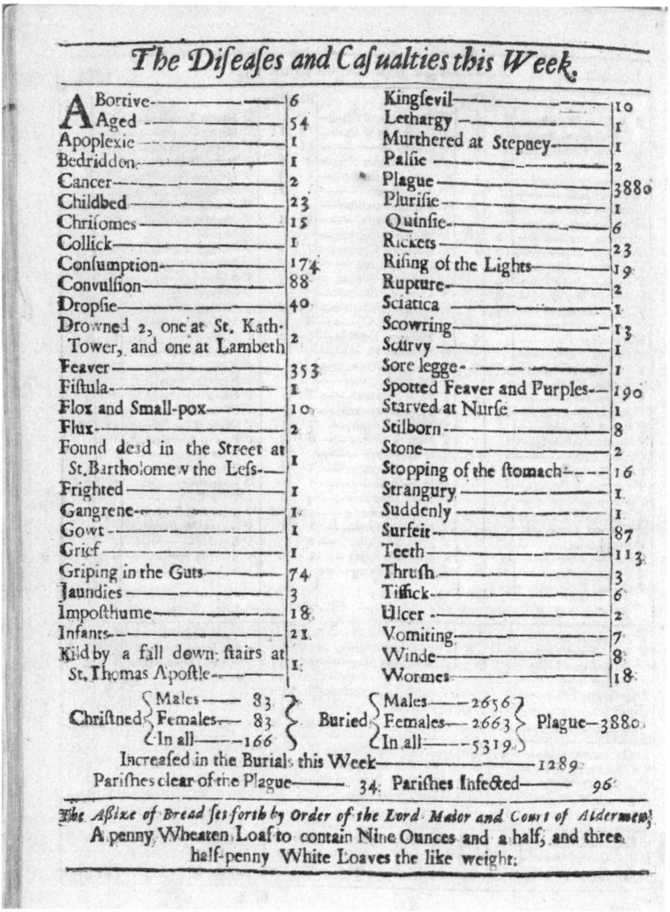

The Diseases and Casualties this Week.

Abortive	6	Kingsevil	10
Aged	54	Lethargy	1
Apoplexie	1	Murthered at Stepney	1
Bedridden	1	Palsie	2
Cancer	2	Plague	3880
Childbed	23	Plurisie	1
Chrisomes	15	Quinsie	6
Collick	1	Rickets	23
Consumption	174	Rising of the Lights	19
Convulsion	88	Rupture	2
Dropsie	40	Sciatica	1
Drowned 2, one at St. Kath-Tower, and one at Lambeth	2	Scowring	13
Feaver	353	Scurvy	1
Fistula	1	Sore legge	1
Flox and Small-pox	10	Spotted Feaver and Purples	190
Flux	2	Starved at Nurse	1
Found dead in the Street at St. Bartholomew the Less	1	Stilborn	8
		Stone	2
Frighted	1	Stopping of the stomach	16
Gangrene	1	Strangury	1
Gowt	1	Suddenly	1
Grief	1	Surfeit	87
Griping in the Guts	74	Teeth	113
Jaundies	3	Thrush	3
Imposthume	18	Tissick	6
Infants	21	Ulcer	2
Kild by a fall down stairs at St. Thomas Apostle	1	Vomiting	7
		Winde	8
		Wormes	18

Christned { Males — 83, Females — 83, In all — 166 }
Buried { Males — 2656, Females — 2663, In all — 5319 } Plague — 3880.

Increased in the Burials this Week — 1289
Parishes clear of the Plague — 34. Parishes Infected — 96

The Assize of Bread set forth by Order of the Lord Maior and Court of Aldermen,
A penny Wheaten Loaf to contain Nine Ounces and a half; and three
half-penny White Loaves the like weight.

Figure 14: Bills of mortality, August 15-22, 1665
Courtesy Wellcome Library, London

7

'A Broom in the Hand of the Almighty'[1]:
The Plague and the Unruly Poor

September 4, 1665... it troubled me to pass by Come Farme, where about 21 people have died of the plague and three or four days since I saw a dead corpse in a Coffin lie in the close unburyed and a watch is constantly kept there, night and day, to keep people in[;] the plague making us cruel as dogs one to another.[2]

Now many houses are shut up where the Plague comes and the inhabitants are shut in, lest coming abroad they should spread infection. It was very dismal to behold the Red Crosses, and read in great letters, LORD HAVE MERCY UPON US, on the doors, and Watchmen standing before them with Halberts, and such a solitude about those places, and people passing by them so gingerly, and with such fearful looks, as if they had been lined with enemies in ambush, that waited to destroy them.[3]

Bubonic plague was only one of many epidemic diseases of the early modern period. Typhus and dysentery were more common, influenza killed many more people, and numerous childhood diseases checked the rate of population.[4] Yet no disease evoked quite the same degree of dread and terror in contemporaries as bubonic plague. In his account of the plague, Thomas Dekker determined that it was awful in three ways: 'in the general spreading; in the quickness of the stroke; and in the terror that waits upon it.'[5] Contemporary medical texts alluded to the fear that the disease evoked. *The Plagues Approved Physitian* began with the premise, 'Of all the diseases whereunto the body of man is subject, the Plague or Pestilence is the most terrible and fearefull.'[6] At the onset of the 1665 epidemic, the president of the Royal College of Physicians, Nathaniel Hodges, noted that in anticipation of an outbreak, people 'terrified each other with remembrances of a former pestilence.'[7] The dread was in part due to the high mortality rate of sufferers, coupled with the swiftness of death and the rapidity of its spread.[8]

As a result, there was a certain terror accompanying outbreaks of plague that was distinct to that disease. This fear led to flight to the countryside for those able to afford it. Lloyd and Dorothy Moote have estimated the cost of fleeing to the countryside at a minimum of five shillings, placing escape far beyond the means of London's skilled craftspersons. Additionally, those who fled risked starvation or shunning by the local inhabitants because of their poor dress and appearance, which would be associated with carrying the plague.[9] With the affected city or town emptied of those with the means to flee, commerce came to a halt, resulting in a large concentration of the poor and idle. The situation was fraught with tension for those forced to stay behind as well as for those entrusted to keep order during precarious times. Rioting by the 'unruly poor' was a particularly acute concern during outbreaks of epidemics, when food, medical help, and employment were in short supply.[10]

Plague has piqued the interest of historians primarily due to the fear and terror associated with outbreaks, coupled with the ensuing displacement and disruption of society in its wake.[11] Rather than depicting early modern people as victims of their circumstances and of biological processes that were beyond their understanding and control, the prevailing interpretation has been that although early modern societies misunderstood its mode of transmission, they were not inactive in times of plague. They enacted household isolation, quarantined ships, and even issued *cordons sanitaires* around entire towns. The clothes and other personal items belonging to the victims of plague were burned, and restrictions were placed on public assemblies and gatherings, even funerals.[12] Since it was widely accepted that foul air was the culprit and human contact spread the disease, in theory it was preventable.[13]

The belief that human measures could prevent or ameliorate the plague led some European countries to enforce strict policies such as household quarantine or laws against vagrancy. For instance, the city-states of Northern Italy produced an activist military style of public health intervention in response to plague. Historians have determined that they were successful in enforcing their continuing and often brutal attempts at social control only after they were supported by a medical rationale that combined contagion theory with the increasing identification of the poor as carriers of the disease.[14] In short, once the spread of plague was associated with the lower orders, government could justify taking action to control the behavior of that segment of society to prevent them from infecting the rest of society.[15] Plague studies that focus on the Continent have found that successful plague policy was repressive, possessed sufficient central government powers to enforce the directives, and enjoyed the support of the elite.[16] England, on the other hand, was not successful in introducing any public precautions against plague until 1518, and even those were scantily enforced. Part of the reason lay with the government. As Paul Slack has argued, England was hampered by a decentralized government that was unable to force its policies on unreceptive localities. By 1578 government-sponsored proclamations, acts, and statutes began to be developed as a set of coherent social policies aimed at controlling plague, but it was not until the 1630s that the monarchy actively strove to enforce obedience to its directives. English plague policy began to take shape and gain momentum due to the proportionally high incidence of plague among the poor and in the relatively unpoliced suburbs, which gave rise to an association of plague with poverty and filth.[17] This chapter will argue that physicians' writing on the role of poverty and lack of cleanliness in spreading the plague helped bolster England's repressive plague policy in the first half of the seventeenth century. Furthermore, physicians' theories regarding the connection between physical and spiritual health offered support for restrictions on places where vice and disorderliness were thought to thrive.

Some historians have depicted bubonic plague as a failure for the physician, one which exposed traditional Galenic medicine as woefully inadequate to deal with the crisis and impugned the College of Physicians as unwilling to jeopardize their personal safety to care for the ill.[18] Margaret Pelling has concluded that it is 'difficult to see the College's contributions to measures against the plague as anything better than reactive and reluctant.'[19] Part of the reasoning behind such a conclusion is due to the exodus of so many physicians during outbreaks. Although London saw more physicians stay on in the outbreak of 1665 than in any previous outbreak, licensed physicians evacuated en masse. Estimates are that four-fifths of the College of Physicians fled, leaving only between 250 to 300 doctors, apothecaries, and surgeons in London, whereas prior to the plague there would have been 500-600 licensed and unlicensed practitioners.[20] Historians have therefore concluded that any gains the profession of medicine might have made during periods of plague outbreaks were negated by the damage to their public perception engendered by their flight.[21]

While physicians' fleeing did hurt their public perception for the few years following an outbreak, they were in good company as the king, parliament, the clergy, and most of those who could afford to do so left as well. It is also important to bear in mind that unlike the Tudor poor law, plague policy originated from central government who then imposed it on the periphery.[22] Because central government was conducted from outside of London during outbreaks, being absent from London when plague raged did not mean that physicians were unable to exert influence. In fact, they did, through their publications and the advice they submitted to the Privy Council on managing plague epidemics.

The violent outbreaks of plague that ravaged seventeenth-century England spurred the development of public health measures, however ineffectual, and spawned the idea of health protection on a national scale. Although it would take until the nineteenth century to fully realize such approaches, the policies conceptualized by government officials in the seventeenth century paved the way for public health measures achieved much later.[23] This chapter will argue that physicians were active participants in the conceptualization of public health measures. They contributed medical theory about the interconnection of physical and spiritual health to a central government that was eager for support of its directives and that was similarly interested in controlling plague through curbing vice and disorder.

The seventeenth century brought increased interest in the natural causes of plague and in human efforts to quantify plague deaths and identify areas hit hardest by plague. Physicians were able to use the increasing awareness that human measures could be employed to control the spread of plague to focus on the lack of cleanliness of the urban poor. Physicians' contagion theories drew a parallel between physical and spiritual filth as factors that encouraged the transmission of plague. The inclusion by physicians of the moral components of disease, which equated spiritual with physical health, impugned the poor and unruly as sinful, and therefore dangerous, to the health of the country. Such theories provided government officials with the necessary rhetorical ammunition to battle plague through the social control of these groups. As early as 1631 physicians were asked by the government for advice on 'political' as well as 'natural' medicines for the plague.[24] They obliged with suggestions that supported the government's quest to keep order among the poor and unruly of society, and in doing so became instrumental in conceptualizing the public health plan to be enacted during times of greatest crisis and for the public health in general.

By the early seventeenth century, it had become a routine metaphor that

God smote sin with sickness, His most potent weapon being plague.[25] Contemporary authors frequently cited biblical passages that made this claim. Richard Younge's, *The Prevention of Poverty* provided biblical examples that led God to '[smite] the people with an exceeding great plague.'[26] William Gouge quoted Ezekial VI. XI on his title page: 'Alas, for all the evill abominations of the house of Israel: for they shall fall by the Sword, by the Famine, and by the Pestilence.' Gouge explained that 'The procuring cause' of plague was 'the sinne of the people,' and 'the inflicting cause was the Lord.'[27] Seventeenth-century sermons repeatedly credited sin as the 'provoking cause' of plague, a disease defined as 'a speciall blowe inflicted on mankind for sinne.'[28]

Outbreaks of plague were consistently associated with God's divine wrath.[29] It had therefore seemed logical over the centuries to combat plague with prayer and collective remorse for sin as well as changing society's sinful ways. Government-declared days of fasting and communal prayer regularly accompanied plague epidemics.[30] During the plague of 1665, Ralph Josselin asked his parishioners to repent their sins and change their sinful ways so that God would preserve them and heal the city.[31] Prayers and meditations were published for the specific purpose of allaying God's wrath, such as the following selection included in *Great Britains Prayers in This dangerous time of Contagion:*

> We pardon crave for all our sinnes committed,
> Good Lord forgive them, let them be remitted,
> Draw back thy plaguing hand, Lord sheath thy sword
> Of vengeance drawn, and comfort us afford.[32]

Londons Lamentations for her Sinnes: And Complaint to the Lord her God offered a selection of prayers 'for private families, for the time of this fearfull Infection,' as did many others.[33] Sermons stressed the reliance on prayer as 'physick' for plague, such as *A Heavenly Cordial for All Those Servants of the Lord That Have Had the Plague.*[34] Plague, then, was routinely associated with sin, and prayer was its natural antidote.

The notion that plague came from God was so ubiquitous that it is difficult to find a publication of any kind, religious or secular in nature, which did not begin with this premise, whether published in 1500 or 1700.[35] However, during the seventeenth century, there was an increasing interest in the 'natural' or 'secondary' causes of plague, evident in publications ranging from physicians' writing to government-issued plague orders. It is important to note that these publications did not refute or even cast doubt on God as the source of plague, nor did they suggest that spiritual means, such as fasts and prayer, were ineffective or unnecessary components for relief from plague. Rather, they focused new energy on the secondary causes God used to smite with plague, causes which in theory, since they were natural, could be ameliorated by human measures.

Physicians' writing on the subject of plague throughout the seventeenth century reflected this interest. Physicians consistently began their works with the acknowledgement that God sent plague and that it must be His choice to relieve mankind's suffering.[36] However, they typically proceeded by stating that the physician was approved by God to administer healing and relief to sufferers. One explained that physicians were the 'Hands of God,' because they were 'the Instruments he often uses in restoring Health, and repairing decayed Nature.' Another asserted that 'no man doubteth that God hath created both physick and the Physician for the help, comfort, and succour of mankinde in sickenesse.' They set themselves up as God's approved healers of plague: 'for into their [physicians'] Hands God has put the Lives of those he lov'd so well.'[37] Such an intimate connection with the Creator assured that He would 'blesse the means of healing which in His mercy he has ordained for the preservation and cure of soule or body.'[38] Even divines asserted that pious physicians would have success in healing because the Lord would 'prosper that which they give for ease and remedy to prolong life.'[39] The association of the physician as God's approved healer for the plague was a positive one for physicians; thus, the customary link between plague and sin went unquestioned in medical writing throughout the early modern period.

Even though physicians never severed the link between God's wrath and plague outbreaks, they began to focus more on the natural causes of plague, which they often termed the 'secondary causes.'[40] Many of their texts followed a similar format to this 1640s plague treatise in prioritizing the causes of plague: 'The Cause is chiefly the sins of Mankind, provoking the great God to send this Pestiferous distemper as a judgment on them for their Impiety. The Cause (next to God's judgment) is a sharp venemous and contagious volatile Salt in the Air.'[41] This treatise is typical of those written by physicians in that the author began with an acknowledgment of God as the source and then launched into the natural causes of plague. John Gadbury relegated God's hand in plague to a caveat in the 'To the Reader' section: 'When I speak of the causes of the Plague, you are to understand that I tacitly acknowledge, God the chief and supreme Cause of all things! And that it is in his power to alter or suspend second Causes, even as he pleaseth.'[42] However, he then mentioned that God hardly ever interfered in secondary causes and had not really bothered to do so since biblical times. The remainder of the document was concerned with natural causes for plague and physician-approved remedies. When the renowned physician Nathaniel Hodges, who served as President of the Royal College of Physicians during the Great Plague of 1665-6 (also one of the few physicians to remain in London during the outbreak), wrote on plague, he unequivocally expressed the relationship between God and the plague that most physicians were tacitly suggesting in their treatises by that point:

> I cannot think that because *God* doth frequently send out the *Plague* as his *severe judgment* to punish mankind, we ought wholly to desist from all manner of search into *natural causes,* on the knowledg of which depends the *Cure,* procured both by our *devotion,* and the *commanded use* of *natural means.*[43]

He thereby acknowledged God's part in the sending of plague, the physician's skill in eradicating it, and God's approval of his doing so, since it was '*by Gods blessing* and the *care* and *skill* of *experienced Physitians* very many recover.'[44] Physicians were meant to work in harmony with God to help alleviate plague.

It was becoming difficult to attribute plague solely to the will of God without considering secondary causes, a thorn in the side of divines. Many clergymen were critical of the increasing stress on natural causes of plague, triggering the lament that there was 'booke upon booke prescribing naturall meanes as for naturall maladies but little said of spirituall meanes for spirituall maladies.'[45] They saw it as folly at best and hubris at worst that men would waste their time on cures and observations rather than on repentance. Early seventeenth-century sermons used physicians' inability to cure plague as proof that it was God's punishment for sin. For example, the minister Henoch Clapham published a sermon during the epidemic of 1603 in which he stated that the plague was a disease 'confessed by our Physitians, to exceed the compasse and reache of all their naturall reason and reasoning.'[46] Thomas Brooke's 1665 sermon reproached physicians for looking only at the 'second' or 'natural' causes of plague at the expense of losing sight of the primary cause: God.[47] Divines feared that the emphasis placed on natural remedies would divert attention away from sinners repenting in order to stay plague.

Their complaints were legitimate in that the abundance of available information, from physicians' writing on plague to the bills of mortality, collectively altered the manner in which people viewed plague by the latter half of the seventeenth century, although not to the extent that some clergymen feared. For many, dealing with plague throughout the seventeenth century consisted of a combination of prayer and preventative measures. Henry Oldenburg, the secretary of the Royal Society who stayed behind in the plague of 1665, expressed this point explicitly: 'I strive to banish both fear and overconfidence, leading a regular life and avoiding infected places as much as I can, leaving the rest to God.'[48] The new attempts to quantify plague fatalities did not necessarily remove the hand of God from plague, but they did demonstrate that the poor suffered more than the rich did.

The availability of secular works that discussed the secondary causes of plague was rapidly increasing. Between 1486 and 1604 there were twenty-three books published in England dealing exclusively with plague, although many more included sections on plague.[49] By 1665, there were at minimum an additional forty-six publications concerned with plague with many more publications devoting sections to the disease. There was also myriad broadsheets offering many different remedies and preservatives, some of which were distributed in bulk to all churchwardens in order to be passed along to any householder who might request one.[50] These were often, though not always, written by physicians. As a group, they posited the view that plague was a contagion spread by infected people and that public authority could prevent the spread of infection or ameliorate its consequences. Over the course of the seventeenth century, plague pamphlets began to list natural causes for the plague, such as heat, filth, and overcrowding. By 1644 a plague pamphlet noted that the ancients 'not knowing the great cause of corruption in the bloud' referred it to the Gods for their sinnes,' in contrast with the present-day understanding of plague.[51] While many authors of plague pamphlets continued to caution that God was punishing sin through plague, the focus now was on the secondary causes God was using, which could be studied and were in theory controllable.[52]

There were also attempts to quantify plague fatalities, such as newspapers that listed weekly burial totals and the locations of deaths as well as the bills of mortality. The latter were abstracts from Parish Registers showing the numbers of those who died in each parish or place during certain intervals of times, weekly, monthly, or yearly.[53] By breaking down plague deaths according to parish and listing the number dead for each area week by week, the bills helped readers note the regular seasonal periodicity of plague and act accordingly. Quantification provided a means of tracing patterns of plague epidemics and their progression. It is worth noting that as this chapter will illustrate, increasing confidence in secondary causes and the efforts at quantification associated with them did not diminish the belief that God punished sin with plague, at least not in the seventeenth century. However, it did highlight the fact that plague was disproportionately present in the poor areas of town.

The bills of mortality, in particular, helped cement an already-present understanding of the link between plague and poverty by illustrating numerically that plague deaths were concentrated in the suburbs and hence among the poor.[54] The publications that reprinted the bills frequently drew upon the theme that all humanity was susceptible to God's wrath, reminding readers that the bills were meant to confer a '*uniforme* and *cordial repentance*, that every one of us may search out the *plague* of his own *heart* and *brain*, and purge ourselves, by His gracious assistance, from all filthiness of flesh and spirit; so that He may…restore health to our habitations.'[55] Yet by breaking down plague deaths according to parish and listing the number dead for each area week by week, the bills allowed people to make informed decisions about whether they could safely remain in London. Rather than focusing on repentance, the bills gave those wealthy enough to flee the information to aid them in their decision-making process. For instance, during the Great Plague of 1665, Samuel Pepys used the bills to chart his movements through the city, to determine when he should send his wife away, and ultimately when he himself should flee.[56]

By the Great Plague, and arguably sooner, it had become clear that in general the rich 'flie from the stroke, the Poor fall under it. They are shut up in their Houses, as sheep for the slaughter.'[57] Fleeing the plague had become a commonplace for those with the means to do so, as remarked upon by Pepys who found 'all the town going out of town, the coaches and carriages being all full of people going into the country.'[58] In another account of the plague, the author noted a similar situation: 'Most of the rich are now gone and the middle sort will not stay behind; but the poor are forced (through poverty) to stay, and abide the storm.'[59] Because the poor remained after the exodus, they consequently suffered from plague disproportionately.

The concentration of deaths in the poor suburbs helped contemporaries view plague as a social problem. The stress on eradicating it would shift from days of communal prayers and fasting to more tangible measures aimed at controlling the spread of plague among the poor. There were even those among the lay population who welcomed plague as a 'broom in the hands of the Almighty with which he sweepeth the most nasty and uncomely corners of the universe.'[60] The divine Robert Harris termed plague a 'blessing' since its chief victims were 'of the baser and poorer sort, such whose lives were burdensome, whose deaths are beneficial' to the rest of society.[61] The minister William Gouge assumed that God deemed the poor to die in greater numbers from plague because 'they are not of such use' and 'may better be spared.'[62] Although not everyone espoused such a harsh view, the link between plague and poverty became the focal point of both physicians' theories on plague and government's efforts to control it.

The cumulative effect of these publications, with their systematic approach to reporting plague deaths and locations, in essence quantified plague. In doing so, they paved the way for physicians and government officials to justify the ordering of lower classes as a means of protecting the whole of society against infection, ushering in new changes, and fostering new concepts of public health. This trend toward scientific observation and the attempt to control plague through human intervention allowed physicians to take a greater part in the government's efforts to combat plague. Government officials asked their advice, thereby giving them a voice in official publications related to the eradication of plague. Perhaps most significantly, physicians would prove themselves able, as a profession, to continue melding lingering religious concerns about plague as punishment sent from God with the new-found optimism that tangible steps could be taken from a public health point of view to ease plague outbreaks and help prevent them altogether.

By the seventeenth century, it had become clear to observers that poor areas were more prone to plague and that the poor died in greater numbers from outbreaks. One explanation for this was that a lack of cleanliness and crowded living conditions allowed the disease to spread more quickly. However, in their writing about plague, physicians suggested an additional link between poverty and plague: that the unclean living conditions of the poor *created* plague as well as spread it. In addition, they expanded the connotation of 'cleanliness' to incorporate spiritual as well as physical aspects, thereby suggesting that the actions of the poor in plague-prone areas could engender and spread plague as well.

When physicians hypothesized about the spread of plague, they often utilized miasma theory of 'bad air.' The theory held that air could become dangerous if corrupted with poisonous vapors or mists. According to miasma theory, a lack of cleanliness resulted in dangerous air.[63] As early as 1625, the anonymous *The Red Crosse*, a popular plague publication, asserted 'It is no

225

doubt, that the corruption of the Aire, together with uncleanly and unwholsome keeping of the dwelling…at times when the Aire is infected, are great occasions to increase, corrupt, and produce pestilent Diseases.'[64] Thomas Cogan's *Haven of Health* in 1636 noted that 'Plague doth come of corruption of the ayre.'[65] *The Plague's Approved Physitian*, published in 1665, cited lack of cleanliness as 'the Naturall Causes of the Infection of the Ayre.'[66] Dangerous miasma was an essential component of medical theories about plague and its spread.

For the Galenist, plague was a fever in which victims inhaled corrupt air that putrefied the body as if the air were an instantaneous poison.[67] For the practitioner of chemical medicine, disease-forming substances entering the body through the air caused plague.[68] Although physicians may not have been in agreement regarding the exact cause of plague, no matter whether they advocated traditional Galenic theory or were adherents to the newer chemical medicine, they incorporated corrupt air as a natural cause of plague into their theories.[69]

Corrupt air, therefore, was of the utmost importance as a factor in spreading plague, and since lack of sanitation was thought to corrupt air, cleanliness became an important means of controlling outbreaks. In *A Treatise Concerning the Plague and the Pox,* the author, a physician, listed the three chief preventatives of plague as 'Order, Diet and Physicall helps.' Significantly, he defined order in terms of cleanliness: 'first you shall have a care that your houses be kept clean and sweet, not suffering any foule and filthy clothes or stinking things to remain in or about the same.'[70] Physicians lamented the hygiene of the poor, particularly as those in urban areas often lived crowded together. Living conditions associated with the urban poor were observed to be the places where plague was harbored, 'by thrusting a great company of people into a close, narrow, or streight room…and in narrow and close lanes and streets, where many people doe dwell together, and the places not orderly kept clean and sweet.'[71] Contemporaries had already noticed that these were the places where plague outbreaks tended to begin and where plague tended to spread the fastest.

The unclean lower orders posed a health risk to the entire population, as dangerous miasma was not necessarily contained within their areas. The poor corrupted the very air that everyone had to breathe. Miasma theory therefore made plague into a problem of broader public health. Individual physicians addressed this issue by publishing tracts and pamphlets on plague for the 'meaner sort' that sought to educate that segment of the population on ways to guard against contagion.[72] For instance, the author of *The Charitable Pest-master* claimed to have been prompted to publish by the 'great distresses of the Poore' as he observed them to be 'altogether ignorant' in the ways of avoiding the plague.[73] By doing so, physicians claimed to be protecting the 'health of the country,' a phrase employed regularly in physicians' writing on the subject.[74] Many physicians distributed their plague advice free of charge as an act of charity to the poor, to be delivered to them by 'the publick authority,' usually through churchwardens to their parishioners.[75] Basic sanitary advice on keeping one's dwelling and clothing fresh addressed one form of cleanliness. However, cleanliness in seventeenth-century terms denoted both a literal and figurative state, and physicians considered both in their theories. Air could become corrupt through a variety of factors, including dissolute behavior. Disorder and unruliness of all kinds were commonly conceived to be both physical and moral sources of disease, and plague was no exception.[76]

Physicians' theories on plague, therefore, equated the lack of cleanliness associated with poverty with disorder, unruliness, and moral incontinency. Nathaniel Hodges, medical adviser to the city of London during the Great Plague of 1665, decried the common but abhorred practice of shutting up the infected in their houses on the grounds that it kept the poorer sort from working, so that they consequently 'have nothing to do but to commit those sins, which certainly *deserve*, and infallibly *bring* the Plague upon them.'[77] Hodges specifically mentioned the sins of rioting and drunkenness, both of which were associated with disorder. It is also significant that when the Royal College of Physicians published approved medicines for the plague, they did not confine their suggestions to earthly remedies. They divided their text into two parts. The first, titled 'the Kings Medicine against the Plague of the Body,' included a standard recipe for plague medicine that included a mixture of sage, rue, and wormwood. The second section was devoted to 'The Kings Medicine, for this present year, against the Plague of the Soul, and the effect thereof.' It was fashioned after a medicinal recipe but mixed together a metaphoric one based upon virtue, Christ's grace, and humility. They stressed the importance of this part of the preventative in order to aid the more temporal recipes they had previously suggested. Their remedies were published for each major outbreak of plague in the seventeenth century.[78]

As discussed in previous chapters, the parallel of literal and figurative cleanliness in terms of spiritual and moral health was one that physicians incorporated into their ideas about medicine and health. That viewpoint would be particularly useful in their theories about plague. By stressing the ways in which people could avoid plague, spiritual as well as physical, physicians were taking definitive action and offering practical advice. Therefore, in addition to advising avoidance of the infected and their belongings, physicians also advised avoidance of the sinful and their vices. The medical treatise *Levamen infirmi: or, cordial counsel to the sick and diseased* began with the premise that when it came to remedies for the plague, the need to be spiritually clean was foremost. To bolster this point the author, David Irish, quoted scripture: '*My son, in thy sickness be not negligent: but pray unto the Lord, and he will make thee whole,*' (Eccles. 38. 9). Irish also emphasized the connection between sin and bodily disease with scripture, by declaring, 'God saith, *He will put away their Diseases, and heal them, if they keep his Commandments, it should go well with them, and they should be free from Diseases.*' (Exod. 15.26). Irish used scripture in his medical treatise to convey the message that being prayerful and repentant were necessary precursors for good health.[79] His use of scripture to support his medical advice was not uncommon for seventeenth-century physicians who often included biblical quotations on their title pages.[80]

As a result, many medical tracts closely resembled plague sermons published by divines. There were numerous biblical passages to confirm the idea that 'a life led in Religion, vertue, and the fear of God, doth conduce much to the health of Body, and also length of dayes.'[81] Divines were quick to cite them. Plague sermons noted the importance of reforming one's 'irregular disordered affections' in order to 'shake off sinnes, and liue vnto righteousnesse.'[82] Doing so protected a person's physical as well as spiritual health since sin was considered to be a '*Disease* to the *Body*' in that it 'wasts our *Strength*, and either makes the *Candle* of our Life to burn *dim*, or *blazes* it out into an untimely Period.'[83] Immoral behavior led to many diseases, and plague was no exception. Sinners, therefore, had reason to feel terror when plague ravaged, as depicted in Thomas Vincent's account of the Great Plague of 1665:

> The old drunkards, and swearers, and unclean persons are brought into great straits; they look on the right hand, and on the left, and Death is marching towards them from every part…and they see many fellow sinners fall before their faces, expecting every hour themselves to be smitten.[84]

The 'unclean persons' described in the above passage represented a dual meaning of both physical and spiritual filth that clergy acknowledged in similar fashion to physicians. Plague sermons noted that while it helped to have clean hands, one must also have a clean heart in order to escape plague.[85] As one sermon avowed, cleanliness 'is very much encourag'd and commended in Sacred Scripture, according to the words of Esau: "Be glad and be clean, and take away the evil of your thoughts."' Uncleanness, conversely, 'corrupts, and defiles, and infects man.'[86] Cleanliness, whether denoting a physical or spiritual state (or more commonly, both), was essential in avoiding plague.

In spite of some differences of opinion regarding the stress on secondary causes, physicians and divines were actually quite similar in their outlook on plague. With plague, as with most illness, seventeenth-century physicians did not sever the connection between physical and spiritual health when explaining disease and suggesting preventative health measures. This proved a logical way of viewing plague, as physicians' theories and advice regarding plague evolved in a time when disease and death rates were rising ominously, and when contemporaries often blamed poverty, drunkenness, and depravity in cities for outbreaks of epidemic disease.[87]

There were, for instance, contemporary accounts of the disease cropping up in places where disorderly and sinful living occurred. In Cranbrook in 1597, plague was spotted in a house 'out of which much theivery was committed,' and in the home of a couple 'noted much for incontinency.'[88] Plague was carried by 'lewd women' into York and Hitchin, and spread in a 'lawless' alehouse in Hampshire and Somerset.[89] 'Lawlessness' in fact proved a telling description, as contemporaries noted that God was prompted to punish with plague, sins which magistrates should have punished with the rule of law. Inns and alehouses were places 'of great misorder: so that God did seem to punish that himself which officers did neglect.'[90] Disorder, or a failure to enforce order, was a motivating factor in God's decision to send plague.

The places most likely to incur the wrath of God were the suburbs of London, which Thomas Dekker described as 'sinfully polluted,'[91] a notion echoed by the physician Nathaniel Hodges, who noted that such areas were brimming with 'unruly poor.'[92] There was a circular motion to the fear of the disorderly poor because they were also the group feared to become the most disorderly during periods of plague outbreaks. In the Great Plague of 1665, a city marshal of London complained that the 'meaner sort' were particularly likely to defy orders against public gatherings and to attack any officer who attempted to stop them. The magistrate John Ivie complained he felt threatened during an epidemic by 'all the drunkards, whoremasters, and lewd fellows' and concluded his first priority must be to control the 'great unjust rude rabble.' The mayor of York fretted that 'the Poorer sort will not be ruled,' and a town clerk of Norwich commented 'we are in greater fear of the poor than of the plague.'[93] Controlling the disorderly poor during times of epidemics was a serious and pressing problem for authorities. *The Shutting Up Infected Houses as it is practiced in England Soberly Debated* (1665) warned against shutting up houses not just because it was cruel and un-neighborly, but because it kept the poor from employment. The poor needed to work so that 'they would not meet in heards as they do, they would not surfet with rioting and drunkness; but they would securely stick to their work, keep their bodies by exercise and temperance in a good frame, and provide themselves wholsome dyet and Physick.'[94] Considerations of order for the poor occupied a prime concern when deciding the best course of action during outbreaks.

One effort to control the populace during plague epidemics was the issuing of plague orders by the Privy Council. Titled *Orders Thought Meet by Her Majestie, and Her Privie Councell, to Be Executed Throughout the Counties of This Realme in such…places as are…infected with the plague*, the *Orders* were first issued in 1578 as an attempt to devise a uniform policy for public health for the whole kingdom. They were reissued with modifications in all later epidemics. The blaming of the poor for spreading the plague, whether in physicians' writings on the dangers of miasma resulting from spiritual and physical lack of cleanliness, clerical sermons depicting the physical effects of sin, or lay associations of the disorderly poor with spreading the plague, informed the plague orders issued by the Privy Council. The *Orders* rested upon the deep-seated assumption that disease was the product of disorder. This idea, coupled with the association of the poor and unruly with the physical and moral prerequisites for contagion, led to the belief that humanity could conquer plague only by cleansing society of such physical and moral ills as poverty, popular disturbance, drunkenness, and filth of all kinds.[95] The idea of a sick, disorderly poor responsible for spreading plague became instrumental in shaping concepts of public health to be enacted during outbreaks.

Efforts had been made as early as 1518 to mark infected houses and quarantine their inmates to prevent further contagion. The basic tenet of the plague orders was isolation. When plague was discovered, the house of the victim was shut up, along with all members of that household, whether or not they showed signs of infection. The length of time quarantine was imposed varied, but at best, confinement lasted several weeks. If pest houses were available, the infected might be confined there, while their families were isolated at home. In areas where infection was particularly rife, whole streets could be cordoned off, with watchmen assigned to keep people from leaving. In some instances, entire towns were isolated. Other precautions included destroying the clothes and possessions of those who died of plague, restricting public assemblies at funerals and plays, cleaning the streets, and expelling vagrants from the city.[96]

The *Orders* were unequivocally focused on the poor, as their stated intent was to provide for the 'charitable relief and *ordering* of Persons infected with the Plague' (emphasis added). They end with the justification that their directives were necessary due to the lack of order already exhibited by that segment of society:

> And of these things above mentioned, the Justices shall take great care, as of a matter specially directed and commanded by his Majesty upon the princely and natural care he hath conceived towards the preservation of his Subjects, who by very disorder, and for lacke of direction do in many parts wilfully procure the increase of this generall Contagion.[97]

They continued by threatening punishment for anyone who criticized them as 'uncharitable,' suggesting that even the authors of the document realized that though the stated aims were charity and ordering, the latter took priority.[98]

The *Orders* contained a special section devoted to 'loose Persons and idle Assemblies.' The first subsection was dedicated to the problem of beggars, acknowledging that 'nothing is more complained of then the multitude of Rogues and wandering Beggers that swarm in every place about the City, being a great cause of the spreading of the Infection.' They also empowered householders to act against such people:

> That all Householders of whose persons, or at whose houses any such Vagrants shall be taken begging, doe apprehend, or cause them to be apprehended, and caried to the next Constable, or other Officer to be punished, according to the Lawes. And that they forbeare to relieve them, thereby to give them incouragement to continue in their wicked course of life.[99]

The *Orders'* insistence that such people were under no circumstances to be suffered on the streets supported the belief that the unruly poor needed to

231

be contained if plague outbreaks were to be curbed.

The *Orders* were responsive to ideas about the threat to order that the idle poor posed, and they were in line with physicians' theories about plague, as physicians contributed to the plague orders from their inception.[100] The College of Physicians was founded in 1518, during an epidemic of plague, as a source of advice on matters of public health.[101] In fact, the original idea for the plague orders came from a physician, Cesare Adelmare, who in 1578 summarized the methods used in foreign cities to control epidemic disease and argued that similar central direction should be established in England.[102] The College of Physicians contributed to the first national plague orders of 1578 and continued to contribute to the directives contained within the plague orders, and often as a separate addendum labeled *An Advice set down…by the best learned in Physic within this Realm, containing sundry good rules and easy medicines* throughout the seventeenth century. Their advice has been described as 'trite and conservative,' and in terms of recommending remedies for the plague, it was.[103] They suggested the use of perfumes to counteract poisonous air, standard remedies such as mithridatium, rue, wormwood and vinegar, and that clothing and bedding should be changed frequently. By and large their advice remained unchanged until 1630, when an emergency public health subcommittee of the king's council called on the College of Physicians 'to put a stop to that evil as far as [they] could by some remedies.'[104] They obliged, at first offering medicines suggested during previous outbreaks.[105] However, it is significant that the government then asked for further guidance, this time specifically requesting advice on 'political' as well as 'natural' medicines.[106]

In the ensuing recommendations, the College was speaking of the public health of the nation and the conditions that they feared posed a significant danger to it. Their advice was inspired by Theodore De Mayerne, the king's Hugenot physician, who had been trying to improve health care in England. Mayerne had served as court physician in Paris at the beginning of the century when Henry IV was interested in public health initiatives there. Mayerne submitted a lengthy report to Charles I in 1631 on the precautions necessary to prevent plague in London. It began with the premise that 'order is the life and soul of all things,' and made it clear that plague was a threat brought by 'unprofitable and wasteful' vagrants, by 'idle and naughty' assemblies and alehouses, in short by the 'unruly, base sort of people.' He described the conditions of overcrowding and poverty, which endangered public health in London, and included the vices commonly associated with the poor, such as drunkenness and disorderliness, and pegged them as hazards to the 'public health of all.' He suggested the establishment of a permanent 'commission or office of health' that would cover the whole metropolis of London so that it could deal with both epidemics and the conditions which produced them: vagrancy, overcrowding, bad hygiene, and inadequate food supplies. It must have the power to 'suppress all opposition,' and it should rule over all authorities in the metropolis from Richmond to Greenwich. His suggestions reflected 'the admirable practices of Paris, Venice, Padua, and many other cities' in proposing much greater control by the central government over quarantine (which he recommended should include separating the sick from their healthy relatives) and *cordons sanitaires*. The advice given to the Privy Council pulled heavily from Mayerne's report and was reflected in the Privy Council's plague orders issued in 1636.[107]

Physicians based their recommendations upon their own theories on the natural causes and spread of plague, and they seemed logical in the context of contemporary knowledge. However, the suggestions also harmonized well with the aims and concerns of government officials in times of plague (and at other times as well) of maintaining public order and curbing undesirable behavior. Not all of the College of Physicians' recommendations were instituted. Large-scale isolation of the healthy from the sick was never implemented, nor was a permanent board of health established. However, these failures were due to the lack of a central government powerful enough to push through initiatives rather than an indifference to making changes.[108]

The resulting orders issued by the Privy Council were more far reaching than any that had come before. Along with the standard commands of obliging people to keep the areas in front of their houses clean were directives regarding behavior suggested by the Royal College of Physicians. People should avoid drinking and 'lying in company,' as these resulted in a situation where 'pure complexions and cleane bloods are defiled with such as are putrified.' All public gatherings short of attending special plague services at the cathedral, abbey, and parish churches were proscribed.[109] Taverns and inns had long been suspected of acting as breeding grounds for plague, and consequently all vintners, inn holders, sellers of strong waters, alehouse and coffeehouse keepers were forbidden to entertain customers.[110] Only traveling guests could be accommodated on the premises 'with sobriety and moderation.' During the outbreak of 1665, the mayor of London ordered the high parish authorities to clamp down on disorderly tippling, gaming, and rowing on the river, along with other offences, especially on Sundays.[111] These restrictions and closures addressed both spiritual and moral corruption while simultaneously reaffirming the justification for many, which physicians had been theorizing, that moral as well as social order should be imposed in plague times, as disorder of any kind weakened man's defenses against plague and provoked God.

Throughout the century, plague policy plainly linked moral ills to the plague. For example, the 1665 *Orders* was subtitled 'Health better than Gold' and contained a reprint of the popular sermon *The Plague of the Heart*. The sermon focused on God's divine justice in punishing the sins of the people with plague, but it specifically targeted certain sins associated with the type of behavior the government considered threatening to order: 'the vitious Vices of Whoredom, Drunkenness, Sabbath-breaking.'[112] The *Orders* impugned places that housed such activities, such as ale-houses, as being 'disorderly,' since they harbored the 'common sinne of this time.' They were therefore considered the 'greatest occasions of dispersing the Plague.'[113] The message conveyed in the *Orders* was that the controlling of certain behaviors and certain segments of the population provided necessary protection for the health of the whole.

Paul Slack has argued that many of the measures employed to combat plague affected the poor disproportionately since the disease often arrived in and was confined to the poorer districts. The poor typically resided in the back alleys and suburbs (which were also the areas associated with vagrancy and unruly behavior) that were sealed off from the rest of society. Since flight was not an option for the poor, they were forced to stay and endure the restrictions, all of which bred social conflict and resentment of the rich.[114] The outcome was often a partial revolt with the threat of a far more serious uprising in the background. Alan Dyer has suggested that the similarity of quarantine to imprisonment, the breaking up of families by removal to pest houses, the injustice of the escape of the rich, and the collapse of the economic and administrative structure that came on the heels of flight by the rich and isolation of the poor produced an explosive mixture in an atmosphere highly charged with nervous tension.[115]

Such tension made it even more imperative to keep order by imposing restrictions on the poor during outbreaks of plague. Approaching plague policy from the point of view of ongoing efforts to keep order helps to explain the punitive nature of household isolation both as it was delineated in the plague orders and supported by statute in the 1604 Plague Act. Paul Slack has noted that isolation of the infected in English towns was unusually strict. The Plague Act provided for local rates for the sick, but it also had a deliberately disciplinary purpose in providing the first penal sanctions behind the policy of isolation. The Act gave watchmen the legal authority to use violence to keep people shut up in their houses. Anyone with a plague sore found wandering outside in the company of others was guilty of felony and could be hanged; anyone who broke quarantine could be whipped as a vagrant rogue. In effect, the Act of 1604 treated the disorderly sick as vagrants, a fact made even more evident to contemporaries considering the first expense for municipal finances during an epidemic was often a whipping post.[116]

Punitive measures delineated by the Plague Orders were in line with other contemporary legislation, such as the Vagrancy Act of 1609. The Act empowered Justices of the Peace to issue privy search warrants requiring constables within their jurisdiction to seek out and bring before them 'rogues, vagabonds, and sturdy beggars, and all such persons as are suspected to keep bawdy houses, and the frequenters thereof, and also all disturbers of the peace.'[117] This type of punitive legislation has led Michael Braddick to surmise that from 1550-1640, some rapid and radical extension of state activity over the lives of individuals took place in order to preserve social order, particularly in relation to poverty. It was during this period that local governors were given the power to whip and brand vagrants and to shut up houses of plague victims. In addition, there were attempts to deal with perceived threats to the social order such as regulating sexual activity, punishing crimes against property, and licensing and controlling popular drinking places.[118] The restrictions that circumscribed the lives of those who remained during plague epidemics were part of broader notions of public health: what some reformers believed should be enacted at all times in order to keep a town clean, ordered, and therefore healthy.

The Societies for the Reformation of Manners offer one example of the movement to reform the behavior of certain segments of the population for the good of the whole. The Societies' organization and activities are discussed in chapter six, but it is worth revisiting them in the context of the desire of civic authorities and physicians alike to curb dissolute behavior in times of acute threat from epidemic diseases such as bubonic plague. The Societies were dedicated to the suppression of immorality on the premise that abiding a disorderly or dissolute segment of the population affected the health of the whole. This notion was forwarded by Josiah Woodward, the first historian-cum-publicist for the Reformation of Manners Societies: 'National sins deserve national Judgements,' thus, society needed to 'endeavour,

by a General Reformation, to appease the Wrath of God.'[119] Reformation
Societies have usually been explained in religious terms by historians, as have
been various campaigns against vice, but Robert Shoemaker has argued for
viewing them as a response to concerns about social problems such as poverty, crime, and disorder in England's cities, especially London.

Although the Societies were not formed until 1690, well after the last
major plague outbreak in England, they were part of a much earlier Puritan
desire for a reformation of manners in the late sixteenth and early seventeenth centuries that centered upon the need to control the disorderly poor.[120]
Shoemaker has contended that the supporters of such projects were motivated not solely by spiritual considerations, but also by concerns to maintain
social order. One of the main reasons why the inhabitants of late Stuart and
early Hanoverian London welcomed a campaign against vice was it provided
a method of clearing the streets of prostitutes, beggars, street merchants,
and other 'loose idle and disorderly people.'[121] The reformation of manners
campaigns, therefore, were as much about social reform as religious reform.
The campaigns also reflected entrenched concerns that were the result of
major social problems arising from rapid urban growth, particularly regarding the urban poor. It should not be surprising that they began in London
and were more active in the urban areas since wickedness was considered to
be concentrated in the cities, as was population.[122]

Kevin Siena has outlined the medical practitioner's role in moral reform campaigns as part of the ongoing attempt by physicians to control the
spread and damage of disease. By portraying certain behaviors as hazardous
and advising against them, physicians were participating in their capacity as
regulators of social behavior.[123] Such a combination of moral regeneration
for the sake of disease prevention was not unique to physicians of the late
seventeenth century. For example, the Puritan physician and surgeon William Clowes at the end of the sixteenth century strongly advised respectable people to avoid alehouses because he considered them not only to be
unsanitary but also to harbor plague and syphilis.[124] The idea of prevention
through moral reform is at the core of Clowes's writing, as poverty and moral
depravity fit hand-in-glove. For Clowes, disease was a manifestation of sin,
and therefore avoidance of sin, or morality, was a powerful physical preservative.[125] Clowes argued that because diseases like plague and the pox were contagious, the innocent could be infected if they failed to avoid the company of
the godless.[126] He suggested that alehouses be shut down not just for moral
reasons but also for medical ones, because in such places 'dis-ordered per-

sons, some other of better disposition, are many times infected.' He warned that the Lord would soon poison the whole land unless magistrates punished vice and people repented their ungodly life.[127] His ideas reflected previous ones within the medical community about transmission of disease in such places. Clowes's vision of public health was in line with that of other medical practitioners in that it promoted the idea that those in authority had the responsibility to compel individuals to reform their sinful ways for the good of the whole.

Clowes's warnings meshed nicely with larger anti-alehouse campaigns, supported mainly by Puritans, who used the threat of disease to bolster their argument that alehouses were inherently dangerous places where innocent people could be infected.[128] Physicians were at times complicit in these reform projects, as their writing used disease to help create and enforce danger beliefs aimed at policing behavior.[129] Attacking sinful actions and places where sinful behavior was likely to occur was a natural extension of physicians' views on plague prevention and general health.

There were, of course, differences between Puritan reform efforts earlier in the century and the end-of-century reformation societies; the key difference was a more temporal tone of later movements. These reformers stressed the explicitly temporal benefits of a moral populace, in which they equated sin with lawlessness.[130] Their supporters shaped their case for moral reform into a more secularized understanding of the scope of political action, arguing that reform of manners was 'the surest way to revive our Trade, prolong our Peace, and recover England's glory.'[131] The necessity of ensuring a collective health played into the argument as well, since the health of all individuals mattered: 'If ungodly Persons did hurt only themselves, there might be some pretext for indulging, and conniving, at them...but the case is otherwise, they do real harm to the Community, of which they are Members.'[132] Such an argument paralleled notions that all must be clean and continent in order to escape plague. Although God balanced an individual's moral account in the afterlife, governments paid for the toleration of citizens' sins. Supporters cast even divine retribution as a secular concern and contended that the promotion of popular morality served the temporal interest of English society and, for this reason, lay well within the legislative province of civil authority.[133]

Physicians' arguments that suggested the poor were prone to infection (whether the plague or any other disease) because they were prone to disorder are in line with reforming movements that sought to improve the health

of the whole through reforming the habits and manners of the most susceptible to both disease and disorder in society. Physicians advocated disease
prevention as the most important factor in health, a logical emphasis given
the limited efficacy of their treatments. When the physician Steven Bradwell
penned the 'To the reader' section on his book about plague, he stressed the
preventative role of the physician in relation to plague:

> I must labour to preserue the sound; because by profession I am a
> Physition. Therefore I call this Booke, *A Watch-man for the Pest*, because
> it doth onely (as if it were a Warder) stand at the dore without, and
> deliver things necessary for preservation to those within; but neither
> enters the infected house, nor meddles with the Cure of the Conta-
> gious.[134]

Considering Bradwell was convinced that the epidemic was the result of 'the
All-mightie God of Heaven and Earth [who] in wrath & justice sendeth this
Plague upon us,' it should not be surprising that his preventatives included
spiritual cleansing along with practical tips for purifying the infected air.[135]
The physician Robert Johnson suggested that because the chief cause of
the plague was 'the sins of Mankind, provoking the great God to send this
Pestiferous distemper as a judgment on them for their Impiety,' the first line
of defense against it should be prayer and repentance, as well as purifying
the 'infected air.' Additionally, he stressed the need to alter one's behavior by
avoiding 'all passions, watchings, and immoderate exercise and venery.'[136] Dr.
Edwards included a similar message in his tract. Since the first step was to
preserve oneself, Edwards began by describing the 'forewarnings and tokens
[that] are given us before hand of the coming thereof, thereby the better to
prevent the same by prayer and repentance.' If the reader suspected that
he or she was coming down with plague, the first step in counteracting the
disease should be prayer and repentance. He followed this suggestion with
advice to flee infected areas and to 'order' oneself through proper behavior
and diet.[137] The basic elements of the physician's approach to plague was the
same as any disease and incorporated the components that reformers were
emphasizing regarding the maintenance of health: repentance, prayer, and
eschewing sinful behavior.

For government officials and physicians alike, plague policy was never
just about curbing disease--it was about curbing behavior thought to bring
about disease, and this included both filth in the sense of overcrowding, poor

sanitation, and dirt, as well as the lack of cleanliness associated with disorder and vice, as both were thought to encourage the spread of disease. Effective plague policy stressed the need to contain epidemics by imposing order on those deemed to be the most disorderly. If controlling infection in crowded, poor areas meant protecting the health of the greater good, then physicians' writing can be viewed as an attempt to protect society. In linking poverty with disease, and intimating the larger threat that an epidemically ill poor posed to the entire country, physicians' theories on plague supported government efforts to control the spread of infection in poor, densely crowded areas. Public health as conceived by physicians fit hand in glove with public order, a preoccupation of public officials at all times, especially during plague.

Physicians' writing about plague is consistent with their overarching approach to the prevention of disease in general. They emphasized the interconnection of physical and spiritual health, an approach that both defined their offering as pious physicians and was complementary to the preoccupation with order of the government. In times of plague crisis, magistrates and civic authorities were not the only ones envisioning 'cities of God' that could ward off disease; physicians were advocating a congruent vision.

Over the course of the seventeenth century, there arose a new interest in human intervention to prevent or control outbreaks of plague. Intervention included not only sanitary measures but curbing dissolute behavior as well. Despite the fact that physicians could offer no medical cure for plague, they were able to offer social remedies that far exceeded the scope of physic. Their suggestions, though meant to protect the population at large from plague, targeted the poor, and in doing so aided efforts by secular authorities to impose order during precarious times. Physicians' theories such as miasma and the connection between spiritual and physical health may not have been new to the seventeenth century, but they were new to the field of disease management in that they were incorporated into government policy in a way they had not been before.

Physicians' role in curbing plague epidemics aided their profession as a whole because they were able to establish themselves not just as Christ's approved physician, as previous chapters have demonstrated, but as "The Plague's Approved Physician."[138] Their publications carefully melded spiritual and physical health in a way that, in spite of the increasing stress on the natural causes of plague, made God and the physician work in tandem for the public health of all. Such thinking is perhaps best summed up in the physician Richard Barker's publication on plague, which asserted that no matter how bad He may smite England with plague, God would send physicians to offer relief: 'the Lord even in the midst of his Anger being not forgetful of his Mercy, it behoveth…those of our Profession…[to] become Instruments to allay his Wrath, and procure his Mercy.'[139] In the great scourge, as with most other ailments, physicians endeavored to distinguish themselves as a profession through the link between morality and medicine.

Plague provides a vivid example of the nexus between medicine and morality that proved so crucial to the success of the physician in gaining public recognition of his authority and expertise in the seventeenth century. The necessity of keeping society clean, both in a literal and metaphorical sense, in order to keep it healthy was what made the physician's job distinct from all other types of healers. He alone was capable of curing the whole person, both body and soul, and therefore ensuring the health of the nation.

Notes

1   Cited in B. Capp, *Astrology and the Popular Press.* (Boston: Faber and Faber, 1979), 112.

2   R. Latham (ed.), *The Shorter Pepys* (Berkeley: University of California Press, 1985).

3   T. Vincent, *God's Terrible Voice in the City* (1667), 6.

4   A. Dyer, 'The Influence of Bubonic Plague in England, 1550-1667,' *Medical History* 22, no. 3 (1978), 308.

5   F. Wilson (ed.), *Plague Pamphlets of Thomas Dekker* (Oxford: Clarendon Press, 1925), 144.

6   Anon., *The Plague's Approved Physitian, Shewing the Naturall Causes of the Infection of the Ayre, and of the Plague. With Divers Observations to Bee Used, Preserving from the Plague, and Signes to Know the Infected Therewith. Also Many True and Approved Medicines for the Perfect Cure Thereof. Chiefly, a Godly and Penitent Prayer Unto Almighty God, for Our Preservation, and Deliverance Therefrom* (1665).

7   N. Hodges, *Loimologia* (1720), 3.

8   Mortality rates could reach 50% in England and tended to be even higher in warmer European climates. J.F.D. Shrewsbury, *A History of*

Bubonic Plague in the British Isles (London: Cambridge University Press, 1970).

9   A.L. Moote and D. Moote, *The Great Plague: The Story of London's Most Deadly Year* (Baltimore, MD: Johns Hopkins University Press, 2004).

10   A. Dyer, 'The Influence of Bubonic Plague in England, 1550-1667,' 309.

11   On the importance of the bubonic plague to social history, see J. Hays, *The Burdens of Disease: Epidemics and Human Response in Western History* (New Brunswick, NJ: Rutgers University Press, 1998). B.L. Grigsby discusses the importance of bubonic plague in altering man's relationship with disease, or at least his interpretation of that relationship. B.L. Grigsby (ed.), *Pestilence in Medieval and Early Modern English Literature*, Studies in Medieval History and Culture (New York: Routledge, 2004).

12   See H. Zinsser, *Rats, Lice, and History; Being a Study in Biography, Which, after Twelve Preliminary Chapters Indispensable for the Preparation of the Lay Reader, Deals with the Life History of Typhus Fever* (Boston: Pub. for the Atlantic Monthly Press by Little, Brown, and Company, 1935) and S. Gottfried, *The Black Death: Natural and Human Disaster in Medieval Europe* (New York: Collier Macmillan, 1983). The degree to which human intervention was successful in combating and eradicating plague continues to be debated by historians. See for example D.S. Reher, *Town and Country in Pre-Industrial Spain: Cuenca, 1550-1870* (Cambridge: Cambridge University Press, 1990), 164-5 and O.J. Benedictow, 'Morbidity in Historical Plague Epidemics,' *Population Studies* 41, No. 3 (Nov 1987), 41. On climactic change, see J. Post, 'Famine, Mortality, and Epidemic Disease in the Process of Modernization,' *Economic History Review* 29 (1976). On the overall debate, see A. Appleby, 'Famine, Mortality, and Epidemic Disease: A Comment,' *Economic History Review* 30 (1977); A. Appleby, 'The Disappearance of Plague: A Continuing Puzzle,' *Economic History Review* (May 1980); and P. Slack, 'The Disappearance of Plague: An Alternative View,' *Economic History Review* 34 (1984).

13   See for example R. Horrox (ed.), *The Black Death* (New York: Manchester University Press, 1994).

14   See A.G. Carmichael, *Plague and the Poor in Renaissance Florence* (Cambridge: Cambridge University Press, 1986) and J. Arrizabalaga, *Facing the Black Death: Perceptions and Reactions of University Medical*

Practitioners (1994). For a more generalized history of the medical profession in Italy, see C.M. Cipolla, *Public Health and the Medical Profession in the Renaissance* (Cambridge: Cambridge University Press, 1976).

15 S. Watts, *Epidemics and History: Disease, Power, and Imperialism* (New Haven: Yale University Press, 1997).

16 T. Ranger and P. Slack (eds), *Epidemics and Ideas: Essays on the Historical Perception of Pestilence* (New York: Cambridge University Press, 1992). This has been found to be the case in Scotland, as well. See C. Mullett, 'Plague Policy in Scotland, 16th-17th Centuries,' *Osiris* 9 (1950).

17 P. Slack, 'Metropolitan Government in Crisis: The Response to Plague,' in A.L. Beier and R. Finlay (eds), *London 1500-1700: The Making of the Metropolis* (New York: Longman, 1986); P. Slack, 'Books of Orders: The Making of English Social Policy, 1577-1631,' *Transactions of the Royal Historical Society, 5th Series* 30 (1980); and P. Slack, *The Impact of Plague in Tudor and Stuart England* (London: Routledge & K. Paul, 1985).

18 See for example C. Webster, 'The College of Physicians: "Solomon's House" in Commonwealth England,' *Bulletin of the History of Medicine* 51, no. 5 (2003); H. Cook, 'Policing the Health of London: The College of Physicians and the Early Stuart Monarchy,' *Social History of Medicine* 2 (1989), 22; and O.P. Grell, 'Plague in Elizabethan and Stuart London: The Dutch Response,' *Medical History* 34 (1990), 429, 435-6.

19 M. Pelling, *Medical Conflicts in Early Modern London: Patronage, Physicians, and Irregular Practitioners, 1550-1640* (Oxford: Clarendon Press, 2003), 54.

20 A.L. Moote and D. Moote, *The Great Plague: The Story of London's Most Deadly Year* 143-144; A. Wear, *Knowledge and Practice;* and T.D. Whittet, *The Apothecaries in the Great Plague of London in 1665* (London: Society of Apothecaries, 1965). Those that did stay faced an uphill battle, and many died in the attempt. Lloyd and Dorothy Moote estimates that 50 percent of the medical professionals who stayed may have died in either public or private practice—25 percent of the total cohort of licensed and unlicensed practitioners serving London in normal times. Samuel Pepys commented that 'in Westminster there is never a physitian, and but one apothecary left, all being dead.' R. Latham (ed.), *The Shorter Pepys.* 6:268 Oct. 16, 1665.

21 See M. Pelling, *Medical Conflicts in Early Modern London: Patronage, Physicians, and Irregular Practitioners, 1550-1640*, 48-49; O.P. Grell,

'Conflicting Duties: Plague and the Obligations of Early Modern Physicians toward Patients and Commonwealth in England and the Netherlands,' in A. Wear, J. Geyer-Kordesch, and R. French (eds), *Doctors and Ethics: The Earlier Historical Setting of Professional Ethics,* Clio Medica 24 (Amsterdam: Rodopi, 1993); F.P. Wilson, *The Plague in Shakespeare's London* (Oxford: Clarendon Press, 1927), 100-5; N. Sirasi, *Medieval and Early Renaissance Medicine: An Introduction to Knowledge and Practice* (Chicago: University of Chicago Press, 1990), 42-3; and P. Wallis, 'Plagues, Morality and the Place of Medicine in Early Modern England ' *English Historical Review* 121, no. 490 (February 2006).

22 P. Slack, *The Impact of Plague in Tudor and Stuart England,* 200.

23 C. Mullett, *The Bubonic Plague and England; an Essay in the History of Preventive Medicine* (Lexington: University of Kentucky Press, 1956).

24 Royal College of Physicians of London, *Certain Necessary Directions, Aswell for the Cure of the Plague as for Preuenting the Infection; with Many Easie Medicines of Small Charge, Very Profitable to His Maiesties Subiects / Set Downe by the Colledge of Physicians by the Kings Maiesties Speciall Command ; with Sundry Orders Thought Meet by His Maiestie, and His Priuie Councell, to Be Carefully Executed for Preuention of the Plague ; Also Certaine Select Statutes Commanded by His Maiestie to Be Put in Execution by All Iustices, and Other Officers of the Peace Throughout the Realme ; Together with His Maiesties Proclamation for Further Direction Therein, and a Decree in Starre-Chamber, Concerning Buildings and in-Mates* (1636).

25 R. Palmer, 'The Church, Leprosy and Plague in Medieval and Early Modern Europe' in W.J. Sheils (ed.), *The Church and Healing* (Oxford: Basil Blackwell, 1982), 88. See for example H.C., *Londons Vacation, and the Countries Tearme. Or, a Lamentable Relation of Severall Remarkable Passages Which It Hath Pleased the Lord to Shew on This Present Visitation, 1636...*(1637), which contains two poems illustrating that sin leads to divine punishment. See also J. Cragge, *Great Britains Prayers in This Dangerous Time of Contagion* (1641).

26 R. Younge, *The Prevention of Poverty, Together with the Cure of Melancholy, Alias Discontent. Or the Best and Surest Way to Wealth and Happiness Being Subjects Very Seasonable for These Times; Wherein All Are Poor, or Not Pleased, or Both; When They Need Be Neither* (1682).

27 W. Gouge, *God's Three Arrowes: Plague, Famine, Sword* (1636), B.

28 H. Clapham, *An Epistle Discoursing Upon the Present Pestilence* (1603), B1. See also B. There are numerous examples, including Anon., *Voice to the*

City, or, a Loud Cry from Heaven to London, Setting before Her Her Sins, Her Sickness, Her Remedies (1665), whose title page included the following quotation: 'The Lords Voice cryeth to the City, hear the Rod, and who hath appointed it. Mich. 6. 9,' and Anon., *Flagellum Dei: Or a Collection of the Several Fires, Plagues, and Pestilential Diseases That Have Hapned in London Especially, and Other Parts of This Nation, from the Norman Conquest to The Present, 1668* (1668), which looked to Divine Wrath to explain plague along with other disasters that have befallen London.

29   See R. Palmer, 'The Church, Leprosy and Plague in Medieval and Early Modern Europe,' 83 and V. Nutton, 'Seeds of Disease. An Explanation of Contagion and Infection from the Greeks to the Renaissance,' *Medical History* 27 (1983), and Alexandra Walsham, *Providence in Early Modern England* (Oxford: Oxford University Press, 1999).

30   See the collection of J. Cragge, *Great Britains Prayers in This Dangerous Time of Contagion* (1641) and W.C., *Londons Lamentations for Her Sinnes: And Complaint to the Lord Her God* (1625), both of which make reference to government-commanded fasting and prayers. Samuel Pepys makes note of the public fast ordered on August 2, 1665. R. Latham and W. Matthews (eds), *The Diary of Samuel Pepys*, 11 vols. (London: Bell & Hyman, 1970-83).

31   A. MacFarlane (ed.), *Diary of Ralph Josselin 1616-1683* (London: Oxford University Press, New Series, 1976), 519, entry for 2 July.

32   J. Cragge, *Great Britains Prayers in This Dangerous Time of Contagion,* A2.

33   W.C., *Londons Lamentations for Her Sinnes: And Complaint to the Lord Her God.* See for example Anon., 'A Christian Meditation or Praier to Be Sayed by All Tymes Whensoever God Shall Vyset Us Wyth Anye Mortall Plague or Sicnesse' (1551) and Anon., *A Praier Very Comfortable and Necessary to Be Used of All Christians Every Morning and Evening Amongst Heir Families, That It Would Please the Lord God to Be Appeased in Is Wrath, and So Withdraw His Heavy Hand an Greevous Visitations from Amongst Us* (no date given).

34   T. Brooks, *A Heavenly Cordial for All Those Servants of the Lord That Have Had the Plague … , or, Thirteen Divine Maximes, or Conclusions, in Respect of the Pestilence* (1666). See also D.D. Perrinchief, *A Sermon Preached before the Honourable House of Commons, at St. Margarets Westminster, Nov. 7 Being the Fast-Day Appointed for the Plague of Pestilence* (1666) and W. Muggins, *Londons Mourning Garment, or Funerall Teares Worne and Shed for the Death of Her Wealthy Cittizens, and Other Her Inhabitants. To Which Is Added, a*

*Zealous and Feruent Prayer, with a True Relation How Many Haue Dyed of
All Diseases, in Euery Particuler Parish within London, the Liberties, and out
Parishes Neere Adioyning from the 14 of Iuly 1603. To the 17 of Nouember.
Following* (1603). During the plague of 1665, Ralph Josselin recorded
asking his parishioners to repent their sins and change their sinful ways
so that God would preserve them and heal the city. A. MacFarlane
(ed.), *Diary of Ralph Josselin 1616-1683* (London: Oxford University
Press, New Series, 1976), 519, entry for 2 July.

35   This would continue into the eighteenth century. When Britons feared
another plague outbreak in 1720, a national fast was declared on 16
December of that year. Sermons focusing on the sins of the times
were rushed into print in early 1721. Paul Slack asserts 'The approach
of plague was a clear call to the nation to repent.' P. Slack, *The Impact of
Plague in Tudor and Stuart England,* 328.

36   See the physician Stephen Bradwell's book on plague that posits the
idea that the immediate cause of plague was God 'in wrath and justice'
S. Bradwell, *A Watch-Man for the Pest Teaching the True Rules of Preservation
from the Pestilent Contagion, at This Time Fearefully over-Flowing This Famous
Cittie of London. Collected out of the Best Authors, Mixed with Auncient
Experience, and Moulded into a New and Most Plaine Method* (1625).

37   D. Irish, *Levamen Infirmi: Or, Cordial Counsel to the Sick and Diseased
Containing I. Advice Concerning Physick, and What a Physician Ought to
Be; with an Account of the Author's Remedies, and How to Take Them. Ii.
Concerning Melancholy, Frensie, and Madness; in Which, Amongst Other Things,
Is Shew'd, How Far They Differ from a Conscience Opprest with the Sense of Sin,
and Likewise How They Differ among Themselves. Iii. A Miscellany of Pious
Discourses, Concerning the Attributes of God; with Ejaculations and Prayers,
According to Scripture Rule. Likewise an Account of Many Things Which Have
Happen'd since the Creation. To Which Are Added Several Predictions of What
May Happen to the End of the World. The Whole Being Enrich'd with Physical,
Pious, Moral & Historical Observations, Delightful to Read, & Necessary to
Know* (1700). See also T. Cogan, *The Haven of Health Chiefly Gathered for
the Comfort of Students, and Consequently of All Those That Have a Care of
Their Health, Amplified Upon Five Words of Hippocrates, Written Epid. 6.
Labour, Cibus, Potio, Somnus, Venus. Hereunto Is Added a Preservation from
the Pestilence, with a Short Censure of the Late Sicknes at Oxford* (1636).

38   Anon., *The Plagues Approved Physitian. Shewing the Naturall Causes of the
Infection of the Ayre, and of the Plague. With Divers Observations to Bee Used,*

245

Preserving from the Plague, and Signes to Know the Infected Therewith. Also Many True and Approved Medicines for the Perfect Cure Thereof (1665).

39   J. Harris, *The Divine Physician, Prescribing Rules for the Prevention, and Cure of Most Diseases, as Well of the Body, as the Soul Demonstrating by Natural Reason, and Also Divine and Humane Testimony, That, as Vicious and Irregular Actions and Affections Prove Often Occasions of Most Bodily Diseases, and Shortness of Life, So the Contrary Do Conduce to the Preservation of Health, and Prolongation of Life: In Two Parts* (1676).

40   What plague pamphlets began to list as natural causes of plague were heat, filth, and overcrowding. They were in general agreement that plague was a contagion spread by infected people and that it was, in theory, controllable.

41   R. Johnson, *Enchiridion Medicum, or, a Manual of Physick Being a Compendium of the Whole Art, in Three Parts... : Wherein Is Briefly Shewed 1. The Names, 2. The Derivation, 3. The Causes, 4. The Signs, 5. The Prognosticks, and 6. A Rational Method of Cure* (1684).

42   J. Gadbury, 'London's Deliverance Predicted' (1665), A6.

43   N. Hodges, *Vindiciae Medicinae & Medicorum: Or an Apology for the Profession and Professors of Physick in Answer to the Several Pleas of Illegal Practitioners; Wherein Their Positions Are Examined, Their Cheats Discovered, and Their Danger to the Nation Asserted. As Also an Account of the Present Pest, in Answer to a Letter* (1666).

44   N. Hodges, *Vindiciae Medicinae & Medicorum: Or an Apology for the Profession and Professors of Physick in Answer to the Several Pleas of Illegal Practitioners; Wherein Their Positions Are Examined, Their Cheats Discovered, and Their Danger to the Nation Asserted. As Also an Account of the Present Pest, in Answer to a Letter* (1666).

45   H. Clapham, *An Epistle Discoursing Upon the Present Pestilence*. See also J. Godskall, *The King's Medicine for This Present Yeere 1604* (1604).

46   H. Clapham, *An Epistle Discoursing Vpon the Present Pestilence* (1603), B1.

47   T. Brooks, *A Heavenly Cordial for All Those Servants of the Lord That Have Had the Plague ..., or, Thirteen Divine Maximes, or Conclusions, in Respect of the Pestilence* (1666), 3-4.

48   A.R. and M.B. Hall (eds), *The Correspondence of Henry Oldenburg* (Madison, Wisconsin: 1965-73), II 479, 527. This idea was echoed in a tract published early in the century, *Certain Prayers...to be used in the present Visitation* (1603): 'If we make a mock of all preservatives of Art: if we neglect all evil and infectious savours and refuse the

benefit of purer air: if we run desperately and disorderly into all places and amongst all persons and pretend our faith and trust in God's providence, saying: "If he will save me, he will save me, and if I die, I die"—this is not faith in God but a gross, ignorant and foolhardy… presumption.'

49   See P. Slack, 'Demographic crises and subsistence crises in France, 1650-1725' in J. Walter and R. Schofield (eds), *Famine, Disease and the Social Order in Early Modern Society* (Cambridge: Cambridge University Press, 1989), 23-24.

50   A sampling of those published include T. Willis, *A Plain and Easie Method for Preserving (by God's Blessing) Those That Are Well from the Infection of the Plague, or Any Contagious Distemper in City, Camp, Fleet, &C. And for Curing Such as Are Infected with It: Written in the Year 1666 by Tho. Willis…; with a Poem on the Virtue of a Laurel Leaf for Curing of a Rheumatism* (1691), T. Thayre, *An Excellent and Best Approoued Treatise of the Plague Containing, the Nature, Signes, and Accidents of the Same. With the Certaine and Absolute Cure of the Feuers, Botches, and Carbuncles, That Raigne in These Times; and Aboue All Things, Most Singular Experiments in the Same: Gathered by the Obseruations of Diuers Worthy Travilers, and Selected out of the Best Learned Physitions in This Age. Likewise Is Taught, the True and Perfect Cure of the Plague, with Secret and Vnknowne Preseruatiues against All Infection; and How So Withstand the Most Dangerous Accidents, Which May Happen This Fearefull Contagious Time. Generall Rules of Life to Be Obserued by All Men This Plague Time. Directions for the Commons, Country-Men and Strangers That Be Necessitated to Come into the City* (1625) and T. Wharton, *Directions for the Prevention and Cure of the Plague Fitted for the Poorer Sort* (1665).

51   Anon., *Concerning the Constitution of an Aire Infected. And How to Know Plague-Sores from Carbuncles* (1644), 4.

52   B.L. Grigsby, *Pestilence in Medieval and Early Modern English Literature*, Francis Gentry (ed.), Studies in Medieval History and Culture (New York: Routledge, 2004).

53   The information contained in the Bills of Mortality were gleaned from the reports of the Searchers, given to the Parish Clerk, published and distributed to the families who paid 4s per annum for them. They were first published for public distribution in 1594 by the Company of Parish Clerks. Cornelius Walford, 'Early Bills of Mortality,' *Transactions of the Royal Historical Society* 7 (1878), 212, 214, 216, 226.

54   P. Slack, *The Impact of Plague in Tudor and Stuart England,* 239.

55   Anon., *London's Dreadful Visitation* (1665).

56   Pepys refered regularly to the bills throughout the summer of 1665, commenting on their increasing or decreasing numbers, and discussing them with others. R. Latham and W. Matthews (eds), *The Diary of Samuel Pepys,* VI 128, 149, 174.

57   T. Willis, *A Help for the Poor Who Are Visited with the Plague: To Be Communicated to Them by the Rich* (London: 1666), A3; and Anon., *Lord Have Mercy Upon Us* (1665).

58   August 21. John Graunt estimated that 200,000 people left London during the plague of 1665. J. Graunt, *Natural and Political Observations Made Upon the Bills of Mortality* W. Willcox (ed.), (Baltimore: Johns Hopkins University Press, 1939). Another contemporary source estimated that 494,000 people remained in and around London. Anon., *Reflections on the Weekly Bills of Mortality for the Cities of London and Westminster...So Far as It Relates to Plague* (1665).

59   T. Vincent, *God's Terrible Voice in the City* (1667), 7. Even if they could manage to flee the city, they risked a hostile reception in the country. For examples of cruelty against less affluent people fleeing to the countryside during the plague, see Anon., *Londoners Their Entertainment in the Countrie. Or the Whipping of Runnawayes. Wherein Is Described, Londons Miserie, the Countries Crueltie, and Mans Inhumantie* (1604); H.C., *Londons Vacation, and the Countries Tearme.* (1637); Benjamin Spenser, *Vox Ciuitatis, or Londons Complaint against Her Children in the Countrie* (1636); and Anon., *A Dialogue Betwixt a Citizen, and a Poore Countrey Man and His Wife, in the Country, Where the Citizen Remaineth Now in This Time of Sicknesse* (1636).

60   Cited in B. Capp, *Astrology and the Popular Press* (Boston: Faber and Faber, 1979), 112.

61   R. Harris, *Hezekiah's Recovery* (1626), 42.

62   W. Gouge, *God's Three Arrowes,* 25. Cited in P. Slack, *The Impact of Plague in Tudor and Stuart England,* 239-240.

63   F.P. Wilson, *The Plague in Shakespeare's London* (Oxford: Clarendon Press, 1927) and J.F.D. Shrewsbury, *A History of Bubonic Plague in the British Isles* (London: Cambridge University Press, 1970).

64   Anon., *The Red Crosse: Or, Englands Lord Haue Mercy Upon Us.* (1625), P1.

65   T. Cogan, *The Haven of Health Chiefly Gathered for the Comfort of Students,*

and Consequently of All Those That Have a Care of Their Health, Amplified Upon Five Words of Hippocrates, Written Epid. 6. Labour, Cibus, Potio, Somnus, Venus. Hereunto Is Added a Preservation from the Pestilence, with a Short Censure of the Late Sicknes at Oxford,' (1636). See also R. Younge, *The Prevention of Poverty, Together with the Cure of Melancholy, Alias Discontent. Or the Best and Surest Way to Wealth and Happiness Being Subjects Very Seasonable for These Times; Wherein All Are Poor, or Not Pleased, or Both; When They Need Be Neither.* 'Plague or Pestilence is not caused, but through the breathing in of pestilent and corrupt Ayre.'

66   Anon., *The Plague's Approved Physitian, Shewing the Naturall Causes of the Infection of the Ayre, and of the Plague. With Divers Observations to Bee Used, Preserving from the Plague, and Signes to Know the Infected Therewith. Also Many True and Approved Medicines for the Perfect Cure Thereof. Chiefely, a Godly and Penitent Prayer Unto Almighty God, for Our Preservation, and Deliverance Therefrom.* A3; Bradwell, *A Watch-Man for the Pest Teaching the True Rules of Preservation from the Pestilent Contagion, at This Time Fearefully over-Flowing This Famous Cittie of London. Collected out of the Best Authors, Mixed with Auncient Experience, and Moulded into a New and Most Plaine Method.*

67   I. Pantin, 'Fracastoro's De Contagione and Medieval Reflection on "Action at a Distance": Old and New Trends in Renaissance Discourse on the Plague,' in C. Carlin (ed.), *Imagining Contagion in Early Modern Europe* (New York: Palgrave Macmillan, 2005). Evidence that plague was considered by most healers to be a fever lies in the plague's categorization under the heading of 'fever' in larger compendiums of disease. See for example N. Culpeper, *The English Physitian, or an Astrologo-Physical Discourse of the Vulgar Herbs of This Nation Being a Compleat Method of Physick, Whereby a Man May Preserve His Body in Health, or Cure Himself Being Sick for Three Pence Charge, with Such Things Only as Grow in England* (1652) and T. Shirley, MD, Written in Latine by Dr. A. Valentinus Molimbrochius of Lipswick. Englished by Tho. Sherley, MD and physician in ordinary to His present Majesty. *Cochlearia Curiosa: Or the Curiosities of Scurvygrass. Being an Exact Scrutiny and Careful Description of the Nature and Medicinal Vertue of Scurvygrass. In Which Is Exhibited to Publick Use the Most and Best Preparations of Medicines, Both Galenical and Chymical; Either for Internal or External Use, in Which That Plant, or Any Part Thereof Is Imployed* (1676). For one of many contemporary sources making this direct claim, see Anon., *A Treatise*

Concerning the Plague and Pox (1652).

68   A. Debus, 'Chemists, Physicians, and Changing Perspectives on the Scientific Revolution,' *Isis* 89 (1998), 73 and A. Debus, *The English Paracelsians* (London: Oldbourne, 1965). For a discussion of both Chemical and Galenic disease theories, see J. Walter and R. Schofield, 'Famine, Disease and Crisis Mortality in Early Modern Society,' in J. Walter and R. Schofield (eds), *Famine, Disease and the Social Order in Early Modern Society* (New Yrok: Cambridge University Press, 1989), 23-24.

69   I. Pantin, 'Fracastoro's De Contagione and Medieval Reflection on "Action at a Distance": Old and New Trends in Renaissance Discourse on the Plague,' in C. Carlin (ed.), *Imagining Contagion in Early Modern Europe* (New York: Palgrave Macmillan, 2005), 4 and A.L. Moote and D. Moote, *The Great Plague: The Story of London's Most Deadly Year* (Baltimore, MD: Johns Hopkins University Press, 2004), 98, 141. For explanations of plague from the chemical point of view see Anon., *An Advertisement from the Society of Chymical Physitians Touching Medicines... For the Prevention, and the Cure of the Plague* (1665). W. Simpson, *Zenexton Ante-Pestilentiale. Or, a Short Discourse of the Plague* (1665), A3, and G. Thomson, *Loimologia* (1665), 1, 3-4.

70   Edwards, *A Treatise Concerning the Plague and the Pox Discovering as Well the Meanes How to Preserve from the Danger of These Infectious Contagions, as Also How to Cure Those Which Are Infected with Either of Them* (1652).

71   Edwards, *A Treatise Concerning the Plague and the Pox Discovering as Well the Meanes How to Preserve from the Danger of These Infectious Contagions, as Also How to Cure Those Which Are Infected with Either of Them* (1652). See also T. Wharton, *Directions for the Prevention and Cure of the Plague Fitted for the Poorer Sort,* (1665) in which the author stated that physicians were in agreement that the plague was spread in crowded places.

72   Physicians had long been publishing for the benefit of the poor. Dr. George Thomson claimed to be compelled by charity to share his secret and powerful chemical remedies to cure the plague. G. Thomson, *Loimologia,* 1, 3-4. A similar sentiment was expressed in W. Simpson, *Zenexton Ante-Pestilentiale. Or, a Short Discourse of the Plague,* A3; R. Fletcher, *A Character of a True Physician, or, a True Chymist Compared with a Goose-Quill Pedant with a Short View of the Frauds and Abuses in Physick, Committed by the Confederate Prescribing Doctoral Methodists, with Their Combinators the Apothecaries ... : Being a Vindication of Such Physicians as Follow Not Their Method but Make and Administer Their Own Medicines,*

Being the Honestest, Safest, Cheapest, and Speediest Way of Practice, Both for Physician and Patient (1676).

73 See T. Sherwood, *The Charitable Pestmaster*, 1, 3-4. A similar sentiment was expressed in F.L. Herring, *Certaine Rules, Directions, or Aduertisments for This Time of Pestilentiall Contagion* (1625) and W. J. Gent, *A Collection of Seven and Fifty Approved Receipts Good against the Plague. Taken out of the Five Books of That Renowned Dr. Don Alexes Secrets, for the Benefit of the Poorer Sort of People of These Nations* (1665).

74 Anon., *Present Remedies against the Plague* (1603), A3; R. Fletcher, *A Character of a True Physician, or, a True Chymist Compared with a Goose-Quill Pedant with a Short View of the Frauds and Abuses in Physick, Committed by the Confederate Prescribing Doctoral Methodists, with Their Combinators the Apothecaries...: Being a Vindication of Such Physicians as Follow Not Their Method but Make and Administer Their Own Medicines, Being the Honestest, Safest, Cheapest, and Speediest Way of Practice, Both for Physician and Patient* (1676). Even those who did not identify themselves as physicians stated similar claims of publishing for the public good, especially for the poorer sort, such as T. Wharton, *Directions for the Prevention and Cure of the Plague* (1665); Anon., *Famous and Effectual Medicine to Cure the Plague* (1670); and M.R., *The Meanes of Preventing, and Preserving from, and Curing of That Most Contagious Disease, Called the Plague* (1665), A3.

75 See T. Cock, *Advice for the Poor by Way of Cure and Caution* (1665). These publications appeared in similar forms, reprinted for every major outbreak of plague throughout the century. Examples of various titles include Anon., *Medicines against the Pest, or an Advice Set Down by the Best Learned in Physick within the Kingdome of England* (1645). They were also included in plague orders issued during outbreaks. See for example Anon., *Orders Thought Meet by His Majestie, and His Privie Councell, to Be Executed Throughout the Counties of This Realme* (1625) and Royal College of Physicians of London, *Certain Necessary Directions, Aswell for the Cure of the Plague as for Preuenting the Infection; with Many Easie Medicines of Small Charge, Very Profitable to His Maiesties Subiects / Set Downe by the Colledge of Physicians by the Kings Maiesties Speciall Command ; with Sundry Orders Thought Meet by His Maiestie, and His Priuie Councell, to Be Carefully Executed for Preuention of the Plague ; Also Certaine Select Statutes Commanded by His Maiestie to Be Put in Execution by All Iustices, and Other Officers of the Peace Throughout the Realme ; Together with His Maiesties Proclamation for Further Direction Therein, and a Decree in Starre-Chamber, Concerning*

Buildings and in-Mates (1636).

76 P. Slack, *The Impact of Plague in Tudor and Stuart England*, 304.

77 Anon, *The Shutting up Infected Houses as It Is Practised in England Soberly Debated by Way of Address from the Poor Souls That Are Visited, to Their Brethren That Are Free. With Observations on the Wayes Whereby the Present Infection Hath Spread. As Also a Certain Method of Diet, Attendance, Lodging and Physick, Experimented in the Recovery of Many Sick Persons* (1665).

78 Anon, *The King's Medicines for the Plague. Prescribed in the Year 1604 by the Whole Collodge of Physitians, Both Spiritual and Temporal* (1665), A3-A4.

79 D. Irish, *Levamen Infirmi: Or, Cordial Counsel to the Sick and Diseased Containing I. Advice Concerning Physick, and What a Physician Ought to Be; with an Account of the Author's Remedies, and How to Take Them. Ii. Concerning Melancholy, Frensie, and Madness; in Which, Amongst Other Things, Is Shew'd, How Far They Differ from a Conscience Opprest with the Sense of Sin, and Likewise How They Differ among Themselves. Iii. A Miscellany of Pious Discourses, Concerning the Attributes of God; with Ejaculations and Prayers, According to Scripture Rule. Likewise an Account of Many Things Which Have Happen'd since the Creation. To Which Are Added Several Predictions of What May Happen to the End of the World. The Whole Being Enrich'd with Physical, Pious, Moral & Historical Observations, Delightful to Read, & Necessary to Know.*

80 For examples of scriptural references in medical documents related to plague, see Anon, *The Plague's Approved Physitian, Shewing the Naturall Causes of the Infection of the Ayre, and of the Plague. With Divers Observations to Bee Used, Preserving from the Plague, and Signes to Know the Infected Therewith. Also Many True and Approved Medicines for the Perfect Cure Thereof. Chiefely, a Godly and Penitent Prayer Unto Almighty God, for Our Preservation, and Deliverance Therefrom* (1665); R. Barker, *Consilium Anti-Pestilentiale: Or, Seasonable Advice, Concerning Sure, Safe, Specifick, and Experimented Medicines, Both for the Preservation from, and Cure of This Present Plague* (1665); and T. Willis, *A Help for the Poor Who Are Visited with the Plague: To Be Communicated to Them by the Rich* (1666).

81 J. Harris, *The Divine Physician, Prescribing Rules for the Prevention, and Cure of Most Diseases, as Well of the Body, as the Soul Demonstrating by Natural Reason, and Also Divine and Humane Testimony, That, as Vicious and Irregular Actions and Affections Prove Often Occasions of Most Bodily Diseases, and Shortness of Life, So the Contrary Do Conduce to the Preservation of Health, and Prolongation of Life : In Two Parts. Harris lists the following scriptural passages:* 'Ye shall serve the Lord your God,---and I will take sickness away from

the midst of thee, Exod. 23. 25. 'Long life is promised as a blessing unto them that keep the Commandments in these ensuing words,---*That he turn not aside from the Commandment, to the right hand, or to the left: to the end that he may prolong his dayes in his Kingdom,'* Deut. 17. 20. Also in these: *That thou mayest love the Lord thy God, and that thou mayest obey his voice, and that thou mayest cleave unto him: for he is thy life, and the length of thy dayes,* Cap. 30. vers. 20. Again health was promised upon like conditions: *Be not wise in thine own eyes* (saith *Solomon) fear the Lord and depart from evil: It shall be health to thy navel, and marrow to thy bones,* Pro. 3. 7, 8.' He concluded: 'Thus Jesus Christ, the grand Exemplar of innocency and integrity, was without sin, and therefore without sickness.'

82 W. Muggins, *Londons Mourning Garment, or Funerall Teares Worne and Shed for the Death of Her Wealthy Cittizens, and Other Her Inhabitants. To Which Is Added, a Zealous and Feruent Prayer, with a True Relation How Many Haue Dyed of All Diseases, in Euery Particuler Parish within London, the Liberties, and out Parishes Neere Adioyning from the 14 of Iuly 1603. To the 17 of Nouember. Following* (1603). A similar notion of the importance of keeping order, in the physical and spiritual sense, was echoed in the sermon *A Short Rule of Good Life,* which was intended to lead devout Christians in a 'regular and orderly course' so that they could avoid sin, which 'maketh our soules more vgly, then the plague · leprosy, or any other moste filthy disease doth the body.' R. Southwell, *A Short Rule of Good Life to Direct the Deuout Christian in a Regular and Orderly Course* (1622).

83 J. Scott, *The Christian Life Part Iii. Wherein the Great Duties of Justice, Mercy, and Mortification Are Fully Explained and Inforced. Vol. Iv* (1696). See also W. Austin, *Epiloimia Epe, or, the Anatomy of the Pestilence a Poem in Three Parts : Describing the Deplorable Condition of the City of London under Its Merciless Dominion, 1665 : What the Plague Is, Together with the Causes of It : As Also, the Prognosticks and Most Effectual Means of Safety, Both Preservative and Curative* (1666).

84 T. Vincent, *God's Terrible Voice in the City.* The popular publications that combined prayers with the current Bills of Mortality and cures for plague consistently linked plague to sin, such as this one printed in 1665: 'My sins are cause of all Gods Judgements that upon this Land do fall... Say to thyself, this Plague may be removed, if I repent...' Anon., *Londons Lord Have Mercy Upon Us* (1665).

85 For sermons stressing the need for a clean heart to stave off plague,

see T. Adams, *God's Anger; and, Man's Comfort Two Sermons* (1652) and J. Alleine, *An Alarme to Unconverted Sinners, in a Serious Treatise ... Whereunto Are Annexed Divers Practical Cases of Conscience Judiciously Resolved* (1672). For an example of the need to be healed from the plague in both body and soul, see the prayer printed with numbers form the Bills of Mortality on Anon., *Lord Have Mercy Upon Us* (1636).

86   A. von Nettesheim and H. Cornelius *The Vanity of Arts and Sciences by Henry Cornelius Agrippa, Knight* (1676).

87   R. Shryock, *The Development of Modern Medicine* (Philadelphia: University of Pennsylvania Press, 1936).

88   P. Slack, *The Impact of Plague in Tudor and Stuart England,* 304.

89   P. Slack, *The Impact of Plague in Tudor and Stuart England,* 304.

90   P. Slack, *The Impact of Plague in Tudor and Stuart England,* 304.

91   T. Dekker, 'The Wonderful Year 1603: Wherein Is Shewed the Picture of London Lying Sick of the Plague,' in *Three Elizabethan Pamphlets,* G.R. Hibbard (ed.), (London: George G. Harrap & Co. Ltd., 1951), 183.

92   N. Hodges, *Loimologia.*

93   Cited in A. Dyer, 'The Influence of Bubonic Plague in England, 1550-1667,' 320.

94   Anon, *The Shutting up Infected Houses as It Is Practised in England Soberly Debated by Way of Address from the Poor Souls That Are Visited, to Their Brethren That Are Free. With Observations on the Wayes Whereby the Present Infection Hath Spread. As Also a Certain Method of Diet, Attendance, Lodging and Physick, Experimented in the Recovery of Many Sick Persons* (1665).

95   Cited in A. Dyer, 'The Influence of Bubonic Plague in England, 1550-1667,' 339.

96   For more on this see A. Dyer, 'The Influence of Bubonic Plague in England, 1550-1667,' 314 and R. Munkhoff, 'Searchers of the Dead: Authority, Marginality, and the Interpretation of the Plague in England 1574-1665,' *Gender & History* 11.1 (1999): 1-29.

97   Anon, *Orders Thought Meet by His Majestie, and His Privie Councell, to Be Executed Throughout the Counties of This Realme* (1625).

98   Anon, *Orders Thought Meet by His Majestie, and His Privie Councell, to Be Executed Throughout the Counties of This Realme.*

99   Anon, *Orders Thought Meet by His Majestie, and His Privie Councell, to Be Executed Throughout the Counties of This Realme.*

100 These *Orders* were part of a larger project for dealing with social

problems, and other Books included ones geared toward famine and poverty. For a consideration of the collective significance of the Books of Orders to social policy during the period, see P. Slack, 'Books of Orders: The Making of English Social Policy, 1577-1631,' *Transactions of the Royal Historical Society, 5th Series* 30 (1980).

101 A.L. Moote and D. Moote, *The Great Plague: The Story of London's Most Deadly Year*, 96.

102 A. Dyer, 'The Influence of Bubonic Plague in England, 1550-1667.'

103 P. Slack, *The Impact of Plague in Tudor and Stuart England*, 209.

104 A.L. Moote and D. Moote, *The Great Plague: The Story of London's Most Deadly Year*, 96.

105 Physicians' remedies were not necessarily different from those employed by lay healers, in part because they tended to be traditional and also because there was much borrowing of ideas back and forth. Both lay and professional texts, for example, espoused sweating, bleeding, chicken soup, plasters, and the more labour-intensive practice of plucking the feathers from the tail of a pigeon or chicken, setting the tail to the sore to draw out the poison, and repeating with new birds until they no longer died. See H. Clapham, *An Epistle Discoursing Upon the Present Pestilence* (1603); T. Cogan, *The Haven of Health Chiefly Gathered for the Comfort of Students, and Consequently of All Those That Have a Care of Their Health, Amplified Upon Five Words of Hippocrates, Written Epid. 6. Labour, Cibus, Potio, Somnus, Venus. Hereunto Is Added a Preservation from the Pestilence, with a Short Censure of the Late Sicknes at Oxford*, and William Bullein, *A Dialogue against the Fever Pestilence* (1564).

106 P. Slack, *The Impact of Plague in Tudor and Stuart England*, 219.

107 College of Physicians, Annals III, ff. 97r, 98, 99r. Reprinted in Royal College of Physicians of London., *Certain Necessary Directions, Aswell for the Cure of the Plague as for Preuenting the Infection; with Many Easie Medicines of Small Charge, Very Profitable to His Maiesties Subiects / Set Downe by the Colledge of Physicians by the Kings Maiesties Speciall Command ; with Sundry Orders Thought Meet by His Maiestie, and His Priuie Councell, to Be Carefully Executed for Preuention of the Plague ; Also Certaine Select Statutes Commanded by His Maiestie to Be Put in Execution by All Iustices, and Other Officers of the Peace Throughout the Realme ; Together with His Maiesties Proclamation for Further Direction Therein, and a Decree in Starre-Chamber, Concerning Buildings and in-Mates*. Cited in P. Slack, *The Impact of Plague in Tudor and Stuart England*, 219.

108 See P. Slack, *The Impact of Plague in Tudor and Stuart England*, 223-226.

109 A.L. Moote and D. Moote, *The Great Plague: The Story of London's Most Deadly Year*, 116-17.

110 For a treatise on the connection between the theatre and plague from a moral perspective, see J. Collier, *A Second Defence of the Short View of the Prophaneness and Immorality of the English Stage, &C. Being a Reply to a Book, Entituled, the Ancient and Modern Stages Surveyed, &C.* (1699).

111 P. Slack, *The Impact of Plague in Tudor and Stuart England*, 306.

112 Anon, *The Orders and Directions, of the Right Honourable the Lord Mayor and Court of Aldermen, to Be Diligently Observed and Kept by the Citizens of London, During the Time of the Present Visitation of the Plague* (1665), 1.

113 Royal College of Physicians of London., *Certain Necessary Directions, Aswell for the Cure of the Plague as for Preuenting the Infection; with Many Easie Medicines of Small Charge, Very Profitable to His Maiesties Subiects / Set Downe by the Colledge of Physicians by the Kings Maiesties Speciall Command ; with Sundry Orders Thought Meet by His Maiestie, and His Priuie Councell, to Be Carefully Executed for Preuention of the Plague ; Also Certaine Select Statutes Commanded by His Maiestie to Be Put in Execution by All Iustices, and Other Officers of the Peace Throughout the Realme ; Together with His Maiesties Proclamation for Further Direction Therein, and a Decree in Starre-Chamber, Concerning Buildings and in-Mates* (1636). There are many similar examples, such as Anon., *An Act for the Charitable Reliefe and Ordering of Persons Infected with the Plague* (1630).

114 From P. Slack, *From Reformation to Improvement: Public Welfare in Early Modern England* (Oxford: Clarendon Press, 1999).

115 A. Dyer, 'The Influence of Bubonic Plague in England, 1550-1667,' 320.

116 P. Slack, *The Impact of Plague in Tudor and Stuart England*, 211 and M. Braddick, 'The Early Modern State and the Question of Differentiation, from 1550 to 1700,' *Comparative Studies in Society and History* 38, no. 1 (May 1996), 96.

117 Cited in T. Henderson, *Disorderly Women in Eighteenth-Century London* (New York: Longman, 1999), 92.

118 M. Braddick, 'The Early Modern State and the Question of Differentiation, from 1550 to 1700,' 96.

119 Cited in M. Fissel, 'Charity Universal? Institutions and Moral Reform in Eighteenth-Century Bristol,' in L. Davison, T. Hitchcock, T. Keirn, R. Shoemaker (eds), *Stilling the Grumbling Hive: The Response to Social and*

Economic Problems in England, 1689-1750 (New York: St. Martin's Press, 1992), 128. On the Reformation of Manners see D. Balhman, *The Moral Revolution of 1688* (New Haven: Yale University Press, 1957); T.C. Curtis and W.A. Speck, 'The Societies of the Reformation of Manners: A Case Study in the Theory and Practice of Moral Reform,' *Literature and History* 3 (1976); and J. Spurr, '"Virtue, Religion, and Government": The Anglican Uses of Providence,' in T. Harris, P. Seaward, and M. Goldie (eds), *The Politics of Religion in Restoration England* (Cambridge, MA: Basil Blackwell, 1990).

120 S. MacFarlane, 'Social Policy and the Poor in the Later Seventeenth Century,' in A.L. Beier and R. Finlay (eds), *London 1500-1700: The Making of the Metropolis* (New York: Longman, 1986), 253. See also E. Duffy, 'Primitive Christianity Revived: Religious Renewal in Augustan England,' in D. Baker (ed.), *Renaissance and Renewal in Christian History* (Oxford: Published for the Ecclesiastical History Society by B. Blackwell, 1977).

121 R. Shoemaker, 'Reforming the City: The Reformation of Manners Campaign in London, 1690-1738,' in L. Davison, T. Hitchcock, T. Keirn, R. Shoemaker (eds), *Stilling the Grumbling Hive: The Response to Social and Economic Problems in England, 1689-1750* (New York: St. Martin's Press, 1992), 100-1.

122 D. Hayton, 'Moral Reform and Country Politics in the Late Seventeenth-Century House of Commons,' *Past and Present* 128 (1990), 51.

123 K. Siena, 'Pandora's Pox: The Medical Presentation of Women in Early Modern Venereological Tracts' Thesis (M.A.)--University Of Rochester, 1993, 100.

124 W. Clowes, *A Briefe and Necessarie Treatise, Touching the Cure of the Disease Called Morbus Gallicus, or Lues Venerea, by Vnctions and Other Approoued Waies of Curing: Nevvlie Corrected and Augmented by William Clowes of London* (1585), fol. 1v. On the connection between sin and alehouses as perceived by Puritan society, see P. Clark, 'The Alehouse and the Alternative Society,' in K. Thomas and D. Pennington (eds), *Puritans and Revolutionaries: Essays Presented to Christopher Hill* (Oxford: Oxford University Press, 1978) and D. Underdown, *Fire from Heaven: The Life of an English Town in the Seventeenth Century* (New Haven : Yale University Press, 1992).

125 W. Schleiner, 'Moral Attitudes toward Syphilis and Its Prevention in the

Renaissance,' *Bulletin of the History of Medicine* 68, no. 3 (1994), 394-396.

126 M. Pelling, 'Appearance and Reality: Barber-Surgeons, the Body and Disease," in A.L. Beier and R. Finlay (eds), *London 1500-1700: The Making of the Metropolis* (New York: Longman, 1986), 99.

127 W. Clowes, *Morbus Gallicus* (1585). Cited in M. Pelling, 'Appearance and Reality: Barber-Surgeons, the Body and Disease,' 100. For similar sixteenth-century medical opinions see A. Boorde, *Brievyary of Helthe: For All Manor of Sycknesses and Diseases* (1547) and J. de Vigo, *The Most Excellent Works of Chirurgerie* (1543).

128 K. Siena, 'Pollution, Promiscuity, and the Pox: English Venereology and the Early Modern Medical Discourse on Social and Sexual Danger,' *Journal of the History of Sexuality* 8, no. 4 (1998), 560-561.

129 M. Douglas, *Purity and Danger: An Analysis of Concepts of Pollution and Taboo* (London: 1966); K. Siena, 'Pollution, Promiscuity, and the Pox: English Venereology and the Early Modern Medical Discourse on Social and Sexual Danger,' *Journal of the History of Sexuality* 8, no. 4 (1998), 553-555.

130 S. Burtt, 'The Societies for the Reformation of Manners: Between John Locke and the Devil in Augustan England' in *The Margins of Orthodoxy: Heterodox Writing and Cultural Response, 1660-1750* (New York: Cambridge University Press, 1995), 155.

131 D. Williams, *A Sermon Preach'd at Salter's Hall to the Societies for the Reformation of Manners* (1699), 53.

132 J. Spademan, *A SermonPreach'd November 14, 1698 and Now Publish'd at the Request of the Societies for Reformation of Manners* (1699), 36.

133 S. Burtt, 'The Societies for the Reformation of Manners: Between John Locke and the Devil in Augustan England,' 161.

134 S. Bradwell, *A Watch-Man for the Pest Teaching the True Rules of Preservation from the Pestilent Contagion, at This Time Fearefully over-Flowing This Famous Cittie of London. Collected out of the Best Authors, Mixed with Auncient Experience, and Moulded into a New and Most Plaine Method* (1625), To the Reader.

135 S. Bradwell, *A Watch-Man for the Pest Teaching the True Rules of Preservation from the Pestilent Contagion, at This Time Fearefully over-Flowing This Famous Cittie of London. Collected out of the Best Authors, Mixed with Auncient Experience, and Moulded into a New and Most Plaine Method* (1625), To the Reader.

136 R. Johnson, *Enchiridion Medicum, or, a Manual of Physick Being a*

Compendium of the Whole Art, in Three Parts…: Wherein Is Briefly Shewed 1. The Names, 2. The Derivation, 3. The Causes, 4. The Signs, 5. The Prognosticks, and 6. A Rational Method of Cure (1684).

137 Edwards, *A Treatise Concerning the Plague and the Pox Discovering as Well the Meanes How to Preserve from the Danger of These Infectious Contagions, as Also How to Cure Those Which Are Infected with Either of Them.* See also R. Younge, *The prevention of poverty*: 'A man falleth into the Pestilence by disordering of himselfe, either in diet, or with other exercises. Therefore, during the time of this contagious sicknesse, hee must have a speciall regard, to keepe himselfe from all outrages, and surfets (to wit) from all excess of meate, drinke, sweating, bathes, letehery, and all other things that open the pores of the body, and causeth the bad ayres to enter, which entring, invenome the lively spirits of man, and infect, and indanger the whole body.'

138 Anon, *The Plagues Approved Physitian. Shewing the Naturall Causes of the Infection of the Ayre, and of the Plague. With Divers Observations to Bee Used, Preserving from the Plague, and Signes to Know the Infected Therewith. Also Many True and Approved Medicines for the Perfect Cure Thereof.*

139 R. Barker, *Consilium Anti-Pestilentiale: Or, Seasonable Advice, Concerning Sure, Safe, Specifick, and Experimented Medicines, Both for the Preservation from, and Cure of This Present Plague.*

Conclusion

This book began by questioning why anyone would see a doctor in the seventeenth century. At first glance, the employment of a physician might seem to defy explanation, yet we know that physicians did come to be entrenched in medical care in the next century, although few major medical advances occurred. Clearly, physicians were successful in differentiating themselves from their competition on other grounds. There was, in fact, another aspect of medicine that went beyond dispensing physic. Physicians self-fashioned an image of themselves as knowledgeable health experts whose education assured good judgment and sage advice and whose interest in the health of their patients surpassed the peddling of a single nostrum to everyone. As Roy Porter has cautioned, historians should question medical history's preoccupying concern with *cures* (even cures that did not work), as it is modern medicine that is cure-fixated. Physicians' treatments went far beyond drug intervention. They were much more interested in fortifying the body and adjusting the whole constitution. Early modern people, patients and practitioners alike, were concerned with positive health and routine health maintenance as much as with sickness, just as they were concerned with prevention rather than with therapeutics alone.[1] Physicians excelled at selling the idea of health to a population who understood the term in a much different way than we do today.

Physicians made certain inroads during the seventeenth century in overcoming their issues of status. They were not necessarily better at healing their patients, but they were successful in conjuring a representation of their profession as distinct from and superior to other types of healers because they alone were educated and therefore possessed the wisdom and knowledge to assist their patients through the quagmire of early modern medicine and therapeutics. In sum, when historians wonder why people chose physicians, they are perhaps not considering the offering of physicians from an early modern perspective but from a modern one. They were able to recommend health maintenance in the form of customized preventative programs, a concept that would remain appealing to patients throughout much of the seventeenth century and would not decline significantly until changes in the medical marketplace brought on by the new consumer economy of the eighteenth century altered the way physicians practiced medicine.

In the seventeenth century, this was not yet the case. Spiritual and physical health remained connected. This connection might lead a modern observer to presume that in such an environment, traditional medicine would have thrived at the expense of professional medicine.[2] However, physicians' consideration of both the physical and spiritual health of their patients was a crucial factor in their ability to survive the seventeenth century. They used the connection to counteract traditional criticism of members of their profession as atheistic and greedy while fashioning an image of themselves as pious physicians, and they emphasized the connection between physical and spiritual health when suggesting public health measures to counteract epidemic diseases.

Physicians saw themselves as offering something unique to their patients: wise counsel on matters of health, based on their learning and moral character. They strove to differentiate themselves from the bevy of other healers who could not offer learned advice, just as they increased their efforts to close ranks against those who had traditionally sought to practice medicine without a university education. They possessed a vision of themselves filling a role in society that was different from others, in that their primary concern was disease prevention based on individual constitution, humoral makeup, and proper lifestyle choices. They emphasized health maintenance first and foremost, along with carefully directed courses of treatment should illness arise.

Physicians capitalized on medicine's association with the divine to establish themselves as morally responsible professionals who worked in tandem with God to do for the body what the minister did for the soul. By doing so, physicians were able to market themselves as moral authorities, which made them distinguishable from all other healers in their unique ability to care for the whole patient, both body and soul. The link between medicine and religion was a positive one in terms of disseminating the idea of the godly physician, which explains why physicians stressed it in their writing and why they prescribed rules for behavior as much as physic in the medical literature they published.[3]

This association was not a far-fetched one because in theoretical terms, medicine and religious healing coexisted rather peacefully due to theories of primary and secondary causation incorporated into seventeenth-century disease theory. God's will to punish was considered an explanation for otherwise inexplicable natural phenomena or for disease outbreaks.[4] Moreover, sermons encouraged people to 'honor thy physician.'[5] Sermons offered an image of the 'learned and godly Physitian' that was in keeping with the way physicians themselves wished the public to view them.[6] By making connections between medicine and the divine, physicians were echoing cultural conceptions imbedded in broader society. It was not the case that medicine and religion were at odds with one another. Conversely, by presenting disease and healing in the same terms, both worked to the advantage of the physician.

Physicians communicated the unique offering of their profession to the public through the printing press, which they used to defend themselves against their competitors. They became adept at impugning other types of healers while more clearly delineating their attributes to a wider audience. In his *Medicas Absolutus* the physician Everard Maynwaring described the learned physician as engaged in a 'grand business,' as opposed to quacks who lead 'a loose idle life,' occupied solely with the 'Manufacture, Buying and Selling' of medicine.[7] Physicians were able to adapt to the printing of medical works in the vernacular to sell their vision of healthcare to the public. By claiming to publish as an act of charity, either to educate unlearned healers or to provide basic information for the poor who would otherwise not have access to a physician, physicians bolstered their authority. They also showed an altruistic side to a segment of the population that they had very little desire to treat as patients.

Throughout most of European history, regular medical attendance and personal health care remained the prerogative of a privileged minority. Johan Goudsblom has suggested that since the days of Hippocrates and Galen, physicians had known that only a miniscule portion of the population could afford to regularly spend a great deal of attention on the preservation of their health. Only those who had sufficient financial means and leisure would be able to put Galen's precepts about personal hygiene into practice or to produce the inner rest and wisdom to follow a life of temperance and moderation.[8] Work on lay healers providing medical care to much of the population who would never have access to a physician supports this notion, as does research on the practices of specific doctors.[9] There had always been a difference between medical care for private, fee-paying patients that entailed the expensive and lengthy cures of the physician and medical care for the rest of society. One was accommodating; the other was restrictive. The pox and plague both manifestly demonstrate this difference.[10] Seventeenth-century physicians in general provided personal care for the former group and advice for the latter.

Their acting as advisors about health care for the poor became more critical with the rise of the urban environment in the late Tudor period. Margaret Pelling has demonstrated that it did not escape contemporary notice that for the city dweller, degeneration of health and premature death seemed omnipresent. Urban living therefore raised an already high level of anxiety about health to the point of obsession and prompted an increasing resort to medical practitioners.[11] Pelling's focus is on lay healers, but urbanization and the ensuing health risks that accompanied it, particularly plague epidemics, proved pivotal in the professionalization of physicians. Their decision to focus on the poor and disorderly as vectors of infection, along with their suggestions for sanitary measures that affected the poor more so than the rich, clearly aligned physicians with elite authority. Physicians, in effect, gained in authority by supporting authority.

It was essential to the success of the medical profession that they assumed greater moral control of the realm without alienating affluent patients. They accomplished this by defining public health as a means of regulating the behavior of the poor in order to restrain them from spreading disease to the rest of the population. Such was the vision of public health that physicians were instrumental in developing: one based on control of those elements of society that seemed threatening to social order and stability. As Bruce Boehrer has argued, Renaissance medicine developed not out of liberating impulses but out of a desire to protect 'an aristocratic social order that felt itself threatened from without.' The European medical profession, according to Boehrer's interpretation, was dedicated to the service of the 'ruling elite.'[12] Given their anxiety about status, it was even more imperative for seventeenth-century English physicians to make such alignments in order to protect their precarious position in society and garner additional status.

Supporting the social order by suggesting public health policy became the hallmark of the medical profession by the turn of the eighteenth century. Such an agenda is evident in early eighteenth-century plague policy in anticipation of another epidemic in 1721. The physician Sir John Colbatch noted that barracks for the infected were necessary only for the 'miserable and indigent,' which he considered 'the dangerous classes.' Physicians submitted various proposals to keep order, should the poor prove ungovernable. In short, they made containing the contagious poor in order to protect the rest of society a priority into the eighteenth century.[13]

Guenter Risse has commented that early eighteenth-century medicine

263

'dramatically expanded the scope of its activities under the influence of powerful social and political forces.' Foucault has referred to this expansion of activities as the 'medicalization of society.'[14] It was a trend that not only allowed physicians to reach new sectors of the burgeoning middle class, but for the first time in history, make significant contact with the sectors of the lower classes of society. Physicians made critical inroads essential to the medicalization of society in the seventeenth century, from their publications that claimed to promote proper health care for all to their suggestions for public health measures to curb the spread of epidemics. The philosophy of medicine during the Enlightenment, which regarded health as a positive tenet that could be attained, preserved, and even recovered with the aid of a proper lifestyle, public and personal hygiene, and the aid of medicine, would not have been possible were it not for the efforts of seventeenth-century physicians. They distinguished themselves from other healers and convinced the public to view the physician as an authority on health: a health whose paradigm in the seventeenth century was still relatively untouched by the scientific revolution and was much more in tune with Divine Providence than with the discoveries of Sydenham and Harvey.

Doreen Nagy has used the example of the mid-seventeenth-century critic of the medical profession, Noah Biggs, to represent a vision of the medical profession as antiquated and ineffective. Biggs believed physicians practiced an impotent and ineffective system of medicine. They were taught to 'mouth out the perfection of their Art' even though they knew from their lack of success that they were only 'catching at painted Butterflies.'[15] Nagy has used such criticism to conclude that since professional and popular medicine borrowed remedies from each other, physicians had a hard time justifying their existence and were incapable of demonstrating a clear superiority. Yet we need to look beyond remedies and higher fees to discern why physicians were able to achieve success in the eighteenth century. Assessing the success of medicine's response to a disease is a culturally constructed endeavor, and it is one that shifts over time. Early modern standards did not necessarily require that physicians cure the disease: it was sufficient that the public see them as actively battling it. They did this by focusing their erudite knowledge of the disease on the types of people who most frequently spread contagion and the places where people would most often encounter disease. By focusing on the behavior that precipitated infection, physicians gained greater control over the lives and souls of their patients. We must remember that the primary goal of the seventeenth-century physician was to preserve health and prolong life, not to fight disease.[16] In this context they were not 'catching at painted Butterflies' so much as shouting in Babel: struggling to be heard amidst a confusion of voices. The challenge lay in delivering their message above the clamor of their competition; evidence that they managed this lies in their ability to thrive in the next century.

Notes

1   R. Porter, 'The Patient's View: Doing Medical History from Below,' *Theory and Society* 14, no. 2 (1985), 193.

2   D. Nagy, *Popular Medicine in Seventeenth-Century England* (Bowling Green: Bowling Green State University Popular Press, 1988), 35.

3   For primary source examples see W. Bullein, *A Dialogue against the Fever Pestilence* (1564); Osiander, *How and Wither a Christian Man Ought to Fly the Plague;* A.T., *A Rich Store-House, Vol. Fol.65;* T. Cogan, *The Haven of Health Chiefly Gathered for the Comfort of Students, and Consequently of All Those That Have a Care of Their Health, Amplified Upon Five Words of Hippocrates, Written Epid. 6. Labour, Cibus, Potio, Somnus, Venus. Hereunto Is Added a Preservation from the Pestilence, with a Short Censure of the Late Sicknes at Oxford* (1636); and L. Fuchs, *A worthy practise of the moste learned phisition Maister Leonerd Fuchsius, Doctor in phisicke, moste necessary in this needfull tyme of our visitation, for the comforte of all good and faythfull people, both olde and yonge, bothe for the sicke and for them that woulde auoyde the daunger of the contagion* 1563.

4   R. Palmer, 'The Church, Leprosy and Plague in Medieval and Early Modern Europe' in W.J. Sheils (ed.), *The Church and Healing* (Oxford: Basil Blackwell, 1982), 88. See also K. Thomas, *Religion and the Decline of Magic* (New York: Scribner, 1971).

5   D. Harley, "Medical Metaphors in English Moral Theology, 1560-1660," *Journal of the History of Medicine and Allied Sciences* 48, no. 4 (1993), 423-4.

6   S. Page, *The Broken Heart: Or, Davids Penance Fully Exprest in Holy Meditations Upon the 51 Psalme* (1637), 22.

7   E. Maynwaring, *Medicas Absolutus* (1668).

8   J. Goudsblom, 'Public Health and the Civilizing Process,' *The Milbank Quarterly* 64, no. 2 (1986), 181-2.

9   Doreen Nagy's analysis of the case records of Dr John Symcotts reveal that licensed practitioners drew most of their clientele from small group of about 5-15 % of the population. D. Nagy, *Popular Medicine in Seventeenth-Century England,* 31. On lay healers providing the bulk of medical care in seventeenth-century society, see L. Beier, *Sufferers and Healers: The Experience of Illness in Seventeenth-Century England* (New York: Routledge, 1987); R. Porter, *Disease, Medicine, and Society in England, 1550-1860* (Basingstoke: Macmillan, 1987); and M. Pelling, 'Irregular Practitioners: A Wilderness of Mirrors,' in M. Pelling (ed.), *Medical Conflicts in Early Modern London: Patronage, Physicians, and Irregular Practitioners, 1550-1640* (Oxford: Clarendon Press, 2003).

10 J. Goudsblom, 'Public Health and the Civilizing Process,' *The Milbank Quarterly* 64, no. 2 (1986), 181-2.

11 M. Pelling, 'Appearance and Reality: Barber-Surgeons, the Body and Disease,' in A.L. Beier and R. Finlay (ed.), *London 1500-1700: The Making of the Metropolis* (New York: Longman, 1986), 82.

12 B.T. Boehrer, 'Early Modern Syphilis,' *Journal of the History of Sexuality* 1, no. 2 (October 1990), 200.

13 P. Slack, *The Impact of Plague in Tudor and Stuart England* (London: Routledge & K. Paul, 1985), 334-5.

14 G. Risse, 'Medicine in the Age of Enlightenment,' in A. Wear (ed.), *Medicine in Society: Historical Essays* (Cambridge: Cambridge University Press, 1992), 171, 195.

15 N. Biggs, *Mataeo Technia Medicinae Paxeos or Vanity of the Craft of Physick* (1651), Forward. Cited in D. Nagy, *Popular Medicine in Seventeenth-Century England,* 50.

16 H. Cook, 'Good Advice and Little Medicine: The Professional Authority of Early Modern English Physicians,' *The Journal of British Studies* 33, no. 1 (January 1994), 12.

Bibliography

I
Primary Sources
The city of publication is London unless noted otherwise.

Religious Tracts

A Christian Meditation or Praier to Be Sayed by All Tymes Whensoever God Shall Vyset Us Wyth Anye Mortall Plague or Sicnesse (1551).

A Moral Essay Upon the Soul of Man in Three Parts: I. The Preference Due to the Soul above the Body...Ii. Of Our Duties of Religion and Morality...Iii. Concerning Our Duties of Time and Eternity (1687).

A Praier Very Comfortable and Necessary to Be Used of All Christians Every Morning and Evening Amongst Heir Families, That It Would Please the Lord God to Be Appeased in Is Wrath, and So Withdraw His Heavy Hand an Greevous Visitations from Amongst Us (no date given).

Saint Bernard's Vision (a Brief Discourse Dialogue-Wise) between the Soul and Body Of a Damned Man Newly Deceased, Laying the Faults One Upon Other: With a Speech of the Devils in Hell 1640.

"A Sermon, Containing the Strangeness, Frequency, and Desperate Consequence of Impenitency," in *Six Sermons Preached by the Right Reverend Father in God, Seth Lord Bishop of Sarum* (1672).

T. Adams, *The deuills banket described in foure sermons [brace], 1. The banket propounded, begunne, 2. The second seruice, 3. The breaking vp of the feast, 4. The shot or reckoning, [and] The sinners passing-bell, together with Phisicke from heauen* (1614).

———, *Diseases of the Soule a Discourse Diuine, Morall, and Physicall* (1616).

———, *God's Anger; and, Man's Comfort Two Sermons* (1652).

J. Alleine, *An Alarme to Unconverted Sinners, in a Serious Treatise ... Whereunto Are Annexed Divers Practical Cases of Conscience Judiciously Resolved* (1672).

T. Allefree, *Ephroditus's Sickness and Recovery, in Three Sermons* (1671).

R. Allen, *A Gainful Death at the End of a Truly Christian Life* (1700).

R. Ames, *The Female Fire-Ships. A Satyr Aginst Whoring* (1691).

L. Andrews, *A Sermon of Pestilence, Preached at Chiswick, 1603* (1636).

J.B. *The Journal or Diary of a Thankful Christian* (1656).

F. Bampfield, Francis. *All in One, All Useful Sciences and Profitable Arts in One Book of Jehovah Aelohim, Copied out and Commented Upon in Created Beings, Comprehended and Discovered in the Fulness and Perfection of Scr[I]pture-Knowledges* (1677).

J. Bastwick, *The Confession of the Faithful Witnesse of Christ, Mr. John Bastwick Doctor of Physick* (1641).

W. Bates, *A Funeral Sermon Preached Upon the Death of Mr. Thomas Gouge* (1681).

R. Baxter, *A Christian Directory, or, a Summ of Practical Theologie and Cases of Conscience Directing Christians How to Use Their Knowledge and Faith, How to Improve All Helps and Means, and to Perform All Duties, How to Overcome Temptations, and to Escape or Mortifie Every Sin: In Four Parts* (1673).

————, *The Invaluable Price of an Immortal Soul Shewing the Vanity of Most People in Taking Care for the Body, but Neglect Their Duty as to the Preservation of Their Never-Dying Souls* (1681).

P. Bayne, *A Caveat for Cold Christians Wherein the Common Disease of Christians, with the Remedie, Is Plainly and Excellently Set Downe for All That Will Use It* (1618).

J. Beadle, *The Journal or Diary of a Thankful Christian* (1656).

T. Beard and T. Taylor, *The theatre of Gods judgements wherein is represented the admirable justice of God against all notorious sinners ... /* collected out of sacred, ecclesiasticall, and pagan histories by two most reverend doctors in divinity, Thomas Beard ... and Tho. Taylor ... (1642).

T. Becon, *Prayer for Them That Are Sick* (no date given).

N. Bisbie, *Prosecution No Persecution: Or, the Difference Between Suffering for Disobedience and Faction, and Suffering for Righteousness and Christ's Sake* (1682).

C. Blackwood, *Some Pious Treatises Being 1. A Bridle for the Tongue: Or, a Treatise Directing a Christian How to Order His His [Sic] Words in a Holy Maner. 2. The Present Sweetness, and Future Bitterness of a Delicious Sin. 3. A Christians Groans under the Body of Sin. 4. Proving the Resurrection of the Same Body Committed to the Dust: Also, the Not Dying of the Soul within the Body. 5. Tractatus De Clavibus Ecclesiae* (1654).

R. Bolton, *Instructions for a Right Comforting Afflicted Consciences with Speciall Antidotes against Some Grievous Temptations: Delivered for the Most Part in the Lecture at Kettering in North-Hampton-Shire* (1631).

268

N. Bownd, *A Storehouse of Comfort for the Afflicted in Spirit* (1604).

F. Bugg, *The Pilgrim's Progress, from Quakerism to Christianity* (1700).

F. Bunny, *A Guide Unto Godliness* (1617).

T. Burroughs, *A Soveraign Remedy for All Kinds of Grief* (1662).

M.H. Burton, *A Most Godly Sermon: Preached at St. Albons in Woodstreet on Sunday Last, Being the 10 of October, 1641* (1641).

W.C. *Londons Lamentations for Her Sinnes: And Complaint to the Lord Her God* (1625).

E. Calamy, *The Art of Divine Meditation, or, a Discourse of the Nature, Necessity, and Excellency Thereof with Motives to, and Rules for the Better Performance of That Most Important Christian Duty: In Several Sermons on Gen. 24:63* (1680).

A. Carpenter, *Destructorium Vitiorum, or Destroyer Of Vice* (1429).

E. Carrey, *A Serious Meditation for Sinners Which Is Set Forth in Several Discourses, Which Passed between a Soul at Her Departure, and the Members of the Body* (1688).

N. Caussin, *The Christian Diary* (1648).

W. Charlton, *Darkness of Atheism* (1652).

———, *Immortality of the Human Soul* (1657).

S. Clarke, *The Marrow of Ecclesiastical Historie* (1650).

J. Collier, *A Second Defence of the Short View of the Prophaneness and Immorality of the English Stage, &C. Being a Reply to a Book, Entituled, the Ancient and Modern Stages Surveyed, &C.* (1699).

J. Cragge, *Great Britains Prayers in This Dangerous Time of Contagion* (1641).

W. Cupper, *Certaine Sermons Concerning God's Late Visitation* (1592).

J. Davies and T. Jenner, *A Work for None but Angels...A Book Shewing What the Soule Is, Subsisting and Having Its Operations without the Body* (1658).

K. Digby, *Two Treatises in the One of Which, the Nature of Bodies: In the Other, the Nature of Mans Soul Is Looked into in Way of Discovery of the Immortality of Reasonable Souls* (1658).

G. Downame, *Two Sermons, the One Commending the Ministrie in General: The Other Defending to Office of Bishops in Particular* (1608).

J. Dunton, *The Visions of the Soule, before It Comes into the Body in Several Dialogues* (1692).

J. Edwards, *The Plague of the Heart* (1665).

———, *A Treatise Concerning the Plague and the Pox Discovering as Well the Meanes How to Preserve from the Danger of These Infectious Contagions, as Also*

269

How to Cure Those Which Are Infected with Either of Them (1652).

J.F. *A New Letter, to All Drunkards, Whoremongers, Thieves, Disobedience to Parents, Swearers, Lyers* (1696).

J. Flavel, *Pneumatologia, a Treatise of the Soul of Man Wherein the Divine Original, Excellent and Immortal Nature of the Soul Are Opened, Its Love and Inclination to the Body, with the Necessity of Its Separation from It, Considered and Improved, the Existence, Operations, and States of Separated Souls, Both in Heaven and Hell, Immediately after Death, Asserted, Discussed, and Variously Applyed...* (1685).

H. Gosson, *Christs Teares over Jerusalem. Or, a Caveat for England, to Call to God for Mercy, Lest We Be Plagued for Our Contempt and Wickedness* (1624).

W. Gouge, *God's Three Arrowes: Plague, Famine, Sword* (1636).

R. Harris, *Hezekiah's Recovery* (1626).

E. Heron, *Physicke for Body and Soule Shewing That the Maladies of the One, Proceede from the Sinnes of the Other: With a Remedie against Both, Prescribed by Our Heauenly Physitian Iesus Christ* (1621).

J. Howell, *The Vision or a Dialog between the Soul and the Bodie, Fancid in a Morning-Dream* (1651).

D. King, *A Discovery of Some Troublesome Thoughts Wherewith Many Godly Precious Souls Are Burthened, and Extreamly Pressed: That Like a Canker Eats out All Their Comforts, and Keeps Their Souls under Continuall Fears and Distractions. Together with a Compound of Some Scripture and Experimentall Cordials, for the Refreshing of Those Who Are Sick of Such a Disease; and through the Blessing of God, May Prove Medicinall, to the Cure of Some, and the Comforting of Others* (1651).

———, *Self the Grand Enemy of Jesus Christ, and Mortall Disease of Man. Or, a Treatise Discovering What a Heart-Plague Self Is with Its Mischief and Danger: Also, Special Remedies for Its Cure* (1660).

E. Lawrence, *Christ's Power over Bodily Diseases Preached in Several Sermons* (1662).

G. Lesly, *The Universal Medicine: A Sermon* (1678).

T. Manlove, *The Immortality of the Soul Asserted, and Practically Improved Shewing by Scripture, Reason, and the Testimony of the Ancient Philosophers, That the Soul of Man Is Capable of Subsisting and Acting in a State of Separation from the Body, and How Much It Concerns Us All to Prepare for That State...* (1697).

W. Miller, *A Sermon Preached at the Funerall of the Worshipfull Gilbert Davies, at Christow in Devon* (1621).

T. Oldman, *Gods Rubuke in Taking from Us That Worthy and Honourable Gentleman Sir Edward Lewkenor Knight* (1619).

R. Overton, *Man Wholly Mortal, or, a Treatise Wherein 'Tis Proved Both Theologically and Philosophically, That as Whole Man Sinned, So Whole Man Died Contrary to That Common Distinction of Soul and Body* (1655).

S. Page, *The Broken Heart: Or, Davids Penance Fully Exprest in Holy Meditations Upon the 51 Psalme* (1637).

Paracelsus, *An Excellent Treatise Teaching Howe to Cure the French-Pockes with All Other Diseases Arising and Growing Thereof, and in a Manner All Other Sicknesses. Dravvne out of the Bookes of That Learned Doctor and Prince of Phisitians, Theophrastus Paracelsus. Compiled by the Learned Phillippus Hermanus, Phisition and Chirurgion*, trans. John Hester (1590).

W. Parke, *A Tractat of the Universal Panacaea of Soul and Body* (1665).

S. Patrick, *Jewish Hypocrisie, a Caveat to the Present Generation* (1660).

J. Pearson, *An Exposition of the Creed* (1659).

Perrinchief, *A Sermon Preached before the Honourable House of Commons, at St. Margarets Westminster, Nov. 7 Being the Fast-Day Appointed for the Plague of Pestilence* (1666).

G. Rust, *Funeral Sermon Preached at the Obsequies Of...Jeremy, Lord Bishop of Down*, (1668).

J. Scott, *The Christian Life Part Iii. Wherein the Great Duties of Justice, Mercy, and Mortification Are Fully Explained and Inforced. Vol. Iv*, (1696).

T. Sherwood, *The Charitable Pestmaster* (1641).

R. Sibbes, *The Soules Conflict with It Selfe* (1635).

J. Smith, *Gerochomia vasilike King Solomons portraiture of old age : wherein is contained a sacred anatomy both of soul and body, and a perfect account of the infirmities of age, incident to them both : and all those mystical and aenigmatical symptomes expressed in the six former verses of the 12th chapter of Ecclesiastes, are here paraphrased upon and made plain and easie to a mean capacity* (1666).

R. Southwell, *A Short Rule of Good Life to Direct the Deuout Christian in a Regular and Orderly Course* (1622).

E. Stillingfleet, *The Works of Dr. Edward Stillingfleet. 6 vols. Vol. 1.* (1704).

J. Turner, *Choice Experiences of the Kind Dealings of God* (1653).

R. Venning, *Sin, the Plague of Plagues; or, Sinful Sin the Worst of Evils* (1669).

T. Vincent, *God's Terrible Voice in the City* (1667).

W.W., *The Anchor of Faith. Upon Which, a Christian May Repose in All Manner of Temptations* (1628).

————, *Physick to Cure the Most Dangerous Disease, Desperation* (1607).

R. Walker, *A Learned and Profitable Treatise of God's Providence* (1608).

G. Whitefield, *Christ the Physician of the Soul* (1750).

T. Woolnough, *The Dust Returning to Earth* (1669).

Diaries and Letters

His Majesty's Letter to the Lord Bishop of London (1690).

The Mid-Wives Just Petition: Or, a Complaint of Divers Good Gentlewomen of That Faculty. Shewing the Whole Christian World Their Just Cause of Their Sufferings in These Distracted Times, for Their Want of Trading. Which Said Complaint They Tendered to the House on Monday Last, Being the 23. Of Ian. 1643 (1643).

B. Blackstine (ed.), *The Ferrar Papers*. London: Cambridge University Press (1938).

E. Cellier, *A Letter to Dr. ----* (1680).

E. Dunk, *The Copy of a Letter Written by E.D. Doctour of Physicke to a Gentleman, by Whom It Was Published* (1606).

G.P. Elliot (ed.), *Diary of Dr. Edward Lake* (London: Camden Society, no. 39, 1846).

R. Latham (ed.), *The Shorter Pepys* (Berkeley: University of California Press, 1985).

R. Latham and W. Matthews (eds), *The Diary of Samuel Pepys*. 11 vols. (London: Bell & Hyman, 1970).

Lowther, *Lowther Family Estate Books, 1617-1675*. Vol. 191. C.B. Philips (ed.), (Gateshead: Northumberland Press, 1979).

A. MacFarlane (ed.), *Diary of Ralph Josselin 1616-1683* (London: Oxford University Press, New Series, 1976).

A.R., and M.B. Hall (eds), *The Correspondence of Henry Oldenburg* (Madison, Wisconsin, 1965-73).

C. Severn (ed.), *The Diary of the Reverend John Ward [1648-79]* (London, 1839).

F. Verney, and M.M. Verney (ed.), *The Verney Memoirs. 2 Vols.* (London: Longmans, Green and Company, 1925).

Drama and Literature

The Cruel Midwife. Being a True Account of a Most Sad and Lamentable Discovery That Has Been Lately Made in the Village of Poplar in the Parish of Stepney (1693).

The Murderous Midwife (1673).

The Poor Whore's Lamentation, or, the Fleet-Street Crack's Complaint for Want of Trading to the Tune of the Guinea Wins Her (1685).

The Quack Triumphant: Or, the N-R--Ch Cavalcade. A New Ballad (1733).

T. Bentley, *The Monument of Matrones* (1582).

R. Cawdry, *A treasurie or store-house of similies both pleasaunt, delightfull, and profitable, for all estates of men in generall. Newly collected into heades and common places* (1600).

T. Dekker, *The Gull's Hornbook* (1609).

———. "The Honest Whore.--Part the First," in E. Rhys (ed.), *The Best Plays of the Old Dramatists: Thomas Dekker* (New York: Charles Scribner's Sons, 1900), 89-190.

———. *Newes from Graves-Ende* (1604).

———. *The Pleasant Comedie of Old Fortunatus* (1600).

———. 'The Wonderful Year 1603: Wherein Is Shewed the Picture of London Lying Sick of the Plague,' in G.R. Hibbard (ed.), *Three Elizabethan Pamphlets* (London: George G. Harrap & Co. Ltd., 1951), 160-207.

J. Donne, *Devotions Upon Emergent Occasions* (1623).

J. Ford, *The Lover's Melancholy* (1629).

———. *Perkin Warbeck* (1634).

B. Franklin, *Poor Richard's Almanac* (1744).

T. Heywood, *The Wise-Woman of Hogsden* (1638).

P. Holland, *Cyrupaedia the Institution and Life of Cyrus, the First of That Name, King of Persians. Eight Bookes. Treating of Noble Education, of Princely Exercises, Military Discipline, Warlike Stratagems, Preparations and Expeditions: As Appeareth by the Contents before the Beginning of the First Booke. Written in Greeke by the Sage Xenophon. Translated out of Greeke into English, and Conferred with the Latine and French Translations* (Coventry, 1632).

B. Jonson, *The Poetaster* (1616).

———. *The Silent Woman* (1610).

———. *Volpone* (1606).

T. Lyle, *Campaspe* (1632).

P. Massinger and T. Dekker, *Virgin Martyr* (1622).

273

T. Middleton, *A Fair Quarrel* (1613).

T. Nabbes, *The Bride* (1638).

W. Shakespeare, "Hamlet," in *The Complete Pelican Shakespeare* A. Harbage
(ed.), (New York: Viking Penguin, 1969), 930-76.

———. "The Life of Timon of Athens," in *The Complete Pelican Shakespeare*
A. Harbage (ed.), (New York: Viking Penguin, 1969), 1136-68.

J. Webster, *Duchess of Malfi* (1613).

F.P. Wilson (ed.), *The Plague Pamphlets of Thomas Dekker* (Oxford: Clarendon
Press, 1925).

Political and Social Tracts

'An Account of the Institution of the Lock Asylum; for the reception of
Penitent Female patients, when discharged from the Lock Hospital'
(1793).

An Account of the Societies for the Reformation of Manners in England and Ireland
(1701).

*Antimoixeria: or, the Honest and Joynt-Design of the Tower Hamlets for the
General Suppression of Bawdy-Houses, as Encouraged by the Publick
Magistrates* (18 June 1691).

*Certain Necessary Directions, Aswell for the Cure of the Plague as for Preventing the
Infection; with Many Easie Medicines of Small Charge, Very Profitable to His
Maiesties Subiects / Set Downe by the Colledge of Physicians by the Kings Maies-
ties Speciall Command ; with Sundry Orders Thought Meet by His Maiestie, and
His Priuie Councell, to Be Carefully Executed for Preuention of the Plague ; Also
Certaine Select Statutes Commanded by His Maiestie to Be Put in Execution by
All Iustices, and Other Officers of the Peace Throughout the Realme ; Together
with His Maiesties Proclamation for Further Direction Therein, and a Decree in
Starre-Chamber, Concerning Buildings and in-Mates* (1636).

Character of a Good Woman (1697).

*The Crafty Whore: Or, the Mistery and Iniquity of Bawdy Houses Laid Open, in
a Dialogue between Two Subtle Bawds, Wherein, as in a Mirrour, Our City-
Curtesans May See Their Soul-Destroying Art, and Crafty Devices, Whereby
They Insnare and Beguile Youth, Pourtraied to the Life, by the Pensell of One of
Their Late, (but Now Penitent) Captives, for the Benefit of All, but Especially the
Younger Sort. Whereunto Is Added Dehortations from Lust Drawn from the Sad
and Lamentable Consequences It Produceth* (1658).

A Cure for the State. Or, an Excellent Remedy against the Apostacy of the Times (1659).

A Dialogue Betwixt a Citizen, and a Poore Countrey Man and His Wife, in the Country, Where the Citizen Remaineth Now in This Time of Sicknesse (1636).

The Disease of the House: Or, the State Mountebanck: Administering Physick to a Sick Parliament (1649).

Flagellum Dei: Or a Collection of the Several Fires, Plagues, and Pestilential Diseases That Have Hapned in London Especially, and Other Parts of This Nation, from the Norman Conquest to This present, 1668 (1668).

The Honestie of This Age (1615).

The King's Medicines for the Plague. Prescribed in the Year 1604 by the Whole Collodge of Physitians, Both Spiritual and Temporal (1665).

Londoners Their Entertainment in the Countrie. Or the Whipping of Runnawayes. Wherein Is Described, Londons Miserie, the Countries Crueltie, and Mans Inhumantie (1604).

Londons Lord Have Mercy Upon Us (1665).

Orders Thought Meet by His Majestie, and His Privie Councell, to Be Executed Throughout the Counties of This Realme (1625).

The Parliament Mended or Ended; or, a Philter and Halter for the Two Houses. Prescribed by Their Doctor Mercurius Elenticus (1648).

The Poor Whore's Lamentation, or, the Fleet-Street Crack's Complaint for Want of Trading to the Tune of the Guinea Wins Her (1685).

The Red Crosse: Or, Englands Lord Haue Mercy Upon Us (1625).

A Representation of the State of the Societies for Reformation of Manners, Humbly *Offered to his Majesty* (1715).

The Sad State of the Kingdom, Being an Account of the First Years Charge of Our Reformation (no date given).

P. Aretine, *Strange &Amp; True Nevves from Jack-a-Newberries Six Windmills, or, the Crafty, Impudent, Common-Whore (Turned Bawd) Anatomised and Discovered in the Unparralleld Practises of Mris Fotheringham ... With Five and Twenty Orders Agreeed Upon by Consent of Mris Creswell, Betty Lawrence ... With Divers Others for Establishing Thereof / Published by Way of Admonition to All Persons to Beware of That House of Darkness* (1660).

W. Bridge, *The Diseases That Make a Stoppage to Englands Mercies Discovered, and Attended with Their Remedies* (1642).

———, *Two Sermons: I. The Diseases That Make a Stoppage to Englands Mercies Discovered, and Attended with Their Remedies Ii. A Preparation for Suffering in These Plundering Times* (1642).

275

G. Burnet, *The Plague at Westminster. Or, an Order for the Visitation of a Sick Parliament, Grievously Troubled with a New Disease, Called the Consumption of Their Members* (1609).

H.C. *Londons Vacation, and the Countries Tearme* (1637).

E. Chamberlayne, *Angliae Notitia, or the Present State of England* (1682).

R. Dingley, *Proposals for Establishing a Public Place of Reception for Penitent Prostitutes* (1758).

R. Greene, *A Disputation between a He-Cony--Catcher and a She-Cony--Catcher* (1592).

W.L., *A Medicine for Malignancy: Or, Parliament Pill, Serving to Purge out the Malignant Humours of Men Dis-Affected to the Republick* (1644).

W. Muggins, *Londons Mourning Garment, or Funerall Teares Worne and Shed for the Death of Her Wealthy Cittizens, and Other Her Inhabitants. To Which Is Added, a Zealous and Feruent Prayer, with a True Relation How Many Haue Dyed of All Diseases, in Euery Particuler Parish within London, the Liberties, and out Parishes Neere Adioyning from the 14 of Iuly 1603. To the 17 of Nouember. Following* (1603).

A. von Nettesheim and H. Cornelius, *The Vanity of Arts and Sciences by Henry Cornelius Agrippa, Knight* (1676).

Osiander. *How and whither a Chrysten man ought to flye the horryble plague of the pestilence A sermon out of the Psalme. Qui habitat in adiutorio altissimi. Translated out of hie Almaine into Englishe* (1563).

E. Pool, *A Vision: Wherein Is Manifested the Disease and Cure of the Kingdome* (1648).

Royal College of Physicians of London. *Certain Necessary Directions, Aswell for the Cure of the Plague as for Preuenting the Infection; with Many Easie Medicines of Small Charge, Very Profitable to His Maiesties Subiects / Set Downe by the Colledge of Physicians by the Kings Maiesties Speciall Command ; with Sundry Orders Thought Meet by His Maiestie, and His Priuie Councell, to Be Carefully Executed for Preuention of the Plague ; Also Certaine Select Statutes Commanded by His Maiestie to Be Put in Execution by All Iustices, and Other Officers of the Peace Throughout the Realme ; Together with His Maiesties Proclamation for Further Direction Therein, and a Decree in Starre-Chamber, Concerning Buildings and in-Mates* (1636).

J. Spademan, *A Sermon Preach'd November 14, 1698 and Now Publish'd at the Request of the Societies for Reformation of Manners* (1699).

W. Stampe, *A Treatise of Spiritual Infatuation, Being the Resent Visible Disease of the English Nation. Delivered in Severall Sermons* (1650).

J. Taylor, "A Bawd, a Vertuous Bawd, a Modest Bawd: As She Deserves, Reprove or Else Applaud" (1630).

J. Taylor, *Rare Physick for the Church Sick of an Ague with the Names of Every Particular Disease, and the Manner How She Contracted Them, and by What Means, as Also Prescripts to Remedy the Same. Humbly Commended to the Parliament, Those Admirable Physicians of the Church and State* (1642).

J. Tichborne, *A Triple Antidote against Certaine Very Common Scandals of This Time, Which, Like Infections and Epidemicall Diseases, Have Generally Annoyed Most Sorts of People Amongst Us, Poisoned Also Not a Few, and Divers Waies Plagued and Afflicted the Whole State* (1609).

D. Williams, *A Sermon Preach'd at Salter's Hall to the Societies for the Reformation of Manners* (1699).

Scientific and Medical Treatises

An advertisement at the blew ball in Great Knight-Rider-Street, by Doctors Commons *Back-gate liveth a physician which hath a pill far beyond any medicament yet ever known, or at least published; which cureth those diseases so many pretend to, and so few do understand, called, the French Pox and gonorrhea...*(1675)

An Advertisement from the Society of Chymical Physitians Touching Medicines...For the Prevention, and the Cure of the Plague (1665).

The Character of a Quack Doctor, or, the Abusive Practices of Impudent Illiterate Pretenders to Physick Exposed (1676).

Concerning the Constitution of an Aire Infected. And How to Know Plague-Sores from Carbuncles (1644).

The English Midwife Enlarged, Containing Directions to Midwives; Wherein Is Laid Down Whatever Is Most Requisite for the Safe Practising Her Art (1682).

Every Woman Her Own Midwife (1675).

The Honestie of This Age (1615).

Levinus Lemnius, the Secret Miracles of Nature in Four Books: Learnedly and Moderately Treating of Generation, and the Parts Thereof, the Soul, and Its Immortality, of Plants and Living Creatures, of Diseases, Their Symptoms and Cures, and Many Other Rarities... (1658).

Medicina Flagellata or The Doctor Scarify'd (1721).

A Method of Curing the French Pox (1690).

The Plague's Approved Physitian, Shewing the Naturall Causes of the Infection of the Ayre, and of the Plague. With Divers Observations to Bee Used, Preserving from the Plague, and Signes to Know the Infected Therewith. Also Many True and Approved Medicines for the Perfect Cure Thereof. Chiefely, a Godly and Penitent Prayer Unto Almighty God, for Our Preservation, and Deliverance Therefrom (1665).

The Practical Scheme for the Secret Disease (1728).

The Shutting up Infected Houses as It Is Practised in England Soberly Debated by Way of Address from the Poor Souls That Are Visited, to Their Brethren That Are Free. With Observations on the Wayes Whereby the Present Infection Hath Spread. As Also a Certain Method of Diet, Attendance, Lodging and Physick, Experimented in the Recovery of Many Sick Persons (1665).

Some Reasons of a Member of the Committee, Etc. Of the Trustees of the Infirmary in James Street Westminister, near St. James Park, for His Dividing against the Admission of Venereal Patients (1738).

The Tomb of Venus (1710).

The Treasurie of Commodious Conceits, and Hidden Secretes, Commonlie Called the Good Huswives Closet of Provision, for the Health of Her Houshold... (1591).

The Treasurie of Hidden Secrets (1627).

A Treatise Concerning the Plague and Pox (1652).

Voice to the City, or, a Loud Cry from Heaven to London, Setting before Her Her Sins, Her Sickness, Her Remedies (1665).

The Woman's Counsellor; or the Feminine Physitian. Translated by A. Massaria (1657).

J. Archer, *Every Man His Own Doctor, Compleated with an Herbal Shewing, First, How Every One May Know His Own Constitution and Complexion by Certain Signs : Also, the Nature and Faculties of All Food ...* (1673).

———, *Secrets Disclosed, or, a Treatise of Consumptions; Their Various Causes and Cure* (1693).

J. Astruc, *A Treatise of Venereal Diseases, in Nine Books.* Translated by William Barrowby (1754).

W. Austin, *Epiloimia Epe, or, the Anatomy of the Pestilence a Poem in Three Parts : Describing the Deplorable Condition of the City of London under Its Merciless Dominion, 1665 : What the Plague Is, Together with the Causes of It : As Also, the Prognosticks and Most Effectual Means of Safety, Both Preservative and Curative* (1666).

R. Bannister, *A Treatise of One Hundred and Thirteene Diseases of the Eye* (1622).

F. Bacon, *The Advancement of Learning* G.W. Kitchin (ed.), (London: Everyman, 1965).

R. Barker, *Consilium Anti-Pestilentiale: Or, Seasonable Advice, Concerning Sure, Safe, Specifick, and Experimented Medicines, Both for the Preservation from, and Cure of This Present Plague* (1665).

P. Barrough, "The Sixth Booke Containing the Cure of the Disease Called Morbus Gallicus," in *The Methode of Physicke* (1596).

C. Bartholin, *De Studio Medici* (1628).

J. Bellers, *An Essay Towards the Improvement of Physick* (1714).

N. Biggs, *Mataeo Technia Medicinae Paxeos or Vanity of the Craft of Physick* (1651).

A. Boorde, Andrew, *Brievyary of Helthe: For All Manor of Sycknesses and Diseases* (1547).

S. Bradwell, *A Watch-Man for the Pest Teaching the True Rules of Preservation from the Pestilent Contagion, at This Time Fearefully over-Flowing This Famous Cittie of London. Collected out of the Best Authors, Mixed with Auncient Experience, and Moulded into a New and Most Plaine Method* (1625).

T. Brooks, *A Heavenly Cordial for All Those Servants of the Lord That Have Had the Plague ... , or, Thirteen Divine Maximes, or Conclusions, in Respect of the Pestilence* (1666).

T. Browne, *Religio Medici* (1642).

G. Bruele, *Praxis Medicinae; or, the Physicians Practice* (1639).

T. Brugis, *The Marrow of Physicke. Or, a Learned Discourse of the Severall Parts of Mans Body* (1640).

———, *Vade Mecum; or, a Companion for a Chyrurgion* (1652).

W. Bullein, *A Dialogue against the Fever Pestilence* (1564).

R. Bunworth, *The Doctresse: A Plain and Easie Method of Curing Those Diseases Which Are Peculiar to Women* (1656).

———, *A New Discovery of the French Disease and Running of the Reins Their Causes, Signs, with Plain and Easie Direction of Perfect Curing the Same* (1662).

R. Burton, *The Anatomy of Melancholy, What It Is: With All the Kinds, Causes, Symptomes, Prognostickes, and Several Cures of It. In Three Maine Partitions with Their Several Sections, Members, and Subsections. Philosophically, Historically, Opened and Cut Up* (1621).

T.C., I.D., M.S., and T.B. *The Complear Midwifes Practice* (1656).

J. Cam, *A Rational and Useful Account of the Venereal Disease: With Observations on the Nature, Symptoms, and Cure, and the Bad Consequences That Attend by Ill Management* (1740).

B.a Castro, *Flagellum Calumniantium* (Amsterdam, 1631).

279

H. Clapham, *An Epistle Discoursing Upon the Present Pestilence* (1603).

W. Clowes, *A Briefe and Necessarie Treatise, Touching the Cure of the Disease Called Morbus Gallicus, or Lues Venerea, by Vnctions and Other Approoued Waies of Curing: Newlie Corrected and Augmented by William Clowes of London* (1585).

———, *A Profitable and Necessarie Booke of Observations* (1596).

———, *A Short and Profitable Treatise Touching the Cure of the Disease Called (Morbus Gallicus) by Unctions* (1579).

T. Cock, *Advice for the Poor by Way of Cure and Caution* (1665).

L. Coelson, *The Poor-Mans Physician and Chyrurgion* (1656).

T. Cogan, *The Haven of Health Chiefly Gathered for the Comfort of Students, and Consequently of All Those That Have a Care of Their Health, Amplified Upon Five Words of Hippocrates, Written Epid. 6. Labour, Cibus, Potio, Somnus, Venus. Hereunto Is Added a Preservation from the Pestilence, with a Short Censure of the Late Sicknes at Oxford* (1636).

W. Cole, *A Physico-Medical Essay Concerning the Late Frequency of Apoplexies Together with a General Method of Their Prevention and Cure : In a Letter to a Physician* (1689).

J. Cotta, *A Short Discouerie of Seuerall Sorts of Ignorant and Vnconsiderate Practisers of Physicke in England with Direction for the Safest Election of a Physition in Necessitie* (1619).

N. Culpeper, *Compleat Method of Physick, Whereby a Man May Preserve His Body in Health; or Cure Himself, Being Sick, for Three Pence Charge, with Such Things Only as Grow in England, They Being Most Fit for English Bodies* (1652).

———, *Culpeper's School of Physick* (1659).

———, *A Directory for Midwives: Or a Guide for Women. In Their Conception, Bearing and Suckling Children* (1651).

———, *The English Physitian: Or an Astrologo-Physical Discourse of the Vulgar Herbs of This Nation* (1652).

———, *Pharmacopoeia* (1649).

———, *Physical Receipts; or, the New English Physician* (1690).

N. Culpeper, D. Sennert, and A. Cole, *Two Treatises. The First of the Venereal Pocks. The Second Treatise of the Gout* (1660).

C.D., *Some Reasons, of the Present Decay of the Practise of Physick in Learned and Approved Doctors* (1675).

T. Dawson, *The Good Housewife's Jewel* (1596).

J. Dryander, *Artzenei Speigel* (Frankfurt am Main, 1547).

J. Earle, *Microcosmographie, or a Piece of the Worlds Discovered in Essays and Characters* (1529).

Edwards, *A Treatise Concerning the Plague and the Pox Discovering as Well the Meanes How to Preserve from the Danger of These Infectious Contagions, as Also How to Cure Those Which Are Infected with Either of Them* (1652).

T. Elyot, *The Castle of Helth* (1541).

A.O. Faber, *Alberti Ottonis Fabri Medici Regii Exer. Suec. Paradoxon De Morbo Gallico Libr. Ii, or, a Paradox Concerning the Shameful Disease for a Warning to All against Deceitful Cures / Translated out of the High-Dutch by Johan Kauffman* (1662).

J. Ferrand, *Erotomania or a Treatise Discoursing of the Essence, Causes, Symptomes, Prognosticks, and Cure of Love, or Erotique Melancholy* (1640).

L. Fioravanti, *A Short Discourse of the Excellent Doctor*...Translated by John Hester (1580).

R. Fletcher, *A Character of a True Physician, or, a True Chymist Compared with a Goose-Quill Pedant with a Short View of the Frauds and Abuses in Physick, Committed by the Confederate Prescribing Doctoral Methodists, with Their Combinators the Apothecaries ... : Being a Vindication of Such Physicians as Follow Not Their Method but Make and Administer Their Own Medicines, Being the Honestest, Safest, Cheapest, and Speediest Way of Practice, Both for Physician and Patient* (1676).

G. Fracastoro, *Syphilis Sive Morbus Gallicus.* Translated by Nahum Tate (1686).

L. Fuchs, A worthy practise of the moste learned phisition Maister Leonerd Fuchsius, Doctor in phisicke, moste necessary in this needfull tyme of our visitation, for the comforte of all good and faythfull people, both olde and yonge, bothe for the sicke and for them that woulde auoyde the daunger of the contagion, Printed at London : By Rouland Hall, for Michell Lobley in Poules Churchyeard at the corner shop on the right hand as ye come oute of Chepe (1563).

L. Gatford, *Logos Alexipharmakos, or, Hyperphysicall Directions in Time of Plague. Collected out of the Sole-Authentick Dispensatory of the Chief Physitian Both of Soule and Body, and Disposed More Particularly (Though Not without Some Alteration and Addition) According to the Method of Those Physicall Directions Printed by Command of the Lords of the Councell at Oxford 1644. And Very Requisite to Be Used with Them. Also, Certain Aphorismes, Premised, and Conclusions from Them Deduced, Concerning the Plague, Necessary to Be Knovvn and Observed of All, That Would Either Prevent It, or Get It Cured* (1644).

281

E. Gayton, *The Religion of a Physician: Or, Divine Meditations* (1663).

W.J. Gent, *A Collection of Seven and Fifty Approved Receipts Good against the Plague. Taken out of the Five Books of That Renowned Dr. Don Alexes Secrets, for the Benefit of the Poorer Sort of People of These Nations* (1665).

F. Glisson, G. Bate, and A. Regemorter, *A Treatise of the Rickets Being a Disease Common to Children* (1650).

J. Goddard, *Discourse on the Unhappy Condition of the Practice of Physic in London. And Offering Some Means to Put It into a Better; for the Interest of Patients, No Less, or Rather More, Than of Physicians* (1670).

J. Godskall, *The King's Medicine for This Present Yeere 1604* (1604).

J. Goeurot, *The Regiment of Life*. Translated by T. Phayer (1544).

Graunt, John. *Natural and Political Observations Made Upon the Bills of Mortality.* Edited by Walter Willcox (Baltimore: Johns Hopkins University Press, 1939).

Grey, Elizabeth. *A Choice Manual of Rare Secrets* (1653).

Guillemeau, J. *Childbirth* (1635).

J. Harris, *The Divine Physician, Prescribing Rules for the Prevention, and Cure of Most Diseases, as Well of the Body, as the Soul Demonstrating by Natural Reason, and Also Divine and Humane Testimony, That, as Vicious and Irregular Actions and Affections Prove Often Occasions of Most Bodily Diseases, and Shortness of Life, So the Contrary Do Conduce to the Preservation of Health, and Prolongation of Life : In Two Parts* (1676).

J. Hart, *The Anatomie of Urines* (1625).

———, *The Arraignment of Urines* (1623).

G. Harvey, *Great Venus: A New Method of Curing the French-Pox* (Amsterdam, 1690).

———, *Great Venus Unmasked, or, a More Exact Discovery of the Venereal Evil, or French Disease Comprizing the Opinions of Most Antient and Modern Physicians with the Particular Sentiment of the Author Touching the Rise, Nature, Subject, Causes, Kinds, Progress, Changes, Signs, and Prognosticks of the Said Evil : Together with Luculent Problems, Pregnant Observations, and the Most Practical Cures of That Disease, and Virulent Gonorrhoea, or Running of the Reins* (1672).

———, *Little Venus Unmask'd; or, a Perfect Discovery of the French Pox* (1670).

S. Haworth, *Anthropologia, or, a Philosophic Discourse Concernng Man Being the Anatomy of Both His Soul and Body: Wherein the Natue, Origin, Union, Immateriality, Immortality, Extension, and Faculties of the One and Parts, Tem-*

perament, Complexions, Functions, Sexes, and Ages Respecting the Other Are Concisely Delineated (1680).

P. Hermanni, *An Excellent Treatise Teaching Howe to Cure the French-Pockes.* Translated by Iohn Hester (1590).

F. Herring, *Certaine Rules, Directions, or Aduertisments for This Time of Pestilentiall Contagion* (1625).

N. Hodges, *Loimologia* (1720).

C. Hueber, *A Riche Storehouse or Treasurie, for the Sicke* (1578).

U. von Hutten, *De Morbo Gallico. A Treatise of the French Disease, Publish'd above 200 Years Past* (1730).

D. Irish, *Levamen Infirmi: Or, Cordial Counsel to the Sick and Diseased Containing I. Advice Concerning Physick, and What a Physician Ought to Be; with an Account of the Author's Remedies, and How to Take Them. Ii. Concerning Melancholy, Frensie, and Madness; in Which, Amongst Other Things, Is Shew'd, How Far They Differ from a Conscience Opprest with the Sense of Sin, and Likewise How They Differ among Themselves. Iii. A Miscellany of Pious Discourses, Concerning the Attributes of God; with Ejaculations and Prayers, According to Scripture Rule. Likewise an Account of Many Things Which Have Happen'd since the Creation. To Which Are Added Several Predictions of What May Happen to the End of the World. The Whole Being Enrich'd with Physical, Pious, Moral & Historical Observations, Delightful to Read, & Necessary to Know* (1700).

R.D. de Isla, *Treatise on the Serpentine Malady* (1539).

R. Johnson, *Enchiridion Medicum, or, a Manual of Physick Being a Compendium of the Whole Art, in Three Parts ... : Wherein Is Briefly Shewed 1. The Names, 2. The Derivation, 3. The Causes, 4. The Signs, 5. The Prognosticks, and 6. A Rational Method of Cure* (1684).

J. Jonas, *The Arte and Science of Preserving Bodie and Soule in Healthe, Wisdome, and Catholike Religion: Physically, Philosophically, and Divinely Devised by John Jonas, Physitian* (1579).

L. Joubert, *Populaar Errours.* Translated by G.D. de Rocher (Tuscaloosa: University of Alabama Press, 1989).

L. Lessius, *Hygiasticon: Or, the Right Course of Preserving Life and Health Unto Extream Old Age* (Cambridge, 1634).

P. Levens, *A Right Profitable Booke for All Diseases* (1582).

———, *A Right Profitable Boole for All Diseases Called, the Path-Way to Health* (1632).

P. Lowe, *An Easie, Certaine, and Perfect Method, to Cure and Preuent the Spanish*

Sicknes Wherby the Learned and Skilfull Chirurgian May Heale a Great Many Other Diseases (1596).

W.M. *The Queens Closet Opened. Incomparable Secrets in Physick, Chirurgery, Preserving, Candying, and Cookery* (1655).

J. Marten, *A Treatise of All the Degrees and Symptoms of the Venereal Diseases, in Both Sexes.* London (1708).

F. Mauriceau, *The Accomplisht Midwife, Treating of the Diseases of Women with Child, and in Child-Bed* (1673).

E. Maynwaringe, *The History and Mystery of the Venereal Lues Concisely Abstracted and Modelled (Occasionally) from Serious Strict Perpensions, and Critical Collations of Divers Repugning Sentiments and Contrary Assertions of Eminent Physicians: English, French, German, Dutch, Spanish, and Italian Dissenting Writers. Convincing by Argument and Proof the Traditional Notions Touching This Grand Evil, and Common Reputed Practice Grounded Thereon, as Erroneous and Unfound. Solving the Most Dubious and Important Quaeries Concerning the Abstruse Nature, Difficult and Deceitful Cures of This Popular Malady. With Animadversions Upon Various Methods of Cure, Practised in Those Several Nations* (1673).

------, *Medicus Absolutus. The Compleat Physitian* (1668).

S. Mercurio, *De Gli Errori [Popolari D'italia]* (Venice, 1603).

F. Moryson, *An Itinerary* (1617).

M. Nedham, *Medela Medicinae* (1665).

T. Needham, *A Treatise of a Venereal Consumption and the Venereal Disease: The Signs or Symptoms of the Venereal Infection with Various Methods of Cure* (1700).

I.F. Nicholson, *The Modern Syphilis: Or, the True Method of Curing Every Stage and Symptom of the Venereal Disease* (1718).

J. Oberndoerffer, *The Anatomies of the True Physician and Counterfeit Mountebank.* Translated by Francis Herring (1602).

Pechey, Physitian in the countrey (probably Dr. John Pechey.) *Some Observations Made Upon the Maldiva Nut Shewing Its Admirable Virtue in Giving an Easie, Safe, and Speedy Delivery to Women in Child-Bed/ Written by a Physitian in the Countrey to Dr. Hinton at London, 1663* (1694).

J. Pechy, *The Store-House of Physical Practice* (1695).

C. Peter, *A Description of the Venereal Disease: Declaring the Causes, Signs, and Effects, and Cure Thereof. With a Discourse of the Most Wonderful Antivenereal Pill* (1678).

————, *Observations on the Venereal Disease, with the True Way of Curing the Same* (1686).

J. Primrose, *Popular Errours. Or the Errours of the People in Physick*. Translated by R. Wittie (1651).

M.R. *The Meanes of Preventing, and Preserving from, and Curing of That Most Contagious Disease, Called the Plague* (1665).

A. Read, *The Manuall of the Anatomy or Dissection of the Body of Man Containing the Enumeration, and Description of the Parts of the Same, Which Usually Are Shewed in the Publike Anatomicall Exercises. Enlarged and More Methodically Digested into 6. Books* (1638).

L. Riviere, *The Practice of Physick*. Translated by N. Culpeper, A. Cole and W. Rowland (1655).

N. Robinson, *A Treatise of the Venereal Disease* (1736).

E. Rudio, *De Morbus Occultis Et Venenatis* (Venice, 1604).

J.S., *Children's Diseases, Both Outward and Inward* (1664).

————, *A Short Compendium of Chirurgery Containing Its Grounds & Principles : More Particularly Treating of Imposthumes, Wounds, Ulcers, Fractures & Dislocations : Also a Discourse of the Generation and Birth of Man, Very Necessary to Be Understood by All Midwives and Child-Bearing Women : With the Several Methods of Curing the French Pox, the Cure of Baldness, Inflammation of the Eyes, and Toothach, and an Account of Blood-Letting, Cup-Setting, and Blooding with Leeches* (1678).

L.S., Doctor of Physic. *Prothylantinon, or, Some Considerations of a Notable Expedient to Root out the French Pox from the English Nation with Excellent Defensive Remedies to Preserve Mankind from the Infection of Pocky Women : Also an Advertisement, Wherein Is Discover'd the Dangerous Practices of Ignorant Pretenders to the Cure of the Disease* (1673).

W. Salmon, *The Family-Dictionary, or, Household Companion* (1696).

————, *Iatrica, Seu, Praxis Medendi, the Practice of Curing Being a Medicinal History of above Three Thousand Famous Observations in the Cure of Diseases* (1681).

————, *Pharmacopoeia Londinensis, or, the New London Dispensatory in Vi Books : Translated into English for the Publick Good...As Also, the Praxis of Chymistry, as Its Now Exercised Fitted to the Meanest Capacity* (1682).

————, *Select Physical and Chyrurgical Observations* (1687).

J. Securis, *A Detection and Querimonie of the Daily Enormities Comitted in Physick* (1566).

D. Sennertus, *Practical Physick, or, Five Distinct Treatises of the Most Predominant Diseases of These Times the First of the Scurvy, the Second of the Dropsie, the Third of Feavers and Agues of All Sort, the Fourth of the French Pox, and the Fifth of the Gout, Wherein the Nature, Causes, Symptomes, Various Methods of Cure, and Waies of Preventing Every of the Said Diseases, Are Severally Handled, and Plainly Discovered to the Meanest Capacity* (1676).

J. Sharp, *The Midwives Book* (1671).

W. Simpson, *Zenexton Ante-Pestilentiale. Or, a Short Discourse of the Plague* (1665).

W. Smellie, *A Treatise on the Theory and Practice of Midwifery* Vol. 3 (1779).

L. Sowerby, *The Ladies Dispensatory Containing the Natures, Vertues and Qualities of All Herbs and Simples Usefull in Physick* (1651).

M. Stephens, *The Domestic Midwife* (1795).

T. Sydenham, *The Entire Works of Dr. Thomas Sydenham.* Translated by John Swan. London: R. Cave (1763).

A.T., practitioner in physicke, *A Rich Store-House* Vol. Fol. 65 (1596).

J. Tanner, *The Hidden Treasures of the Art of Physicke: Fully Discovered in Four Books* (1658).

T. Thayre, *An Excellent and Best Approoued Treatise of the Plague Containing, the Nature, Signes, and Accidents of the Same. With the Certaine and Absolute Cure of the Feuers, Botches, and Carbuncles, That Raigne in These Times; and Aboue All Things, Most Singular Experiments in the Same: Gathered by the Obseruations of Diuers Worthy Travilers, and Selected out of the Best Learned Physitions in This Age. Likewise Is Taught, the True and Perfect Cure of the Plague, with Secret and Vnknowne Preseruatiues against All Infection; and How So Withstand the Most Dangerous Accidents, Which May Happen This Fearefull Contagious Time. Generall Rules of Life to Be Obserued by All Men This Plague Time. Directions for the Commons, Country-Men and Strangers That Be Necessitated to Come into the City* (1625).

G. Thomson, *Loimologia* (1665).

T. Tryon, *The Good House-Wife Made a Doctor* (1692).

———, *Healths Grand Preservative: Or the Womens Best Doctor* (1682).

———, *A Pocket-Companion; Containing Things Necessary to Be Known, by All That Values Their Health and Happiness: Being a Plain Way of Nature's Own Prescribing, to Cure Most Diseases in Men, Women and Children, by Kitchen-Physick Only* (1694).

P.P. Valentinus, *Enchiridion Medicum: Containing an Epitome of the Whole Course of Physic* (1608).

W. Vaughan, *Directions for Health* (1617).

T. Venner, *A Plaine Philosophicall Demonstration Of...The Preservation of Health* (1628).

J. de Vigo, *The Whole Worke of That Famous Chirurgion Maister Iohn Vigo.* Translated by B. Traheron (1586).

J. Wesley, *Primitive Physick: Or, an Essay and Natural Method of Curing Most Diseases* (1747).

T. Wharton, *Directions for the Prevention and Cure of the Plague* (1665).

T. Whitaker, *An Elenchus of Opinions Concerning the Cure of the Small Pox Together with Problematicall Questions Concerning the Cure of the French Pest* (1661).

R. Williams, *Physical Rarities* (1652).

T. Willis, *A Help for the Poor Who Are Visited with the Plague: To Be Communicated to Them by the Rich* (1666).

————, *A Plain and Easie Method for Preserving (by God's Blessing) Those That Are Well from the Infection of the Plague, or Any Contagious Distemper in City, Camp, Fleet, &C. And for Curing Such as Are Infected with It : Written in the Year 1666 / by Tho. Willis ... ; with a Poem on the Virtue of a Laurel Leaf for Curing of a Rheumatism* (1691).

P. Willughby, *Observations in Midwifery* (1660's (exact year not known)).

C. Wirtzung, *The General Practise of Physicke* (1605).

R. Wiseman, *Severall Chirurgicall Treatises* (1676).

R. Wittie, *Popular Errours. Or the Errours of the People in Physick* (1651).

O. Wood, *An Alphabetical Book of Physicall Secrets* (1639).

H. Woolley, *The Gentlewomans Companion* (1675).

C. Wirtzung, *The General Practise of Physicke* (1605).

J. Wynell, MD, *Lues Venera, or a perfect cure for the French pox* (1660).

————, *Lues Venera Wherein the Names, Nature, Subject, Causes, Signes, and Cure, Are Handled, Mistakes in These Discovered, Rectified, Doubts and Questions Succinctly Resolved* (1660).

J. Young, *Medicaster Medicatus, or a Remedy for the Itch of Scribling* (1685).

R. Younge, *The Prevention of Poverty, Together with the Cure of Melancholy, Alias Discontent. Or the Best and Surest Way to Wealth and Happiness Being Subjects Very Seasonable for These Times; Wherein All Are Poor, or Not Pleased, or Both; When They Need Be Neither* (1682).

II
Secondary Sources

J.C. Adams, *Shakespeare's Physic, Lore and Love* (Upton-upon-severn: SPA Limited, 1989).

M.W. Adler, 'The Terrible Peril: A Historical Perspective on the Venereal Diseases,' *British Medical Journal* 19 (July 1980), 206-211.

P.L. Allen, *The Wages of Sin: Sex and Disease, Past and Present* (Chicago: University of Chicago Press, 2000).

D. Amundsen, *Medicine, Society, and Faith in the Ancient and Medieval Worlds* (Baltimore: Johns Hopkins University Press, 1996).

D. Amundsen, and R.L. Numbers (eds), *Caring and Curing: Health and Medicine in the Western Religious Traditions* (New York: Macmillan, 1986).

D. Andrew, *Philanthropy and Police* (Princeton, NJ: Princeton University Press, 1989).

R. Anselment, *The Realms of Apollo: Literature and Healing in Seventeenth-Century England* (Newark: University of Delaware Press, 1995).

———, 'Seventeenth-Century Pox: The Medical and Literary Realities of Venereal Disease,' *Seventeenth Century [Great Britain]* 4, no. 2 (1989), 189-211.

A. Appleby, 'The Disappearance of Plague: A Continuing Puzzle,' *Economic History Review* (May 1980), 169-73.

A. Appleby, 'Famine, Mortality, and Epidemic Disease: A Comment,' *Economic History Review* 30 (1977), 508-12.

J. Arrizabalaga, *Facing the Black Death: Perceptions and Reactions of University Medical Practitioners* (1994).

———, 'Syphilis,' in K. Kiple (ed.), *The Cambridge World History of Human Disease* (Cambridge: Cambridge University Press, 1993), 1025-33.

J. Arrizabalaga, J. Henderson, and R. French, *The Great Pox: The French Disease in Renaissance Europe* (New Haven: Yale University Press, 1997).

M. Ashley, *Life in Stuart England* (London: Batsford, 1964).

C. Atkinson, and W. Stoneman, 'These Griping Greefes and Pinching Pangs: Attitudes to Childbirth in Thomas Bentley's the Monument of Matrones (1582),' *Sixteenth Century Journal* 21, no. 2 (1990), 193-203.

J.H. Aveling, *English Midwives: Their History and Prospects* (New York: AMS Press, 1977).

J. Axtell, 'Education and Status in Stuart England: The London Physicians,'

History of Education Quarterly 10, no. 2 (Summer 1970): 141-59.

B. Baker and G. Armelagos, 'The Origin and Antiquity of Syphilis: Paleo-Pathological Diagnosis and Interpretation,' *Current Anthropology* 29, no. 5 (1988), 732-37.

P. Baldwin, *Contagion and the State in Europe, 1830-1930* (Cambridge: Cambridge University Press, 1999).

D. Balhman, *The Moral Revolution of 1688* (New Haven: Yale University Press, 1957).

J. Barry, 'Publicity and the Public Good: Presenting Medicine in Eighteenth-Century Bristol,' in W. Bynum and R. Porter (eds), *Medical Fringe and Medical Orthodoxy, 1750-1850* (London: Croom Helm, 1987), 29-39.

L. Beier, 'In Sickness and in Health: A Seventeenth Century Family's Experience,' in R. Porter (ed.), *Patients and Practitioners: Lay Perceptions of Medicine in Pre-Industrial Society* (Cambridge: Cambridge University Press, 1985), 101-28.

———, *Sufferers and Healers: The Experience of Illness in Seventeenth-Century England* (New York: Routledge, 1987).

O.J. Benedictow, 'Morbidity in Historical Plague Epidemics,' *Population Studies* 41, No. 3 (Nov 1987), 401-431.

J.M. Bennett, 'Feminism and History,' *Gender and History [Great Britain]* 1 (1989), 251-72.

C. Bentley, 'The Rational Physician: Richard Whitlock's Medical Satires,' *Journal of the History of Medicine and Allied Sciences* 29 (1974), 180-95.

R. Berry, *The Shakespearean Metaphor: Studies in Language and Form* (London: Macmillan, 1978).

C. Bicks, 'Midwiving Virility in Early Modern England,' in N. Miller and N. Yavneh (eds), *Maternal Measures: Figuring Caregiving in the Early Modern Period* (Burlington: Ashgate, 2000), 49-64.

T. Birch (ed.), *Robert Boyle, the Works*. Vol. 4 (Hildesheim: George Olms Verlagsbuchhandlung, 1965).

W. Birkin, 'The Royal College of Physicians of London and Its Support of the Parliamentary Cause in the English Civil War,' *The Journal of British Studies* 23, no. 1 (1983), 47-62.

———, 'The Social Problem of the English Physician in the Early Seventeenth Century,' *Medical History* 31 (April 1987), 201-16.

A. Blair and A. Graftton, 'Reassessing Humanism and Science,' *Journal of the History Of Ideas* 53, no. 4 (Oct- Dec 1992), 535-40.

B. Boehrer, 'Early Modern Syphilis,' *Journal of the Hisotory of Sexuality* 1, no.

2 (October 1990), 197-214.

P. Boitani, and A. Torti (eds), *The Body and the Soul in Medieval Literature: The J.A.W. Bennett Memorial Lectures, Tenth Series, Perugia, 1998* (Rochester: D.S. Brewer, 1999).

J. Boulton, and J. Black, '"Those that die by reason of their madness:" Dying Insane in London, 1629-1830,' *History of Psychiatry* 23.1 (March, 2012), 27-39.

M. Braddick, 'The Early Modern State and the Question of Differentiation, from 1550 to 1700,' *Comparative Studies in Society and History* 38, no. 1 (May 1996), 92-111.

R. Braverman, *Plots and Counterplots: Sexual Politics and the Body Politic in English Literature, 1660-1730* (New York: Cambridge University Press, 1993).

J. Brewer, 'Commercialization and Politics,' in N. McKendrick, J. Brewer and J.H. Plumb (eds), *The Birth of a Consumer Society: The Commercialization of Eighteenth-Century England* (Bloomington: Indiana University Press, 1982).

P. Brewster, 'Physician and Surgeon as Depicted in 16th and 17th Century English Literature,' *Osiris* 14 (1962), 13-32.

C. Bridenbaugh, *Vexed and Troubled Englishmen 1590-1642* (London: Oxford University Press, 1976).

S. Brody, *The Disease of the Soul: Leprosy in Medieval Literature* (London: Cornell University Press, 1974).

T. Brown, 'Word Wars: The Debate over the Use of the Vernacular in Medical Writings of the English Renaissance,' *Texas Studies in Literature and Language* 37, no. 1 (Spring 1995), 98-113.

R.C. Burns, 'The Non-Naturals: A Paradox in the Western Concept of Health,' *Journal of Medicine and Philosophy* 3 (1976), 202-11.

S. Burtt, 'The Societies for the Reformation of Manners: Between John Locke and the Devil in Augustan England,' in R. Lund (ed.), *The Margins of Orthodoxy: Heterodox Writing and Cultural Response, 1660-1750* (New York: Cambridge University Press, 1995), 149-68.

W. Bynum, 'Treating the Wages of Sin: Venereal Disease and Specialism in Eighteenth-Century Britain,' in W. Bynum and R. Porter (eds), *Medical Fringe and Medical Orthodoxy, 1750-1850* (London, Croom Helm 1987), 5-28.

B. Capp, *Astrology and the Popular Press* (London: Faber and Faber, 1979).

A. Carmichael, *Plague and the Poor in Renaissance Florence* (Cambridge Cambridge University Press, 1986).

A. Clark, *The Working Life of Women in the Seventeenth Century* (London: Rout-ledge and Paul, 1991).

E. Clarke, 'Whistler and Glisson on Rickets,' *Bull. Hist. Med* 36 (1962), 58.

G. Clark, *History of the Royal College of Physicians of London* (Oxford: Claren-don Press, 1964).

P. Clark, 'The Alehouse and the Alternative Society,' in K. Thomas and D. Pennington (eds), *Puritans and Revolutionaries: Essays Presented to Christo-pher Hill* (Oxford: Oxford University Press, 1978), 47-72.

W. Clemen, *The Development of Shakespeare's Imagery* (London: Methuen, 1987).

J. Coleman, *Medieval Readers and Writers, 1350-1400* (New York: Columbia University Press, 1981).

A. Conway, 'Defoe's Protestant Whore,' *Eighteenth-Century Studies* 35, no. 2 (2002), 215-33.

H. Cook, *The Decline of the Old Medical Regime in Stuart London* (Ithaca: Cor-nell University Press, 1986).

———, 'Good Advice and Little Medicine: The Professional Authority of Early Modern English Physicians,' *The Journal of British Studies* 33, no. 1 (January 1994), 1-31.

———, 'Policing the Health of London: The College of Physicians and the Early Stuart Monarchy,' *Social History of Medicine* 2 (1989), 1-33.

———, *Trials of an Ordinary Doctor: Joannes Groenevelt in Seventeenth-Century London* (Baltimore: Johns Hopkins University Press, 1994).

W.S.C. Copeman, 'Dr. Johnathan Goddard, F.R.S. (1617-1675),' *Notes and Records of the Royal Society of London* 15 (July 1960), 69-77.

S. Covington, *Wounds, Flesh, and Metaphor in Seventeenth-Century England* (New York: Palgrave Macmillan, 2009).

P. Crawford, 'Attitudes to Menstruation in Seventeenth-Century England,' *Past and Present* 91 (1981), 47-73.

———, 'The Construction and Experience of Maternity in Seventeenth-Century England,' in V. Fildes (ed.), *Women as Mothers in Pre-Industrial England. Essays in Memory of Dorothy Mclaren* (London : Routledge, 1990), 3-38.

A. Cunningham, 'Sir Thomas Browne and His *Religio Medici*: Reason, Nature and Religion,' in O.P. Grell and A. Cunningham (eds), *Religio Medici: Medicine and Religion in Seventeenth-Century England* (Aldershot: Scolar Press, 1996), 12-61.

———, 'Thomas Sydenham: Epidemics, Experiment and the "Good Old Cause,"' in R. French and A. Wear (eds), *The Medical Revolution of the Seventeenth Century* (New York: Cambridge University Press, 1989), 164-90.

———, 'Where there are three physicians, there are two atheists,' in O.P. Greall and A. Cunningham (eds), *Medicine and Religion in Enlightenment Europe* (Aldershot: Ashgate, 2007), 1-4.

T.C. Curtis and W.A. Speck, 'The Societies of the Reformation of Manners: A Case Study in the Theory and Practice of Moral Reform,' *Literature and History* 3 (1976), 45-64.

F. Dabhoiwala, 'Sex and Societies for Moral Reform, 1688-1800' *The Journal of British Studies* 46, no. 2 (April 2007), 290-319.

R. Davenport-Hines, *Sex, Death and Punishment: Attitudes toward Sex and Sexuality in Britain since the Renaissance* (London: Collins, 1990).

R. Davidson and L. Hall (eds), *Sex, Sin, and Suffering: Venereal Disease and European Society Since 1870* (London: Routledge, 2001).

F. Dawbarn, 'Patronage and Power: The College of Physicians and the Jacobean Court,' *BJHS* 31 (1998), 1-19.

A. Debus, 'Chemists, Physicians, and Changing Perspectives on the Scientific Revolution,' *Isis* 89 (1998), 66-81.

———, *The English Paracelsians* (London: Oldbourne, 1965).

J. Donnison, *Midwives and Medical Men: A History of Inter-Professional Rivalries and Women's Rights* (London: Heinemann, 1977).

B. Dooley, *The Social History of Skepticism: Experience and Doubt in Early Modern Culture* Vol. 2, *The Johns Hopkins University Studies in Historical and Political Science* (Baltimore: Johns Hopkins University Press, 1999).

M. Douglas, *Purity and Danger: An Analysis of Concepts of Pollution and Taboo* (London: Routledge & Paul, 1966).

E. Duffy, 'Primitive Christianity Revived; Religious Renewal in Augustan England,' in D. Baker (ed.), *Renaissance and Renewal in Christian History* (Oxford: Published for the Ecclesiastical History Society by B. Blackwell, 1977), 287-300.

A. Dyer, 'The Influence of Bubonic Plague in England, 1550-1667,' *Medical History* 22, no. 3 (1978), 308-26.

W. Eamon, *Science and the Secrets of Nature: Books of Secrets in Medieval and Early Modern Culture* (Princeton: Princeton University Press, 1994).

B. Ehrenreich, and D English, *Witches, Midwives, and Nurses: A History of Women Healers* (New York: Feminist Press, 1973).

E. Eisenstein, *The Printing Press as an Agent of Change* Vol. 2 (Cambridge: Cambridge University Press, 1979).

P. Elmer, 'Medicine, Religion and the Puritan Revolution,' in R. French and A. Wear (eds), *The Medical Revolution of the Seventeenth Century* (New York Cambridge University Press, 1989), 10-45.

————, 'Medicine, Science and the Quakers; the "Puritanism-Science" Debate Reconsidered,' *The Journal of the Friends' Historical Society* 54, no. 6 (1981), 265-86.

N. Enssle, 'Patterns of Godly Life: The Ideal Parish Minister in Sixteenth- and Seventeenth-Century English Thought,' *Sixteenth Century Journal* 28 (1997), 3-28.

D. Evenden, 'Gender Differences in the Licensing and Practice of Female and Male Surgeons in Early Modern England,' *Medical History* 42 (1998), 194-216.

J. Fabricius, *Syphilis in Shakespeare's England* (London: Jessica Kingsley Publishers, 1994).

G.B. Ferngren, 'Early Christianity as a Religion of Healing,' *Bulletin of the History of Medicine* 66 (1992), 1-15.

L.A. Ferrell, *Government by Polemic: James I, the King's Preachers, and the Rhetorics of Conformity, 1603-1625* (Stanford: Stanford University Press, 1998).

V. Fildes, *Wet Nursing* (Oxford: Basil Blackwell, 1988).

M. Fissel, 'Charity Universal? Institutions and Moral Reform in Eighteenth-Century Bristol,' in L. Davison, T. Hitchcock, T. Keirn, and R. Shoemaker (eds), *Stilling the Grumbling Hive: The Response to Social and Economic Problems in England, 1689-1750* (New York: St. Martin's Press, 1992), 121-44.

A. Fletcher, *Gender, Sex and Subordination in England, 1550-1800* (New Haven: Yale University Press, 1995).

T. Forbes, *The Midwife and the Witch* (New Haven: Yale University Press, 1966).

R. French, 'The Medical Ethics of Gabriele De Zerbi,' in A. Wear, J. Geyer-Kordesch and R. French (eds), *Doctors and Ethics: The Earlier Historical Setting of Professional Ethics* (Amsterdam: Rodopi, 1993), 72-97.

————, *Medicine Before Science: The Rational and Learned doctor from the Middle Ages to the Enlightenment* (New York: Cambridge University Press, 2003)

R. French and J. Arrizabalaga, 'Coping with the French Disease: University Practitioners' Strategies and Tactics in the Transition from the Fifteenth to the Sixteenth Century,' in R. French, J. Arrizabalaga, A.

Cunningham, and L. Garcia-Ballester (eds), *Medicine from the Black Death to the French Disease* (Aldershot: Ashgate, 1998), 248-87.

C. Gillispie, 'Physick and Philosophy: A Study of the Influence of the College of Physicians of London Upon the Foundation of the Royal Society,' *The Journal of Modern History* 19, no. 3 (September 1947), 210-25.

S. Gilman, *Disease and Representation: Images of Illness from Madness to Aids* (New York: Ithaca, 1988).

S. Gottfried, *The Black Death: Natural and Human Disaster in Medieval Europe* (New York: Collier Macmillan, 1983).

J. Goudsblom, 'Public Health and the Civilizing Process,' *The Milbank Quarterly* 64, no. 2 (1986), 160-88.

L. Gowing, *Common Bodies: Women, Touch, and Power in Seventeenth-Century England* (New Haven: Yale University Press, 2003).

———, *Domestic Dangers: Women, Words, and Sex in Early Modern London* (Oxford: Clarendon Press, 1996).

R. Grassby, 'Social Mobility and Business Enterprise in Seventeenth-Century England,' in D. Pennington (ed.), *Puritans and Revolutionaries* (Oxford: Clarendon Press, 1982), 355-81.

O.P. Grell, 'Caspar Bartholin and the Education of the Pious Physician,' in O,P, Grell and A. Cunningham (eds), *Medicine and the Reformation* (London: Routledge, 1993), 78-100.

———, 'Conflicting Duties: Plague and the Obligations of Early Modern Physicians toward Patients and Commonwealth in England and the Netherlands' in A. Wear, J. Geyer-Kordesch, and R. French (eds), *Doctors and Ethics: The Earlier Historical Setting of Professional Ethics,* Clio Medica 24 (Amsterdam: Rodopi, 1993), 131-52.

———, 'Plague in Elizabethan and Stuart London: The Dutch Response,' *Medical History* 34 (1990), 424-39.

O.P. Grell and A. Cunningham (eds), *Medicine and the Reformation, the Wellcome Institute Series in the History of Medicine* (London: Routledge, 1993).

———, *Religio Medici: Medicine and Religion in Seventeenth-Century England* (Aldershot: Scolar Press, 1996).

S.M. Grieco, 'The Body, Appearance and Sexuality,' in N.Z. Davis and A. Farge (eds), *A History of Women: Renaissance and Enlightenment Paradoxes* (Cambridge, Mass.: Belknap Press, 1993), 46-84.

P. Griffiths, *Lost Londons: Change, Crime and Control in the Capital City, 1550-1660* (New York: Cambridge University Press, 2008).

———, 'The Structure of Prostitution in Elizabethan London,' *Continuity and Change* 8, no. 1 (1993), 39-63.

B.L. Grigsby, *Pestilence in Medieval and Early Modern English Literature* F. Gentry (ed.), *Studies in Medieval History and Culture* (New York: Routledge, 2004).

V. Groebner, *Defaced: The Visual Culture of Violence in the Late Middle Ages* (New York: Zone Books, 2004).

L. Guilhamet, 'Pox and Malice: Some Representations of Venereal Disease in Restoration and Eighteenth-Century Satire,' in Linda Merians (ed.), *The Secret Malady: Venereal Disease in Eighteenth-century Britain and France* (Lexington: University of Kentucky Press, 1996), 196-212.

J.R. Guy, 'The Episcopal Licensing of Physicians, Surgeons, and Midwives,' *Bulletin of the History of Medicine* 56 (1982), 528-42.

B. Hamilton, 'The Medical Professions in the Eighteenth Century,' *The Economic History Review* IV, no. 2 (1951), 141-45.

D. Harley, 'English Archives, Local History, and the Study of Early Modern Midwifery,' *Archives [Great Britain]* 21, no. 92 (1994): 145-54.

———, 'From Providence To Nature: The Moral Theology and Godly Practice of Maternal Breast-Feeding in Stuart England," *Bulletin of the History of Medicine* 69 (1995), 198-223.

———, 'Ignorant Midwives--a Persistent Stereotype,' *Bulletin of the Society for the Social History of Medicine* 28 (1981), 6-9.

———, 'Medical Metaphors in English Moral Theology, 1560-1660,' *Journal of the History of Medicine and Allied Sciences* 48, no. 4 (1993), 396-435.

———, 'Rhetoric and the Social Construction of Sickness and Healing,' *The Society for the Social History of Medicine* (1999), 407-430.

———, 'Spiritual Physic, Providence and English Medicine, 1560-1640,' in O.P. Grell and A. Cunningham (eds), *Medicine and the Reformation* (London: Routledge, 1993), 101-17.

———, 'The Theology of Affliction and the Experience of Sickness in the Godly Family, 1650-1714: The Henrys and the Newcomes,' in O.P. Grell and A. Cunningham (eds), *Religio Medici: Medicine and Religion in Seventeenth-Century England* (Aldershot: Scolar Press, 1996), 273-92.

J.G. Harris, *Foreign Bodies and the Body Politic: Discourses of Social Pathology in Early Modern England* (New York Cambridge University Press, 1998).

J. Hays, *The Burdens of Disease: Epidemics and Human Response in Western History* (New Brunswick, N.J.: Rutgers University Press, 1998).

D. Hayton, 'Moral Reform and Country Politics in the Late Seventeenth-Century House of Commons,' Past and Present 128 (1990), 48-91.

M. Healy, *Fictions of Disease in Early Modern England* (New York: Palgrave, 2001).

J. Hedley, *Power in Verse: Metaphor and Metonymy in the Renaissance Lyric* (University Park: Pennsylvania State University Press, 1988).

T. Henderson, *Disorderly Women in Eighteenth-Century London* (New York: Longman, 1999).

J. Henry, 'The Matter of Souls: Medical Theory and Theology in Seventeenth-Century England,' in R. French and A. Wear (eds), *The Medical Revolution of the Seventeenth Century* (New York: Cambridge University Press, 1989), 87-113.

C. Hill, 'The Medical Profession and Its Radical Critics,' in C. Hill (ed.), *Change and Continuity in Seventeenth-Century England* (London : Weidenfeld and Nicolson, 1974), 157-78.

T. Hitchcock, 'Paupers and Preachers: The SPCK and the Parochial Workhouse Movement,' in L. Davison, T. Hitchcock, T. Keirn, and R. Shoemaker (eds), *Stilling the Grumbling Hive: The Response to Social and Economic Problems in England, 1689-1750* (New York: St. Martin's Press, 1992), 145-166.

M. Hobbs (ed.), *The Sermons of Henry King (1592-1669), Bishop of Chichester* (Cranbury, New Jersey: Associated University Press, 1992).

S. Hull, *Chaste, Silent and Obedient: English Books for Women, 1475-1640* (San Marino: Huntington Library, 1982).

A. Hunt, *Governing Morals: A Social History of Moral Regulation* (Cambridge: Cambridge University Press, 1999).

R. Hutton, *The Restoration: A Political and Religious History of England and Wales 1658-1667* (Oxford: Clarendon Press, 1985).

K. Jackson, 'Bethlem and Bridewell in the "Honest Whore" Plays,' *Studies in English Literature 1500-1900* 43, no. 2 (2003), 395-413.

M. Jenner, 'Quackery and Enthusiasm, or Why Drinking Water Cured the Plague,' in O.P. Grell and A. Cunningham (eds), *Religio Medici: Medicine and Religion in Seventeenth-Century England* (Aldershot: Scolar Press, 1996), 313-340.

L. Jillings, 'The Aggression of the Cured Syphilitic: Ulrich Von Hutten's Projection of His Desease as Metaphor,' *The German Quarterly* 68, no. 1 (1995), 1-18.

R.M. Karras, *Common Women: Prostitution and Sexuality in Medieval England* (New York: Oxford University Press, 1996).

W. Kerwin, 'Where Have You Gone, Margaret Kennix? Seeking the Tradi-

tion of Healing Women in English Renaissance Drama,' In L. Furst
(ed.), *Women Healers and Physicians: Climbing a Long Hill* (Lexington:
University Press of Kentucky, 1997), 93-113.

G. Keynes, (ed.), *The Works of Sir Thomas Browne* 4 vols. (Chicago: University
of Chicago Press, 1964).

D. King-Hele, *Doctor of Revolution: The Life and Genius of Erasmus Darwin*
(London: Faber, 1977).

K. Kiple, (ed.), *The Cambridge World History of Human Disease* (Cambridge:
Cambridge University Press, 1993).

P. Kocher, *Science and Religion in Elizabethan England* (New York: Octogon
Books, 1969).

K. Knight, 'A Precious Medicine: Tradition and Magic in Some Seventeenth-Century Household Remedies,' *Folklore* (London, England) 113,
no. 2 (October 2002), 237-47.

B. Kreps, 'The Paradox of Women: The Legal Position of Early Modern
Wives and Thomas Dekker's "the Honest Whore."' *English Literary History* 69, no. 1 (2002), 83-102.

J. Lane, *The Making of the English Patient* (Stroud: Sutton, 2000).

C. Larner, *Enemies of God: The Witch-Hunt in Scotland* (Baltimore, Md.: Johns
Hopkins University Press, 1981).

R. Latham (ed.), *The Shorter Pepys* (Berkeley: University of California Press,
1985).

S. Lawrence, *Charitable Knowledge: Hospital Pupils and Practitioners in Eighteenth-
Century London* (Cambridge: Cambridge University Press, 1996).

B.F. Leavy, *To Blight with Plague: Studies in a Literary Theme* (New York: New
York University Press, 1992).

R. Lewis and A. McIntosh, *A Descriptive Guide to the Manuscripts of the Prick
of Conscience* (Oxford: Society for the Study of Medieval Languages an
Literatures, 1982).

M. Lindeman, *Medicine and Society in Early Modern Europe* W. Beik and T.C.W.
Blanning (eds), *New Approaches to European History* (Cambridge: Cambridge University Press, 1999).

A.K. Lingo, 'Empirics and Charlatans in Early Modern France: The Genesis
of the Classification of the 'Other' in Medical Practice,' *Journal of Social
History,* Vol. 19, No. 4 (Summer 1986), 583-603.

F. Livingstone, 'On the Origin of Syphilis: An Alternative Hypothesis,' *Current Anthropology* 32, no. 5 (1991), 587-90.

S. Lloyd, '"Pleasure's Golden Bait": Prostitution, Poverty and the Magdalen

Hospital in Eighteenth-Century London,' *History Workshop Journal*, no. 41 (1996), 51-70.

M. MacDonald, *Mystical Bedlam: Madness, Anxiety, and Healing in Seventeenth-Century England* (Cambridge: Cambridge University Press, 1981).

———, 'Psychological Healing in England, 1600-1800,' in W. J. Sheils (ed.), *The Church and Healing* (Oxford: Basil Blackwell, 1982), 101-25.

A. MacFarlane (ed.), *Diary of Ralph Josselin 1616-1683* (London: Oxford University Press, New Series, 1976).

———, *Witchcraft in Tudor and Stuart England* (London: Routledge and Kegan Paul, 1970).

S. MacFarlane, 'Social Policy and the Poor in the Later Seventeenth Century,' in A.L. Beier and R. Finlay (eds), *London 1500-1700: The Making of the Metropolis* (New York: Longman, 1986), 252-77.

A. Mack, (ed.), *In Time of Plague: The History and Social Consequences of Lethal Epidemic Disease* (New York: New School for Social Research, 1988).

H. Marland, *The Art of Midwifery. Early Modern Midwives in Europe* (London: Routledge, 1993).

L. Mayhood, *The Magdalenes: Prostitution in the Nineteenth Century* (London: Routledge, 1990).

D.M. Meads (ed.), *The Diary of Lady Margaret Hoby, 1599-1605* (New York: Houghton Mifflin, 1930).

S. Melzer, and K. Norberg (eds), *From the Royal to the Republican Body: Incorporating the Political in Seventeenth- and Eighteenth-Century France* (Berkeley: University of California Press, 1998).

L. Merians, 'The London Lock Hospital and the Lock Asylum for Women,' in Linda Merians (ed.), *The Secret Malady: Venereal Disease in Eighteenth-century Britain and France* (Lexington: University of Kentucky Press, 1996) 128-148.

R. Merton, 'Science, Technology and Society in Seventeenth-Century England,' *Osiris* IV (1938), 360-632.

H.W. Miller, *Syphilis and Metaphor of Contagion in Early Modern England* (Columbus: Ohio State University, 2000).

N. Moore, *The History of the Study of Medicine in the British Isles* (Oxford: Clarendon Press, 1908).

A.L. Moote and D. Moote. *The Great Plague: The Story of London's Most Deadly Year* (Baltimore, Md.: Johns Hopkins University Press, 2004).

C. Mullett, *The Bubonic Plague and England; an Essay in the History of Preventive Medicine* (Lexington: University of Kentucky Press, 1956).

R. Munger, 'Guaiacum, the Holy Wood from the New World,' *Journal of the History of Medicine* 4 (1949), 196-229.

R. Munkhoff, 'Searchers of the Dead: Authority, Marginality, and the Interpretation of the Plague in England 1574-1665,' *Gender & History* 11.1 (1999), 1-29.

D. Nagy, *Popular Medicine in Seventeenth-Century England,* (Bowling Green: Bowling Green State University Popular Press, 1988).

S. Nash, 'Prostitution and Charity: The Magdalen Hospital, a Case Study,' *Journal of Social History* 17, no. 4 (Summer 1984), 617-28.

M. Nicolson, 'The Metastatic Theory of Pathogenesis and the Professional Interests of the Eighteenth-Century Physician' *Medical History* 32 (1988).

P.H. Niebyl, 'The Non-Naturals,' *Bulletin of the History of Medicine* 454 (1971), 486-92.

W. Notestein, *The English People on the Eve of Colonization 1603-1630* (New York: Harper, 1954).

R. O'Day, *The Professions in Early Modern England, 1450-1800* (New York: Pearson, 2000).

J.D. Oriel, *The Scars of Venus: A History of Venereology* (London: Springer-Verlag, 1994).

R. Palmer, 'The Church, Leprosy and Plague in Medieval and Early Modern Europe,' in W. J. Sheils (ed.), *The Church and Healing* (Oxford: Basil Blackwell, 1982), 79-99.

I. Pantin, 'Fracastoro's De Contagione and Medieval Reflection on "Action at a Distance": Old and New Trends in Renaissance Discourse on the Plague,' in C. Carlin (ed.), *Imagining Contagion in Early Modern Europe* (New York: Palgrave Macmillan, 2005), 3-15.

E. Partridge, *Shakespeare's Bawdy* (London: Routledge, 1956).

M. Pelling, 'Appearance and Reality: Barber-Surgeons, the Body and Disease,' in A.L. Beier and R. Finlay (eds), *London 1500-1700: The Making of the Metropolis* (New York: Longman, 1986), 82-112.

———, *The Common Lot: Sickness, Medical Occupations and the Urban Poor in Early Modern England* (New York: Longman, 1998).

———, 'Compromised by Gender: The Role of the Male Medical Practitioner in Early Modern England,' in H. Marland and M. Pelling (eds), *The Task of Healing: Medicine, Religion and Gender in England and the Netherlands 1450-1800* (Rotterdam: Erasmus Publishing, 1996), 101-34.

———, 'Irregular Practitioners: A Wilderness of Mirrors,' in M. Pelling (ed.), *Medical Conflicts in Early Modern London: Patronage, Physicians, and Irregular Practitioners, 1550-1640* (Oxford: Clarendon Press, 2003).

——, *Medical Conflicts in Early Modern London: Patronage, Physicians, and Irregular Practitioners, 1550-1640* (Oxford: Clarendon Press, 2003).

——, 'Medical Practice in Early Modern England: Trade or Profession?' in W. Prest (ed.), *The Professions in Early Modern England* (London: Croom Helm, 1987), 90-128.

——, 'Medicine and the Environment in Shakespeare's England,' in M. Pelling (ed.), *The Common Lot: Sickness, Medical Occupations and the Urban Poor in Early Modern England* (London: Longman, 1998), 19-37.

——, 'Thoroughly Resented? Older Women and the Medical Role in Early Modern London,' in L. Hunter and S. Hutton (eds), *Women, Science and Medicine 1500-1700* (Gloucestershire: Sutton Publishing, 1997), 63-88.

M. Pelling and C. Webster, 'Medical Practitioners,' in C. Webster (ed.), *Health, Medicine, and Mortality in the Sixteenth Century* (New York: Cambridge University Press, 1979), 165-236.

M.E. Perry, '"Lost Women" In Early Modern Seville: The Politics of Prostitution,' *Feminist Studies* 4, no. 195-214 (Feb. 1978), 195-214.

T. Pollard, '"No Faith in Physic": Masquerades of Medicine Onstage and Off,' in S. Moss and K.Peterson (eds), *Disease, Diagnosis, and Cure on the Early Modern Stage* (Literary and Scientific Cultures of Early Modernity) (Aldeshot: Ashgate, 2004), 29-42.

L. Pollock, 'Childbearing and Female Bonding in Early Modern England,' *Social History* 22, no. 3 (1997), 286-306.

——, 'Embarking on a Rough Passage: The Experience of Pregnancy in Early-Modern Society,' in V. Fildes (ed.), *Women as Mothers in Pre-Industrial England. Essays in Memory of Dorothy Mclaren* (London : Routledge, 1990), 39-67.

——, *With Faith and Physic: The Life of a Tudor Gentlewoman, Lady Grace Mildmay, 1552-1620* (London: Collins and Brown, 1993).

R. Porter, *Bodies Politic: Disease, Death, and Doctors in Britain, 1650-1900* (London: Reaktion Books, 2001).

——, *Disease, Medicine, and Society in England, 1550-1860* (Basingstoke: Macmillan, 1987).

——, *The Greatest Benefit to Mankind* (New York: W.W. Norton & Company, 1997).

————, *Health for Sale: Quackery in England 1660-1850* (Manchester: Manchester University Press, 1989).

————, '"Laying Aside Any Private Advantage": John Marten and Venereal Disease,' in L. Merians (ed.), *The Secret Malady: Venereal Disease in Eighteenth-century Britain and France* (Lexington: University of Kentucky Press, 1996), 51-67.

————, 'The Patient in England, C. 1660- C.1800,' in A. Wear (ed.), *Medicine in Society* (New York: Cambridge University Press, 1992), 91-118.

————, 'The Patient's View: Doing Medical History from Below,' *Theory and Society* 14, no. 2 (1985), 175-98.

————, (ed.), *Patients and Practitioners: Lay Perceptions of Medicine in Pre-Industrial Society* (Cambridge: Cambridge University Press, 1985).

R. Porter and D. Porter, *In Sickness and in Health: The British Experience 1650-1850* (London: Fourth Estate, 1988).

J. Post, 'Famine, Mortality, and Epidemic Disease in the Process of Modernization,' *Economic History Review* 29 (1976), 14-38.

C. Quetel, *History of Syphilis* Translated by J. Braddock and B. Pike (Baltimore: Johns Hopkins University Press, 1990).

W. Radcliffe, *Milestones of Midwifery* (San Francisco: Norman Publishing, 1989).

T. Ranger and P. Slack (eds), *Epidemics and Ideas: Essays on the Historical Perception of Pestilence* (New York: Cambridge University Press, 1992).

L.J. Rather, 'The Six Things "Non-Natural": A Note on the Origins and the Fate of a Doctrine and a Phrase,' *Clio Medica* 3 (1968), 337-47.

J. Redwood, *Reason, Ridicule and Religion* (London: Thames & Hudson, 1976).

G. Risse, 'Medicine in the Age of Enlightenment,' in A. Wear (ed.), *Medicine in Society: Historical Essays* (Cambridge: Cambridge University Press, 1992), 149-195.

R.S. Roberts, 'The Royal College of Physicians of London in the Sixteenth and Seventeenth Centuries,' *History of Science* 5 (1966), 87-100.

J.D. Rolleston, 'Venereal Disease in Literature,' *British Journal of Venereal Diseases* 10 (1934), 147-73.

G.S. Rousseau, 'John Wesley's *Primitive Physic* (1747),' *Harvard Library Bulletin* 16 (1968), 242-56.

H. Sacks, 'Parliament, Liberty, and the Commonweal,' in J.H. Hexter (ed.), *Parliament and Liberty from Queen Elizabeth I to the Civil Wars* (Stanford: Stanford University Press, 1991), 85-121.

W. Schleiner, *The Imagery of John Donne's Sermons* (Providence: Brown University Press, 1970).

———, *Medical Ethics in the Renaissance* (Washington, D.C.: Georgetown University Press, 1995).

———, 'Moral Attitudes toward Syphilis and Its Prevention in the Renaissance,' *Bulletin of the History of Medicine* 68, no. 3 (1994), 389-410.

P. Seaver, *Wallington's World* (Stanford: Stanford University Press, 1985).

S. Shapin, *A Social History of Truth: Civility and Science in Seventeenth-Century England* (Chicago: Chicago University Press, 1994).

S. Shapin and S. Schaffer, *Leviathan and the Air-Pump: Hobbes, Boyle, and the Experimental Life* (Princeton, N.J.: Princeton University Press, 1985).

B. Shapiro, *A Culture of Fact: England, 1550-1720* (Ithaca: Cornell University Press, 2000).

———, 'Law and Science in Seventeenth-Century England,' *Stanford Law Review* 21, no. 4 (April 1969), 727-66.

———, *Probability and Certainty in Seventeenth-Century England: A Study of the Relations between Natural Science, Religion, History, Law, and Literature* (Princeton: Princeton University Press, 1983).

W. Shiels (ed.), *The Church and Healing* (Oxford: Published for the Ecclesiastical History Society by B. Blackwell, 1982).

R. Shoemaker, 'Reforming the City: The Reformation of Manners Campaign in London, 1690-1738,' in L. Davison, T. Hitchcock, T. Keirn, and R. Shoemaker (eds), *Stilling the Grumbling Hive: The Response to Social and Economic Problems in England, 1689-1750* (New York: St. Martin's Press, 1992), 99-120.

E. Shorter, *Women's Bodies: A Social History of Women's Encounter with Health, Ill-Health, and Medicine* (New Brunswick, NJ: Transactions Publications, 1991).

J.F.D. Shrewsbury, *A History of Bubonic Plague in the British Isles* (London: Cambridge University Press, 1970).

R. Shryock, *The Development of Modern Medicine* (Philadelphia: University of Pennsylvania Press, 1936).

K. Siena, 'The Clean and the Foul: Paupers and the Pox in London Hospitals, C. 1550-C.1700,' in K. Siena (ed.), *Sins of the Flesh: Responding to Sexual Disease in Early Modern Europe* (Toronto: Centre for Reformation and Renaissance Studies, 2005), 261-84.

———, 'The "Foul Disease" And Privacy: The Effects of Venereal Disease and Patient Demand on the Medical Marketplace in Early Modern

London,' *Bulletin of the History of Medicine* 75, no. 2 (2001), 199-224.

————, 'Pandora's Pox: The Medical Presentation of Women in Early Modern Venereological Tracts,' Thesis (M.A.)--University Of Rochester, 1993.

————, 'Pollution, Promiscuity, and the Pox: English Venereology and the Early Modern Medical Discourse on Social and Sexual Danger,' *Journal of the History of Sexuality* 8, no. 4 (1998), 553-74.

————, *Venereal Disease, Hospitals and the Urban Poor: London's 'Foul Wards,'* 1600-1800 (Rochester: Rochester Studies in Medical History, University of Rochester Press, 2004).

J. Simmons, 'Publications of 1623,' in *The Library* (1966), 207-22.

N. Sirasi, *Medieval and Early Renaissance Medicine: An Introduction to Knowledge and Practice* (Chicago: University of Chicago Press, 1990).

————, 'Oratory and Rhetoric in Renaissance Medicine,' *Journal of the History of Ideas* 65, 2 (April 2004), 191-211.

H. Skulsky, *Language Recreated: Seventeenth-Century Metaphorists and the Act of Metaphor* (Athens: University of Georgia Press, 1992).

P. Slack, 'Books of Orders: The Making of English Social Policy, 1577-1631,' *Transactions of the Royal Historical Society, 5th Series* 30 (1980), 1-22.

————, 'The Disappearance of Plague: An Alternative View,' *Economic History Review* 34 (1984), 469-76.

————, *From Reformation to Improvement: Public Welfare in Early Modern England* (Oxford: Clarendon Press, 1999).

————, *The Impact of Plague in Tudor and Stuart England* (London: Routledge & K. Paul, 1985).

————, 'Metropolitan Government in Crisis: The Response to Plague,' in A.L. Beier and R. Finlay (eds), *London 1500-1700: The Making of the Metropolis* (New York: Longman, 1986), 60-81.

————, 'Mirrors of Health and Treasures of Poor Men: The Uses of the Vernacular Medical Literature of Tudor England,' in C. Webster (ed.), *Health, Medicine, and Mortality in the Sixteenth Century* (New York: Cambridge University Press, 1979), 237-74.

————, 'The Response to Plague in Early Modern England: Public Policies and their Consequences,' in J. Walter and R. Schofield (eds), Famine, Disease and the Social Order in Early Modern Society (Cambridge: Cambridge University Press, 1989), 167-188.

C.J. Sommerville, *The Secularization of Early Modern England: From Religious*

Culture to Religious Faith (Oxford: Oxford University Press, 1992).

S. Sontag, *Aids and Its Metaphors* (New York: Farrar, Straus, Giroux, 1988).

———, *Illness as Metaphor* (New York: Farrar, Straus, 1977).

B.C. Southgate, '"Forgotten and Lost": Some Reactions to Autonomous Science in the Seventeenth Century,' *Journal of the History Of Ideas* 50, no. 2 (Apr-Jun 1989), 249-68.

W. Spellman, 'Between Death and Judgment: Conflicting Images of the Afterlife in Late Seventeenth-Century English Eulogies,' *The Harvard Theological Review* 87, no. 1 (January 1994), 49-65.

H. Spencer, *The History of British Midwifery from 1650 to 1800* (New York: AMS Press, 1978).

M. Spongburg, *Feminizing Venereal Disease: The Body of the Prostitute in the Nineteenth Century* (London: MacMillan, 1997).

M. Spufford, *Small Books and Pleasant Histories: Popular Fiction and Its Readership in Seventeenth-Century England* (London: Methuen and Company, 1981).

C. Spurgeon, *Shakespeare's Imagery and What It Tells Us* (Cambridge: Cambridge University Press, 1935).

J. Spurr, 'The Church, the Societies and the Moral Revolution of 1688," in J. Walsh and H. Colin (eds), *The Church of England, c. 1689-c. 1833: From Toleration to Tractarianism* (New York: Cambridge University Press, 1993), 127-142.

———, '"Virtue, Religion, and Government": The Anglican Uses of Providence,' in T. Harris, P. Seaward, and M. Goldie (eds), *The Politics of Religion in Restoration England* (Cambridge, MA: Basil Blackwell, 1990), 29-47.

L. Stevenson, '"New Diseases" in the Seventeenth Century,' *Bull. Hist. Med,* 39 (1965), 1-21.

D. Sven, *Town and Country in Pre-Industrial Spain: Cuenca, 1550-1870* (Cambridge: Cambridge University Press, 1990).

O. Temkin, *Hippocrates in a World of Pagans and Christians* (Baltimore: Johns Hopkins University Press, 1991).

———, 'On the History of "Morality and Syphilis,"' in O. Temkin (ed.), *The Double Face of Janus and Other Essays In the History of Medicine* (Baltimore: Johns Hopkins University Press, 1977), 472-486.

———, 'Medicine and the Problem of Moral Responsibility,' in O. Temkin (ed.), *The Double Face of Janus and Other Essays In the History of Medicine* (Baltimore: Johns Hopkins University Press, 1977), 50-67.

————, 'Therapeutic Trends and the Treatment of Syphilis before 1900,' in O. Temkin (ed.), *The Double Face of Janus and Other Essays In the History of Medicine* (Baltimore: Johns Hopkins University Press, 1977), 472-484.

K. Thomas, 'The Puritans and Adultery: The Act of 1650 Reconsidered,' in K. Thomas and D. Pennington (eds), *Puritans and Revolutionaries: Essays Presented to Christopher Hill* (Oxford: Clarendon Press, 1978), 257-81.

------, *Religion and the Decline of Magic* (New York: Scribner, 1971).

A. Thompson, *Shakespeare, Meaning & Metaphor* (Iowa City: University of Iowa Press, 1987).

J. Towler and J. Bramall, *Midwives in History and Society* (London: Croom Helm, 1986).

B.H. Traister, '"Note Her a Little Farther": Doctors and Healers in the Drama of Shakespeare,' in S. Moss and K.Peterson (eds), *Disease, Diagnosis, and Cure on the Early Modern Stage* (Literary and Scientific Cultures of Early Modernity) (Aldershot: Ashgate, 2004), 43-54.

R. Trumbach, *Sex and the Gender Revolution* Vol. 1. *Heterosexuality and the Third Gender in Enlightenment London* (Chicago: University of Chicago Press, 1998).

W. Turnley, *Shakespearean Medicine, Modernized* (New York: Vantage Press, 1968).

D. Underdown, *Fire from Heaven: The Life of an English Town in the Seventeenth Century* (New Haven : Yale University Press, 1992).

C. Walford, 'Early Bills of Mortality.' *Transactions of the Royal Historical Society* 7 (1878), 212-48.

J. Walkowitz, *Prostitution and Victorian Society: Women, Class, and the State* (Cambridge: Cambridge University Press, 1980).

P. Wallis, 'Plagues, Morality and the Place of Medicine in Early Modern England,' *English Historical Review* 121, no. 490 (February 2006), 1-24.

A. Walsham, *Providence in Early Modern England* (Oxford: Oxford University Press, 1999).

J. Walter and R. Schofield, 'Famine, Disease and Crisis Mortality in Early Modern Society,' in J. Walter and R. Schofield (eds), *Famine, Disease and the Social Order in Early Modern Society* (New York: Cambridge University Press, 1989), 1-74.

O. Watkins, *The Puritan Experience* (London: Routledge, 1972).

S. Watts, *Disease, Power, and Imperialism* (New Haven: Yale University Press, 1997).

A. Wear, 'Interfaces: Perceptions of Health and Illness in Early Modern

305

England,' in R. Porter and A. Wear (eds), *Problems and Methods in the History of Medicine* (London: Groom Helm, 1987), 230-255.

———, 'Medical Ethics in Early Modern England,' in A. Wear, J. Geyer-Kordesch, and R. French (eds), *Doctors and Ethics: The Earlier Historical Setting of Professional Ethics* (Amsterdam: Rodopi, 1993), 98-130.

———, 'Puritan Perceptions of Illness in Seventeenth Century England,' R. Porter *Patients and Practitioners: Lay Perceptions of Medicine in Pre-Industrial Society* (Cambridge: Cambridge University Press, 1985), 55-100.

———, 'Religious Beliefs and Medicine in Early Modern England,' in H. Marland and M. Pelling (eds), *The Task of Healing: Medicine, Religion and Gender in England and the Netherlands 1450-1800* (Rotterdam: Erasmus Publishing, 1996), 145-71.

C. Webster, 'The College of Physicians: "Solomon's House" In Commonwealth England,' *Bulletin of the History of Medicine* 51, no. 5 (2003), 393-412.

———, *From Paracelsus to Newton: Magic and the Making of Modern Science* (New York: Cambridge University Press, 1982).

———, *The Great Instauration: Science, Medicine and Reform 1626-1660* (New York: Holmes and Meier Publishers, 1976).

———, ed. *Health, Medicine, and Mortality in the Sixteenth Century* (New York: Cambridge University Press, 1979).

———, ed. *The Intellectual Revolution of the Seventeenth Century* (Boston: Routledge and Kegan Paul, 1974).

A. Weinstein, *Contagion and Infection* (Baltimore, Md: Johns Hopkins University Press, 2003).

C. Whitbeck, 'Causation in Medicine: The Disease Entity Model,' *Philosophy of Science* 44, no. 4 (December 1977), 619-37.

T.D. Whittet, *The Apothecaries in the Great Plague of London in 1665* (London, Society of Apothecaries, 1965).

A. Wilson, 'Participant or Patient? Seventeenth-Century Childbirth from the Mother's Point of View,' in R. Porter (ed.), *Patients and Practitioners: Lay Perceptions of Medicine in Pre-Industrial England* (Cambridge: Cambridge University Press, 1985), 129-44.

F.P. Wilson, *The Plague in Shakespeare's London* (Oxford: Clarendon Press, 1927).

———, (ed.), *Plague Pamphlets of Thomas Dekker* (Oxford: Clarendon Press, 1925).

P. Wilson, 'Exposing the Secret Disease: Recognizing and Treating Syphilis in Daniel Turner's London,' in Linda Merians (ed.), *The Secret Malady: Venereal Disease in Eighteenth-century Britain and France* (Lexington: University of Kentucky Press, 1996), 68-84.

———, *Surgery, Skin, and Syphilis: Daniel Turner's London (1667-1741)* (Amsterdam: Rodopi, 1999).

T. Wright (ed.), *The Autobiography of Joseph Lister, of Bradford in Yorkshire* (London: John Russell Smith, 1842).

K. Wrightson, *English Society, 1580-1680* (London: Hutchinson, 1982).

M. Yearsley, *Doctors in Elizabethan Drama* (London: John Bale, Sons and Denielsson, Ltd, 1933).

H. Zinsser, *Rats, Lice, and History; Being a Study in Biography, Which, after Twelve Preliminary Chapters Indispensable for the Preparation of the Lay Reader, Deals with the Life History of Typhus Fever* (Boston: Pub. for the Atlantic Monthly Press by Little, Brown, and Ccompany, 1935).

Index

Printed in the United States
By Bookmasters